TEXTBOOK
of
HOMOEOPATHY PHILOSOPHY

Vol. I (Kent)

An Explanation with Summary
of Dr. James Tyler Kent's Philosophy.
Includes his Aphorisms & Precepts from
Lesser Writings.

by

Dr. Raju Subramanian
Dr. (Mrs.) Raaji Subramanian

B. JAIN PUBLISHERS (P) LTD.
NEW DELHI

> **NOTE FROM THE PUBLISHERS**
>
> Any information given in this book is not intended to be taken as a replacement for medical advice. Any person with a condition requiring medical attention should consult a qualified practitioner or therapist.

Textbook of Homoeopathy Philosophy

© All rights are reserved

No part of this publication may be reproduced, stored in a retrieval system or transmitted, in any form or by any means, mechanical, photocopying, recording or otherwise, without prior written permission of the publishers.

First Edition : 2003
Reprint edition: 2005

B. JAIN'S SPECIAL PRICE BHMS BOOKS Rs. 159.00

Published by
Kuldeep Jain
for

B. Jain Publishers (P) Ltd.

1921, Chuna Mandi, St. 10th Paharganj,
New Delhi-110 055

Ph : 2358 0800, 2358 1100, 2358 1300, 2358 3100
Fax: 011-2358 0471

Website : www.bjainbooks.com, Email : bjain@vsnl.com

Printed in India by :
J.J. Offset Printers
533, FIE, Patpar Ganj, Delhi-110 092

ISBN : 81-8056-305-7   BOOK CODE : BS-5684

About the Authors

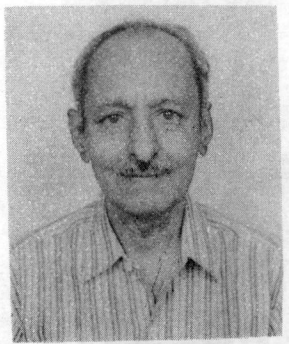
Dr. Raju Subramanian

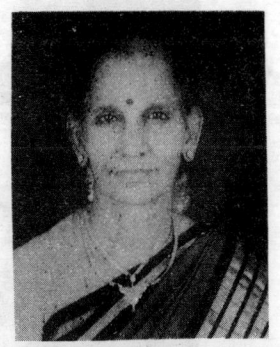
Dr. (Mrs.) Raaji Subramanian

Both have over twenty years' experience in the medical field. They have together conducted many camps under the banners of Rotary Clubs, Lions Clubs and many other Social Organizations. They have given lectures in many Colleges and Schools, in Tamil Nadu, Andhra Pradesh and Karnataka States in India.

Dr. Raju Subramanian is a second-generation of classic practitioners. His parents were classic and ardent practitioners and rendered free treatment to people. The tradition is planted in him well and deep.

Both have appeared in TV programmes and contributed many articles to many magazines. Their interviews have appeared in magazines.

They were Associated Members of the Asian Homoeopathic Medical League.

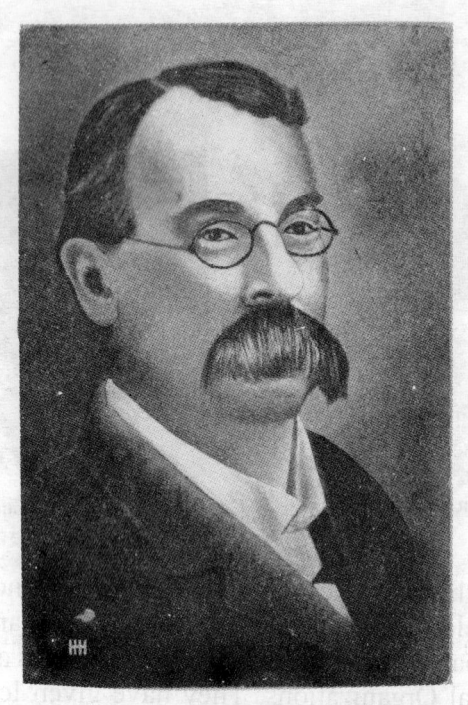

Dr. James Tyler Kent
1849-1910

A Tribute

All hail James Tyler Kent, to all endeared,
Whom, as their chief, his pupils proudly claim,
In ages yet unborn shall be revered.

We, who have groped in ignorance as blind,
Rejoice as those who have received new sight;
This gift we owe to his colossal mind,
And through his teachings revel in the light.

The fire he kindled has been duly fanned
And cannot now be quenched by floods or seas;
The leaping flames spread on through every land,
Restoring health and banishing disease.

Henry B. Blunt, M.D., C.M.

An Appreciation

HAIL KENT!

Prometheus-like thy flame so bright,
Has brought to us a ray of light
From Hahnemann's shining path, so fond
It blazes wondrous realms beyond,
Health, for poor groping human-kind,
A paradise on earth will find,
Dead? No! Thy living law, its seed will sow
That good, diffused, may more abundant grow,
Hail Kent!

A. Eugene Austin, M.D., H.M.

A Salute

Intolerant of sham, firm in the application of the Homeopathic principles, and almost uncanny in his prescience, we can well say with Shakespeare:

"His life was gentle, and the elements
So marked in him, that Nature might stand up
And say to all the world, this was a man."

C. P. Thacher

Preface

We have taken up the burden to execute an easy explanation to Dr. James Tyler Kent's lectures in understandable present-day English. The subject matter is Homoeopathy Philosophy. Dr. Kent has covered one hundred and fifty four paragraphs of Dr. Hahnemann's *Organon* in thirty-four lectures. Lecture thirty five is prognosis, thirty six the second prescription and thirty seven is palliation.

Organon of Dr. Hahnemann is the Bible of all sincere homoeopaths. One has to do some real deep studying of *Organon* when he wants to master homoeopathy. Dr. Kent's lectures on this subject make one's study of *Organon* comparatively easier.

What prompted us to embark on this ambitious project?

Dr. Kent himself has said that when you talk about homoeopathy and Organon, do so in the simplest English so that everyone can understand it easily and any serious homoeopath can contemplate on it without any ambiguity. Dr. Kent's lectures date back to the 1900s. One hundred years back! The English that was in vogue then is not applicable today in the twenty first century!

Further Dr. Kent himself says in his preface that homoeopathy is both a science and an art. "If the art is to remain and progress among men, the science must be better understood than at present."

To meet the above conditions we launched upon this project.

There is one more reason also. Before planning this book, we made several enquiries amidst many practioners, students and those fresh out of the colleges. We had replies, which were more or less identical. Many practitioners continued their practice because of the experience! The student community said that it was mainly for the passing out of the exams they were forced to read it in spite of 'un-understandable' English. Long sentences without any punctuations at times - footnotes confusing, etc. Some freshers said in a lighter view, "we have our certificates, now our job is to earn money - retrieve the expenditure spent on college studies." But a few people did say one thing - and what they said was more or less uniform. They said, "we must have a book that can be understood easily and capable of easy reference at any time." That clinched the deal.

This book is for all homoeopaths - an easy reference work. At the close of each lecture, a summary of that lecture is provided. To enhance the value of the work we have reproduced after each summary (after the fifth lecture) Dr. Kent's Aphorisms and Precepts, as appearing in Dr. Kent's 'Lesser Writings'. In the second part of this book - "Beyond the Lectures" we have gathered and provided the above and two practical chapters on case taking.

Armed with this one book, we are sure one can easily master the principles of homoeopathy. A not so serious reader can just turn to the summary at the end of each chapter. By repeated reference and reading of this work, three things can be achieved:

(1) He can get a good knowledge of homoeopathy philosophy.

(2) Get to know Dr. Kent's Aphorisms and Precepts.

(3) Some more information from other homoeopathy masters.

We thank Dr. V. Narasimhan, President, Trichy District Homoeopathic Doctors' Association for having encouraged us to go through this project.

We also thank Mrs. and Mr. Surianarayanan and Mr. Ravi who have gone out of their way to make this book an excellent presentation.

The authors also thank Mr. Kuldeep Jain for his acceptance to publish this work and his co-operation.

This book is consecrated to the cause of homoeopathy — To Cure Gently, Rapidly and Permanently.

Chennai **The Authors**
5-7-2002

Contents

PART - I

Lectures

Lecture No.	Topics	Page No.
I	The Sick	3
II	The Highest Ideal of a Cure	11
III	What is Curable in Diseases, Curative in Medicine and Their Applications	19
IV	Fixed Principles - Law and Government from Centre	27
V	Discrimination as to Maintaining External Causes and Surgical Cases	35
VI	The Unprejudiced Observer	49
VII	Foot Note - Indispositions and Removal of Their Causes	61
VIII	On Simple Substance	67
IX	Disorder First in Vital Force	85
X	Materialism in Medicine	97
XI	Sickness and Cure on Dynamic Plane	109
XII	The Removal of Totality of Symptoms	121
XIII	The Law of Similars	133
XIV	Susceptibility	143

XV	Protection from Sickness	159
XVI	Oversensitive Patients	169
XVII	The Science and The Art	183
XVIII	Chronic Diseases - Psora	197
XIX	Chronic Diseases - Psora (Contd.)	211
XX	Chronic Diseases - Syphilis	229
XXI	Chronic Diseases - Sycosis	237
XXII	Disease and Drug Study in General	253
XXIII	The Examination of the Patient	267
XXIV	The Examination of the Patient (Contd.)	281
XXV	The Examination of the Patient (Contd.)	299
XXVI	The Examination of the Patient (Contd.)	321
XXVII	Record Keeping	339
XXVIII	The Study of Proving	347
XXIX	Idiosyncrasies	373
XXX	Individualization	389
XXXI	Characteristics	403
XXXII	The Value of Symptoms	417
XXXIII	The Value of Symptoms (Contd.)	435
XXXIV	The Homeopathic Aggravation	447
XXXV	Prognosis after Observing the Action of the Remedy	477
XXXVI	The Second Prescription	515
XXXVII	Difficult and Incurable Cases - Palliation	543

PART - II

Beyond the Lectures

Chapter No.	Topics	Page No.
1.	About Aphorisms and Precepts.	555
2.	Susceptibility.	563
3.	Selection of a Remedy.	567
4.	Value of Symptoms.	575

PART - I
LECTURES

Lecture - I

The Sick

Homoeopathy is governed by principles.

Allopathy accepts nothing but what can be felt with the fingers and seen with the eyes or what is observed through the sense supported by improved instruments. It does not go before or beyond.

In Homoeopathy there is something prior to the results. Every scientific investigation proves that everything that exists does so because of something prior to it. The above helps us to trace the cause and effect, in a series, from beginning to end, and back again from the end to the beginning. By this way, we arrive at a state wherein we do not assume, but in which, we know.

The physician's high and only mission is to restore the sick to health, to cure as it is termed.

Organon - 1

The Homoeopath must abandon the mere expressions of opinion. We should reason out from the facts and not as sometimes they appear. Facts as they appear are expressed as opinions of men, but facts as they are, are facts and truths wherefrom doctrines are evolved and formulated which will interpret or unlock the kingdom of nature, in sickness as well as in health. In science, opinions of men must not be considered; only facts are to be taken.

Dr. Samuel Hahnemann has given us solid principles on which to build up our cases. Laws govern the world and not the opinion of men. We should respect the law. That will be authority.

The Homoeopath knows that crude drugs do not heal the sick, but potentized remedies do. The crude drugs cannot heal the sick and that what changes they do effect are not real, but only apparent.

There can be no cause and no relation between cause and effect without the vital force, without simple substance, without internal or external.

What is meant by 'the sick'? It is the man that is sick and to be restored to health, not his body, nor the tissue.

We find a person coming and telling us that he has gone to various doctors and had underwent all the tests. The doctors had declared that everything was normal. But what is the fact? The fact is that the disease does exist and the person is unwell. So, how do we solve this? By allowing the patient to speak! We should listen to his problems with intense attention and with great care. In the course of his talk the person drops a golden nugget, " I do not sleep well at nights or my bowels do not move and I have pains and aches." There it is! The fact that everything is NOT normal with him is evident. He is sick! Does this condition exist without a cause? Think about it. These symptoms are the language of nature, clearly indicating the internal nature of the sick person.

Let us take a nervous child, as another example. The child has wild dreams, twitching, restless sleep, and hysterical manifestations. On examining the child's organs we find nothing wrong with them. This sickness, which is present, if allowed to go uncured, how would it affect? Several years later this results in tissue change and organs will be affected. At that time they say that the body is sick. But come to think of it for a moment. This individual has been sick from the beginning. So, now it is a question of where we start. If we have material ideas of the disease we will have material ideas of the means of cure.

Remember that nothing exists without a cause. The organs are not the man. The man is prior to the organs. From first to last is the order of sickness as well as the order of cure, from the man to his organs and not from the organs to the man.

The tissues cannot become sick unless something prior to them had been deranged to make them sick. We have got to see here what is there of this person that can be called the internal man? What is there to be removed so that the physical may be left behind?

When a person is dead and we dissect his body, we find all his organs - what is known of the physical man - whatever we can feel with the fingers, touch and see with the eyes. The real sick person, then, is prior to the sick body and our condition must be that the sick man must be somewhere in that portion which is not left behind. What is carried away is primary and what is left behind is ultimate.

Whatever the man feels, sees, tastes, and hears - he thinks his life is just outward manifestations of his thinking. The man lives and understands. A cadaver does not understand. So what departs is that which knows and wills. It is that which can be changed and existed prior to the body.

The will and understanding constitute the man. These make a man's life and activity, they manufacture and cause all things of the body. When the will and understanding operate in order, there we have a healthy man. The man is the will and understanding and the body is the house in which he lives.

We must be scientific Homoeopaths. We should consider from the life to the body and not from body to life. The Homoeopath must understand what cure is. The only mission of a Homoeopath is to heal the sick. His sole duty is not to heal the results of sickness but to heal the sickness itself. When health is restored, harmony is restored in the tissues and in body activities. So, the sole duty of the Homoeopath is to put in order the interior of the economy i.e., of both the will and understanding conjoined. The tissue changes are of the body and are only the results of the disease. The changes are not the disease. Dr. Hahnemann has said, "There are not diseases, but sick people."

The so-called diseases, viz., liver disease, Bright's disease etc., were grosser forms of disease results viz., the appearances of disease. First there is disorder of the government and then this proceeds from within the outward until there are changes in the tissues.

The bacteria are results of diseases. These are scavengers accompanying the disease and they do not cause disease. They are the outcome of disease and are present wherever the disease is. It has been discovered that every pathological result has its corresponding bacteria. The disease cause is very subtle and it cannot be seen through a microscope.

We must remember Dr. Hahnemann's words here. The physician's mission is not, however, to construct so-called systems, by interweaving empty speculations and hypotheses concerning the internal essential nature of the vital process and the mode in which disease originates in the invisible interiors of the organisms, etc.

There is an outgrowth of the old fashioned folly of naming sickness. Except in a few acute diseases no diagnosis can be made and no diagnosis need be made except that the patient is sick. The more one thinks of the name of a disease so called, the more one is beclouded in the search for a remedy, for then the mind is only upon the result of the disease and not upon the image expressed in symptoms.

Lecture - 1

A young patient with gravest inheritances, and with only symptoms to furnish the image of sickness is perfectly curable if treated in time. After the treatment there will be no pathological results. He will go on to old age without any tissue destruction. If for any reason this person is not cured then, the disease results will take on in accordance with the circumstances of his life and inheritances. The housemaid will be subjected to diseases peculiar to housemaid, a chimney sweep, etc.— the patient has the same disease he had when he was born.

So, go back and procure these very symptoms before you can make a prescription. Prescribing for the results of the disease causes changes in the results of the disease but not in the sickness except hurry its progress.

We shall take a family for example. In the same family all are not affected identically. One member has asthma, another cancer, and another eye troubles. Though various members suffer from different problems, the common foundation is the same.

Some people are susceptible to one thing and some to another. A good example is when an epidemic strikes, only some are affected. We should contemplate why some must be affected and some are not. The idiosyncrasies account for this.

The physician's duty is to hunt out the symptoms of the sickness until a remedy is found, that covers the disorder. This remedy which will (produce on healthy person similar symptoms), is the master of the situation. It will overcome the sickness, restore the will and understanding to order and cure the patient.

The investigation has to be made in the most scientific way. Sickness can be learned by the study of the proving of drugs upon the healthy economy.

Mind is the key to the man. The symptoms of the mind are the most important symptoms in a remedy as well as in sickness. Man is what he thinks and what he loves. There is nothing else in the man. If the will and understanding were separated, it means insanity, disorder and death. Every remedy operates upon the will and understanding first. (Sometimes extensively on both). This affects the man in his ability to think or to will and ultimately upon the tissues, the functions and sensations.

Man's highest possible love is for his life. Let us study *Aurum*. *Aurum* affects and disturbs the affections most. *Aurum* destroys this love for his life and he commits suicide. In *Argentum* we see the understanding is destroyed, which results in his being irrational; memory ruined. This we see in every proven remedy in our Materia Medica. We see that first; the man's mind is affected. Proceeding from the mind to the physical economy, to the outer most, to the skin, the hair, the nails are affected. Each remedy has to be studied like this. The Materia Medica has been established on this basis.

Sickness has to be examined by a thorough scrutiny of the elements that make up morbid changes that exists in the likeness of the drug symptoms. We must study sickness with the hope of adjusting remedies to sickness in the man, under the law of similar. Ultimate symptoms, function symptoms, sensorium symptoms and mind symptoms are all useful and none should be over-looked. The idea of sickness in man must be formed from the idea of sickness perceived in our Materia Medica. As we perceive the nature of sickness in a drug image we must perceive the nature of sickness in a human being to be healed.

Our idea of pathology must be adjusted to such a Materia Medica, as we possess. It must be discovered wherein these are similar in order to heal the sick. The totality of the symptoms is all we know of the internal nature of sickness. Then the proper administration of the similar remedy will constitute the art of healing.

Summary

1. This lecture deals with the sick.
2. Homeopathy is governed by principles.
3. In Homoeopathy there is something prior to the results. We investigate from beginning to end and from the end to the beginning. By this process we know, and we do not assume anything.
4. The Homoeopath's only intention must be to cure the sick. The Homoeopath must not take the liberty to stick to the opinions or other's expressions. We should stick to facts only.
5. Law governs everything. It is the authority.
6. Crude drugs do not heal and any change they may bring in will be apparent only.
7. Cause and effect, vital force and simple substance all are interlinked.
8. Treat the individual - not the sickness.
9. Allow the sick to explain his symptom and listen to them carefully and make notes.
10. Will and understanding makes a man.
11. In disease there is a disorder of the economy and when health is restored, this disorder is set right.
12. Dr. Hahnemann said, "There are no diseases, only sick people."
13. Bacteria are results of disease. They are scavengers accompanying the disease.
14. Disease cause is very subtle and cannot be seen by eyes or microscopes.
15. The disease results will take on in accordance with the circumstances.

Lecture - II

The Highest Ideal of a Cure

The highest ideal of a cure is rapid, gentle and permanent restoration of the health, or removal and annihilation of the disease in its whole extent, in the shortest, most reliable and most harmless way, on easily comprehensible principles.

Organon - 2

When I was a student, one of my teachers used to tell us "Let WHO, WHAT, WHEN, WHERE and HOW be your constant questions". Now let us put the questions to the above paragraph of Organon.

WHO said it: None other than the great master Dr. Samuel Hahnemann.

WHAT did he say: Ideal cure is rapid, gentle, permanent restoration of health in whole.

WHEN: In the shortest possible time.

WHERE: In a sick person.

HOW: In the most harmless way on easily comprehensible principles or basis.

It is so simple - Is it not? But how many Homoeopaths stick to the above. —Come think of it.

A good scientific Homoeopath sticks to the law. - Easily comprehensible laws of Homoeopathy and he has got to be successful. No two ways about it.

Now, let us go deeper into the above paragraph and the answers we got for our questions. On carefully going through, the above three points are distinct and noteworthy. Restoration of the health — note this. It is restoration or bringing back — not the removal of the symptoms. What does this restoration of health means to the Homoeopath. What is the picture that flashes or should flash in his mental screen? First of all let us see what this does not mean. It means that it is not removing the symptoms-like the removal of constipation, piles or some swelling etc., or any local manifestation, or the removal of a group of symptoms. Then what is called a cure is a logical question. Where the removal of a symptom is not followed by a restoration to health, it cannot be termed as a cure.

If the words "The physician's sole duty is to heal the sick" is in our minds then removal of a symptom alone does not sustain. Let us go into this further. The removal of a symptom or to change the aspect of the symptom, the appearance of the disease image will end up in the imagination that a cure has been brought, and that, order has been established. Here the physician should remember that every violent change, which he produces in the aspect of disease, aggravates the interior nature of the disease, aggravates the sickness of the man. What happens then? There is an increase in the suffering within him. The patient must be in a position to realize and confirm that he is being restored to health at the removal of each and every symptom. This improvement should correspond with an inward improvement - every time an outward symptom has been wiped out. This can be true only when the order is replaced in the place of chaos, or disease.

From restoration of health, we go to the next step. This is done in the shortest time, gently and permanently. What does this

Lecture - II

shortest time mean? The cure must be quick and speedy at the same time it must be gentle, continuous or permanent. Let us take an example - a case of constipation. The patient is not able to move the bowels. So, what does an average physician do in this case? He resorts to cathartics and the bowel is moved - constipation relieved. Now look into this carefully. Health is restored, but was it gentle? Will this solution be permanent? Think of these things. It might have been a prompt cure - but is this in accordance with the law? It is concentrated alkaloid that cleared the constipation by its violent action. Whenever violent drugs are resorted to, there is nothing mild in the action or the reaction that must follow. Today's drugs are very powerful and extremely violent in action. These drugs are very dangerous in the sense that they do more harm as they attack the mind. Further, the apparent benefits produced by these drugs are never permanent. They may appear permanent in some cases. This is because a new and most insidious disease has been engrafted on the economy. This new disease is subtler and more tenacious then the manifestation that was upon the externals. Due to its tenacity the original symptoms remain away. Here the disease in its nature, its *esse*, has not been changed; it is still very much there, thus causing the internal destruction of the man. Only its manifestations have changed. Let us go into this a little further. To this change, now a drug induced disease is also added. The entire case has now become more serious than the previous condition.

Have you ever seen water flowing? It flows from a higher level to lower level in the path of least resistance. Similarly the cure can be mild only if it flows in the stream of most natural direction. The order will be established and the disease removed. Here a picture comes to my mind. In it a boy is pulling a black cat uphill by its tail. The cat is whining, with all four legs outstretched with the claws trying to dig into the earth, creating maximum resistance against the pull. Got the picture? Well it is the same with a drug with violent action.

Coming back to our subject, a gentle or mild treatment, which can be permanent, flows with the stream. There is scarcely any ripple at all. All internal disorders are adjusted and the outermost of the man is returned back to order. In this case everything is changed to orderliness from the interior. The curative medicine does not act violently upon the human economy. It establishes its action in a mild manner; but while its action is mild and gentle, very often it is followed by a reaction. This reaction is a turmoil when the work of a previously administered traditional medicine is undone and the original state of well being is re-established.

After this comes the point "on easily comprehensible principles". Easily comprehensible principles mean it is plain and intelligible. This means the law built on fixed principals. There is a certainty about it, no guesswork, no roundabout methods. The Homoeopathy principles have never changed - they have always been the same and they will remain the same.

The Homoeopath should become well acquainted with the doctrines and principles, with fixed knowledge, with exactitude or method; to become well acquainted with medicines which never change in their properties and to become well acquainted with their action, is the most important aim in homoeopathic study. The Homoeopath becomes stronger and brighter when he has learned these principles thoroughly and also practices them. These fixed principles or laws are the only royal roads to the restoration to health, mildly, promptly and permanently. There are no short cuts or compromises.

Coming to Homoeopathic way of healing - in sickness it is the interior of the man that is primarily disordered; so first the interior must be set in order and the exterior last. The first of man is his voluntary and the second of man is his understanding and the last of man is his outermost. Here we learn the famous theory - the man is healed from the centre to circumference. The cure proceeds

Lecture - II

from the centre to circumference.

The above famous theory is the cure is from above downward, from within outward. This means from more important to lesser important organs, from head to hands and feet. Every Homoeopath knows for certain when cure is got in these directions the cure is permanent. The Homeopath is also aware that when the symptoms, which disappear in the reverse order of their appearance, are also removed for permanent. This way of cure proves only one thing. The patient was not "just cured" or get well in spite of treatment - he was cured by the action of the remedy. In a patient if the Homoeopath observes that things have not moved as above, he knows for certain one thing - he has goofed; he will have little to do with the converse of things.

If, on the other hand where he observes, after the administration of his medicine, that the symptoms take a reversal course he knows his medicine has acted as expected, since if the disease was allowed to run its course this could not have been accomplished.

The chronic disease progresses from the surface to the centre. All chronic diseases first manifest upon the outer surface and from there the progress is inwards, to the innermost man. Coming to our law of cure we should note how the patient recovers which will be obvious from the proportion in which it is thrown back to the surface. We spoke earlier of the gentle, mild ways of setting things in order, which was also followed by turmoil. The homoeopath would have explained all this to the patient - but the patient does not desire their old symptoms returning. This is in spite of the patient knowing there is no other way out.

Complaints of heart, chest and head must be thrown out upon the surface, the skin, the extremities, etc. Where there is a rheumatic heart, the patient's recovery can be seen from the fact now there is a rheumatic knee. The patient in this case will say or complain that due to the swollen knee he is unable to walk, even inside the house. Here the homoeopath has to be cautious. He should understand the situation and not prescribe for the swollen knee, for, if he does so it will go back to the heart.

It may be impossible to cure certain cases entirely. Then the patient may experience great suffering (in spite of mild means) in the evolution of his disease. In acute diseases so much distress is not observed after the medicine. The return of the outward manifestation upon the extremities is observed where suppression has taken place.

The patient has to wait for the medicine to act. A homoeopath also should wait. If on the contrary he rushes to give another medicine to the patient, the homoeopath has grossly violated the law.

The homoeopath has to have high integrity. This is what you learn from "on principles that are at once plain and intelligible". The homoeopath has to lead an orderly life, inculcate good habits and honesty and be sincere. The physician, who is otherwise, cannot be relied upon.

To summarize this chapter, the homoeopath must first find out the disorder - bring back order and restore the patient to health. This alone will be a perfect cure, which must be accomplished by mild and gentle methods so that order is restored in a most streamlined way. The homoeopath must also apply the law and fixed principle in his practice.

Lecture - II

Summary

1. This lecture deals with the highest ideal of cure - paragraph two of the *Organon*.
2. The cure to be ideal must be rapid, gentle and permanent.
3. Cure means the restoration of health - not the removal of symptoms.
4. The improvement should correspond with the internal improvement.
5. Removal of a symptom may appear like a cure. It is only apparent and not permanent.
6. A curative drug does not act violently upon the human economy. It establishes its action mildly and gently.
7. All homoeopathic laws and principles are easily comprehensible, plain and intelligible. There is no guesswork. The law does not change.
8. It is the interior of the man that is primarily disordered.
9. The man is healed from centre to circumference - from above downward.
10. Where the symptoms take a reversal course after the administration of a drug, the drug is the correct one.
11. We should wait for the action of the medicine to take hold.

Lecture - III

What is curable in Disease, Curative in Medicine and Their Applications

If the physician clearly perceives what is to be cured in disease, that is to say, in every individual case of disease; if he clearly perceives what is curative in medicines, that is to say, in each individual medicine; and if he knows how to adopt, according to clearly-defined principles, what is curative in medicines to what he has discovered to be undoubtedly morbid in the patient, so that recovery must ensue - to adapt it as well in respect to the suitability of the medicine most appropriate according to the mode of action to the case before him, as also in respect to the exact mode of preparation and quantity of it required, and the proper period for repeating the dose; if finally he knows the obstacles to recovery in each case and is aware how to remove them so that the restoration may be permanent; then he understands how to treat judiciously and rationally, he is a true practioner of the healing art.

Organon - 3

In this paragraph Dr. Hahnemann clearly defines who will be a true practitioner of the healing art. We have seen that homoeopathy is based on very clear principles and fixed laws. Thus there is place only for facts - not for guesswork or for opinions. Now remembering this let us go to analyze this paragraph, point by point.

Certain words are very very powerful in splashing or flashing their meanings from rooftops. But certain words are so subtle that one has to contemplate on it for some time to get its proper meaning and the role it has in the point of application. Such a word in the paragraph is "perceives".

The Twentieth Century Dictionary defines perceives as follows: - "To become aware of through the senses; to get knowledge by the mind; to understand; to discern. It is not just seeing, not to pass a casual glance, but deeply see into, get the knowledge by the mind; apprehend with the mind and understanding".

Dr. Hahnemann did not look upon the pathological changes or morbid anatomy as that which constitutes the curative indication in a disease. The homoeopath must perceive what is to be cured in a disease. This curative indication is the totality of symptoms in each particular disease. What is this totality of the symptoms? It is not the *esse* of the disease. It only means the disorder of the internal economy. The manifestations in the tissues will help them arrange themselves and present the internal disorder to the physician. The arrangement of the tissues and their presentation is external.

When we take up a case, the first thing that we should consider what is the curative indications in it. See what indications or symptoms call the physician's attention as symptoms that can be cured. We can understand here that there will be certain symptoms that are curable and others not curable. In chronic disease, the resultant tissue changes, like tumors, cancerous changes, etc., are not curative. But there will be symptoms, which are curable - which can be changed by the administration of suitable remedies. The physician should know this.

Lecture - III

The homoeopath must have a sound knowledge of the human economy and law. He must remember the disease action is from centre to circumference - from the innermost to the outermost. Observe a spider in its web. The web itself is constructed radially from the centre. The spider works from the centre. That is the picture. Have you ever seen two spiders ruling from a single web? So, that is that, there cannot be two governments from one centre.

In science for every standard there is only one unit. In humans the cerebrum is that which is the seat of the government. From here, every nerve cell is governed. Everything begins from here, be it disease or the healing process. Man becomes diseased from causes in himself. The homoeopath must have this idea firmly planted in his mind. Then only he will get the true perception of the disease. All disorders in the vital economy are the primary state of affairs. These disorders manifest themselves by signs and symptoms.

Getting back to where we diverted, what is to be cured in a disease the homoeopath has to proceed from generals to particulars. He must study the disease in its most general features - not as seen upon one particular individual, but upon the whole human race.

We shall take up an example and arrange it for a therapeutic examination. We can take cholera, scarlet fever, measles or such epidemics. Where the epidemic is entirely different from what has hitherto victimized the humanity, at first it will be confusing. The physician gets very vague idea of the disease from the initial few cases. When the epidemic spreads and there are many patients. Once the homoeopath records the symptoms of each case in a schematic form from 'mind, head, eyes, nose, face..........' and review his case sheets he will get the symptoms of that epidemic. He will have that particular disease now, in a schematic form. Thus the homoeopath is able to perceive how this new disease -

the epidemic - affects the human race. He will also be able to identify the generals and particulars. The symptoms, which are common to all, are pathognomonic symptoms. There will be some symptoms that will be rare in each patient and these will be the peculiarities of the different patients. From this totality the homoeopath gets a picture of the disease as close as possible to its nature.

The next step is to pick out the general remedies that will correspond to this epidemic. For this purpose the repertory is used. Now, the homoeopath will have a list of remedies. A scrutiny of this list will show some remedies repeated again and again. These drugs will indicate the epidemic remedies - with these remedies the homoeopath will be able to cure nearly all his cases.

Homeopathy is a case of individualization from the alphabet 'A'. Here also now we take the remedy for each case. When the homoeopath finds that none of the remedies already selected fits a particular patient, the homoeopath should investigate the past history of that particular patient. He may be able to find another remedy that will fit the patient, from the list of his epidemic remedies.

Each remedy has within it a certain state of peculiarities that individualizes or identifies it. The patient also has some peculiarities that identify him. The remedy must fit the patient. No remedy must be given just like that because it is present in the list.

By maintaining a record - of both the symptoms and the medicine that suit there is always a ready reference. After some usage of this list, there may be no need for it.

For making out a proper prescription, the homoeopath must be completely conversant with the nature of the sickness. First he sees the disease in general as to its nature; then he sees the peculiarities that the patient has in the peculiar features of that disease.

Lecture - III

The homoeopath must be in the habit of studying the slightest shades of difference between patients the little pointers that indicate the remedy. Every little peculiarities manifested by every individual patient through his inner life, through everything he thinks, that the homoeopath is enabled to individualize.

The homoeopath must clearly perceive what is curative in each medicine. Here also the physician moves from general to particular. Well, that is the law. Only by this careful study of each medicine like this he will become acquainted with the action of the medicines.

The proving of the medicine must be gone through carefully. The same general features would run through this class of provers, but each individual will have his own peculiarities. For example, No. 1 might bring out mental symptoms more clearly than No. 2 prover. No. 2 might bring out the symptoms of the bowels more clearly than No. 1. The No. 3 prover might bring out head symptoms very strongly - like that. We collect all these symptoms and make a complete list as if one man had all these symptoms. There now, we have got the image of that medicine.

The proving is recorded as per the schema given by Dr. Hahnemann. Each remedy thus recorded and only when it has recorded all the sickness in all regions of the body. Then only, we say that this medicine is proved.

The miasms and their nature should be studied and proceeded. The chronic conditions proceeded exactly as in acute conditions - that is the law. For Dr. Hannemann it took eleven years to record these symptoms of psora from patients who were most certainly psoric. Then he published the anti-psoric remedies based on this - which in their nature have a similarity to psora. The master has shown us the way. There are no short cuts or compromises. We must also follow the master in his footsteps to be successful. Procedure is the same for syphilis or sycosis.

Constant use of the above principles will make it easy for the homoeopath to see the nature of sickness in disease and cure, easily. So, from *Organon* paragraph 3, we learn that we can clearly perceive the nature of the disease as well as the nature of the remedy. By constant practice and close careful observation or by perception we can see the nature of the sickness and healing with a lot more of understanding. This will take us closer to success. Only when the homoeopath does understand clearly without any ambiguity the nature of the disease and the remedy can be skillful and efficient or result oriented.

Summary

1. Lecture III deals with what is curable in disease, curative in medicine and their application. Paragraph three of *Organon* speaks about this.
2. Here Dr. Hahnemann explains a true practitioner and also homoeopathy principles. He says there is no room for opinions - place for facts only.
3. The paragraph explains what the physician has got to perceive.
4. In any disease the totality of the symptoms is to be dealt with.
5. The indications that should draw the physician's attention are symptoms that can be cured.
6. In chronic diseases the resultant tissue changes like tumor or cancerous changes may not be curable - but there will be curable symptoms when searched.
7. The physician must have a sound knowledge of the human economy and law.
8. For any standard, in science, there can be only one unit.
9. The physician must be able to see generals and particulars as such.
10. Homoeopathy is individualization, all the way.

Lecture - III

11. Each remedy has within it certain peculiarities that individualize it. Similarly, the patient will have some peculiarities in his symptoms.
12. The remedy must fit the patient.
13. The homoeopath must be completely conversant with the nature of disease.
14. No symptom can be ignored or considered insignificant.
15. Move from generals to particulars.
16. While proving a drug, the same general features would be common among the provers. But each prover will have his own peculiarities too.
17. The law for acute or chronic conditions is the same.
18. There are no short cuts or compromises in homoeopathy.

Both the nature of the disease and the cure must be studied and understood. This comes by constant perception. Then only he can be skillful.

Lecture - IV

Fixed Principles - Law and Government from Centre

In Organon paragraph 3, we saw it covered the following: -
The physician must understand,

(a) What is curable in disease in general and in each individual case in particular.

(b) What is curative in the remedy in general and in each individual remedy in particular.

(c) How to apply in a clear-cut way, what is curative in the drugs to what is curable in disease.

i.e. proper matching of the remedy to sickness, proper and correct administration of dose and when it is suitable to repeat the dose.

(d) How to remove any obstacles in the way of recovery by recognizing them as such.

We shall now cover here the last part of this paragraph 3 of Organon. This portion gives us the fixed principles by which a homoeopath must be guided. Remember it is a law to be adhered to firmly. We repeat here that there are no shortcuts or compromises. Just sail with the law.

The homoeopath must have an open mind to receive the doctrines. He must catch the true conception of the law and doctrine, order and government. Only by this he would be wise enough to see clearly what is the truth and what is folly.

Experience does count. It has its place in Science. But then experience is only confirmatory. Experience can confirm only what has been discovered through principles and law. Experience can guide us in the right direction. You do not discover anything with experience. But, when man is fully indoctrinated in principle, his experience will or may confirm things that are consistent with law.

One who has no doctrines, no truth, no law and who does not rely on law for everything, imagines that he discovers by experience, there being no fixed law, doctrines etc. his inventions do not take a specific route or path. It is haywire - running in all possible directions. Because of this unhappy haphazard condition no two talkers agree and the debate continues.

The medical science must be firmly built on true foundation. The man has to steadfastly observe - then only he can be sure. There is a difference between true observation in science according to law and principles, and the experience of a person who has no law and no principle.

The homoeopath must necessarily know about the internal government of a man. Only then he can know how the disease develops and travels. There is but one central government that controls and that is the Supreme. In humans, this seat of the central government is in the cerebrum and in the highest portion of the gray matter. Everything in man and everything that takes place in man is prescribed over, primarily by this centre. So you can see, from "centre to circumference".

Let us take the case of an injury. Let us take it as a finger injury. This injury does not disturb the constitutional government of the body. The constitutional government repairs this injury and restores the finger back to operation. This injury is not a disease

Lecture - IV

and it does not rack the whole frame. There is a slight disturbance in the government, and it is got over soon.

A disease is not like that. A disease shakes the whole economy, or rocks the economy, disturbing the government. See the difference? A loss of a limb may affect his functions, but it does not disturb the system. But consider a bout of measles. It flows out from the centre and the whole economy is shattered.

From centre to circumference - that is the point. What comes in the direction of law, what comes from principle always come from the centre. This flow according to the order and experience confirms it. Whatever we have learnt from the use of the law of homoeopathy, whatever we observe after learning that law and the related doctrines and all our subsequent experience does confirm the principles.

With each experience with every remedy our conviction of that medicine grows stronger and stronger and becomes firmly established.

A person who relies on his experience to guide him never knows. His mind changes constantly, it is never settled, and it has no validity. Validity is very very important to science. The homoeopath must rely only upon validity and not on man's opinion. In homoeopathy, only the principles are valid. Whatever is not in accordance with the principle must not be admitted.

Now, we come to potentization. All the causes are so refined in character and very subtle in their nature that they can operate from centre to circumference and from the interior to the very exterior. The coarser things cannot permeate the skin. Man's skin is an envelope. It protects him against contagion from coarser materials; but he is protected only when in perfect health against the immaterial substance. When he is unguarded he suffers. We have to follow this out to find the very house man lives in and his cells are becoming deranged.

Changes occur as a result of disorder and it ends in breakdown, degeneration, etc. Pus cells and the various disorders are only the result of disorder. As long as the order and harmony are maintained, and as long as the tissues are in a state of good health, the metamorphosis is healthy. The tissue change is healthy and is normal; the physiological stand is maintained.

How to comprehend the nature of the disease? This can be done by going back to its beginning. The tissue changes are the result of the disease. The homoeopath knows and understands that the tissue changes are the result of the disease - it is not the disease. According to homoeopathy, the morbid anatomy, no matter where it occurs, is considered as the result of the sickness.

All curable diseases make themselves obvious to the homoeopath by their signs and symptoms. When there are no signs and symptom, and the disease progress in the interior, the man is in a precarious condition. Often the incurable conditions of the body do not have any external signs or symptoms.

Organon fourth paragraph says: " The physician is likewise a preserver of health if he knows the things that derange health and cause disease and how to remove them from the persons in health".

If the homoeopath believes that causes are external, if he believes that the material changes in the body are the things that disturb the health, are the fundamental causes of sickness, the homoeopath will undertake to remove these. The homoeopath sees these in signs and symptoms. If the physician attempts to wipe out the external symptoms by means of local application, it will surmount to suppression. This will complicate the issues further.

The disorder is from the interior, but many disturbances that aggravate the disorders are external. The cause of disorder is internal. It affects the government from the interior. The coarser things that can disturb more especially the body are improperly selected food, living in damp houses, etc. The homoeopath will have to educate the patient and eliminate these things.

Lecture - IV

The fifth paragraph of Organon says:

Useful to the physician in assisting him to cure are the particulars of the most probable exciting cause of acute disease, etc. The probable exciting cause is the in-flow of cause as an invisible immaterial substance. This substance having fixed or fastened upon the interior, flows from the centre to the circumference of the economy, creating additional disorder. These miasms need time to operate before they can affect the external man. This is known as the prodormal stage.

The influx of the miasms is upon the innermost of the physical man - this is not apparent. When it starts to operate upon his nerves and tissues and affects his outermost, the influx become apparent. Each miasm produces upon the human economy its own characteristics. Thus each remedy also produces its own characteristics upon the human economy. The homoeopath must make himself well familiar with the disease cause, its manifestations as well as the drug manifestations. Only then, will he be able to remove the cause of disease and that too in perfect accordance with the fixed and certain homoeopathic principles. From this we are able to see that there is no room for any opinions, no hypothesis. Everything is to be based on facts only.

The nature of the case as a malady should be carefully considered in both acute as well as chronic cases. The homoeopath should know well all the details of the case. This knowledge is obtained by observing the symptoms of many cases. When he has this knowledge there springs to his mind a clear picture of the nature of the case he is about to handle.

Once the homoeopath is thorough with his knowledge of the diseases and then he should study the Materia Medica with great care. He will find out that all the imitations of the miasms are also found in drugs. There is no miasm of the human race, which does not have its imitation in the drugs.

The homoeopathic drugs are from the vegetable, mineral and animal kingdoms. Where the homoeopath is well conversant with these three kingdoms, he can virtually treat the entire human race.

A homoeopath must be well versed and conversant with all the aspects of the diseases. He should be so conversant that the moment he sees a patient all the aspects of the disease should flash in his mind. This can occur only by constant study, observation and application.

Symptomatology is a very important matter. Only the symptoms present to us the disease - for the symptoms are the language of the disease. In his book "Watson's Practice" the author has given details of sickness, and what the patient looks like in sickness. This is a book every homoeopath should study well and also possess. Chambers also relates with accuracy the appearance of a patient. The homoeopath must bring out the smallest detail of the disease - only then he will be able to cure. When we are thorough with all the details sickness we need not worry as to what the sickness will do. We can confidently hand it over to the drug. So knowing the nature of the disease is very important.

Summary

1. This lecture deals with the fixed principles of homoeopathy. This is a continuation of paragraph three of Organon - the last part.

2. The homoeopath must have an open mind, to receive the doctrines.

3. Though experience has its place in science, it is only confirmatory.

4. The medical science must be built on a true and strong foundation.

5. The homoeopath must be aware of the internal economy of man. He should know how the disease develops.

Lecture - IV

6. The seat of the government in a man's economy is in the cerebrum. Every command is from here. All governments act from centre to state. So it is with human economy also - from centre to circumference.

7. A disease shakes the economy - from centre to circumference.

8. Validity is very very important to science. Opinions of men are different from person to person. So, opinions cannot be valid in science.

9. All causes are very refined and subtle. They act from the interior to the exterior.

10. Changes occur as a result of disease, and ends in breakdown. Tissue changes are only the result of disease.

11. All curable diseases make themselves known by signs and symptoms.

12. A homoeopath must know what deranges the health and how to remove them.

13. The disorder is interior. There are many external, coarser things that can aggravate. They are, living in unhealthy surrounding, eating improper food, leading a disorderly life, etc.

14. The influx of miasms is upon the innermost of the physical man. It is not apparent till it starts acting upon his tissues and nerves.

15. Each miasm has its own characteristics.

16. The homoeopath must make familiar the manifestations of a disease cause as well as a drug. He should know the facts.

17. Acute or chronic, the cases are to be treated under the same law.

18. It can be seen from the Materia Medica that all the imitations of miasms are all found in drugs. There is no exception.
19. The homoeopathic drugs are from the vegetable kingdom, animal and mineral kingdoms.
20. Symptomatology is a very important subject. A serious homoeopathic student must study "Watson's Practice" and Chamber's Guide. These two books give with great accuracy the appearance of a patient.

Lecture - V

Discrimination as to Maintaining External Causes and Surgical Cases

We still contemplate on Organon's fourth paragraph here also.

It reads: "The physician is likewise a preserver of health, if he knows the things that derange health and cause disease, and to remove them from person in health."

The paragraph is repeated so that it will stay in our minds.

A homoeopath must discriminate. The adage "Render unto Caeser the things that are Caeser's" holds good in homoeopathy as well. The homoeopath must keep everything in order.

People become sick from bad habits. Once the bad habits are removed, they stay away from overflowing sewerages and take care of hygienic living, a great percentage of their getting sick probably, are removed. Avoiding stimulants like coffee, etc., will also preserve health.

We said the homoeopath must be able to discriminate. It is very important. A sick person needs to be attended by a physician. A person suffering from conscience does not need a surgeon.

The homoeopath must discriminate between the man and his house. When does a man need a medicine? When the man's gross exterior conditions, which are brought on from, exterior causes are complicated with the interior man then medicine is required.

Signs and symptoms indicate the language of the disease. These come from the interior to the exterior. Where the condition is brought out by external causes, the physician must delay his action and wait.

The homoeopath must know what deranges the health and remove them. The basic aim of the homoeopath must be to remove any external cause, which can cause an internal disorder. For e.g. if there is a splinter that presses against a nerve causing discomfort, the homoeopath must remove the splinter and remove the discomfort. It will be foolish to wait under these circumstances.

A patient could be taking food that is not suitable to him. There is no point in going on prescribing *Nux vomica* in this case. Here the external cause has got to be removed. This is what is meant by: the homoeopath has to discriminate. The homoeopath must remove vicious living, living in damp, humid houses and such externals, as they may be a cause for sickness.

When the patient lives comfortable in a well-aired house, has good healthy food and has clean and hygienic living habits and still falls ill, the patient has to be treated from within.

We have covered the fourth paragraph of Organon well enough. The homoeopath must know to discriminate - know the nature of disease in all its aspects and his aim must be to relieve the patient of his discomfort, using his discretion. We shall now proceed further to the fifth paragraph of Organon.

"Useful to the physician in assisting him to cure are the particulars of the most probable existing cause of the acute disease; as also the most significant points in the whole history of the chronic disease to enable him to discover the fundamental cause which is generally due to a chronic miasm. In those investigations the

Lecture - V

ascertainable physical constitution of the patient (especially when the disease is chronic), his moral and intellectual character, his occupation, mode of living and habits, his social and domestic relations, his sexual functions, etc., is to be taken into consideration."

Let us break the above paragraph down for better understanding. What points are useful to the physician to assist him to cure?

The particulars of the most probable existing cause of the acute disease - Here let us take an acute case of diarrhea. We should ascertain from the patient what he consumed to cause diarrhea. Supposing the patient says he consumed some fruit - say jackfruit in large quantities then the cause is known. We can suggest him to be moderate in future and suitably medicate him as well. Assume the patient says he consumed a small quantity of jackfruit and every time he took it the result was diarrhea. In such a case the history of the chronic disease and its fundamental cause is also known.

What other points assist the physician? The homoeopath must go into the constitutional make up of the patient - especially when there is a chronic disease. The Homeopath must, further, ascertain the patient's moral and intellectual character - what the patient does for his living or his occupation, how the patient lives, his habits, how his relationship with the others in the house and in his environment is, even his sexual functions. All these points when gone into the minutest detail will assist the homoeopath to cure.

We shall go into details now. If we contemplate on the real existing causes little is known. The acute diseases are divided into true miasmatic disease and a shadow of it, which may be termed as the mimicking disease.

When the exciting cause is an external cause and when this cause is removed, the patient recovers. To illustrate the point a tailor was doing his marking and cutting on his worktable, standing throughout the day. He got pains and cramps in the night in both the legs. Sometimes there was a slight swelling. He was advised to do his work sitting on a high stool with proper rests to place his feet comfortably during the day. Presto! His pains and discomforts vanished and he became the active smiling friendly tailor to his customers. This is removal of the external exciting causes.

The external cause could be many. Living in improperly ventilated houses, living in damp and humid environments, living in constant grief, non hygienic living, poor habits and junk food, etc., etc. The list can go on and on.

We shall proceed to acute miasm. The homoeopath must remember that the acute miasm have a distinct course to run. We spoke of prodromal period earlier. These have a prodromal period, a period of progress and a period of decline. This is indicated by chart 1.

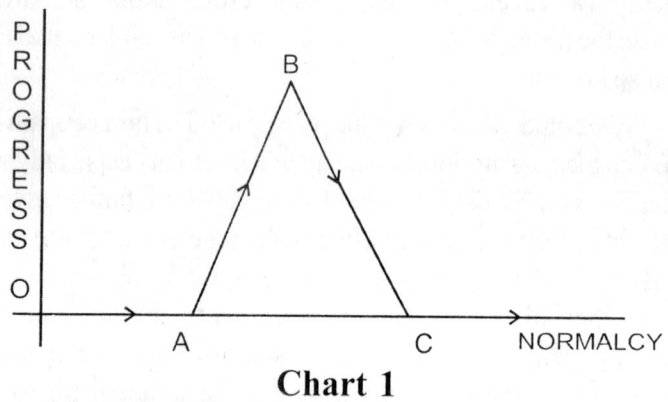

Chart 1

OA - Prodromal period, where the miasm takes its time to operate before affecting external man.

AB - Period of progress

BC - The decline of miasmatic disease

C onwards - Normalcy sets in

Here it is assumed that the acute miasmatic disease is non-fatal.

Measles, scarlet fever, whooping cough, small pox, etc., are examples of acute miasms. The homoeopath must be well acquainted with acute miasms and also the chronic ones like psora, syphilis and sycosis. We can add psuedo-psora in this list.

The chronic miasms also have a prodromal stage or period. They have a period of progress but they do not have a period of decline.

See chart 2.

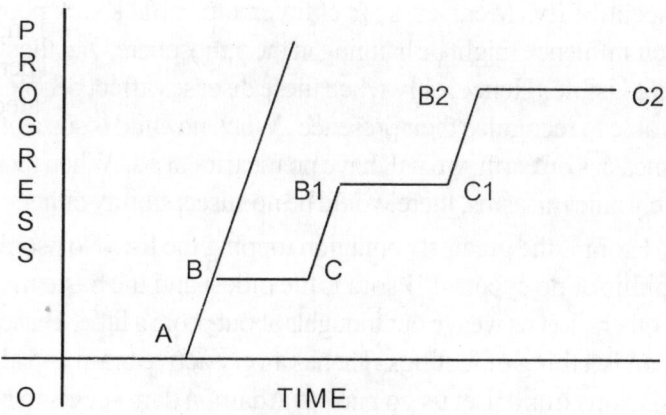

Chart 2

OA - Prodromal period

BC, B1C1, B2C2 - When the time is adverse for the progress of the chronic miasm

CB1, C1B2, etc. - When the conditions are favorable for chronic miasmatic disease progresses further

From the chart it could be seen that the chronic miasm does not progress steadily. When the conditions for its progress are adverse it lies low and when the conditions for its progress is favorable it progresses. At every arousal the condition is worse than the earliest exacerbation. Observe there is no decline here.

Dr. Hahneman says that the chronic miasms are the fundamental cause for acute miasms. That means if there is no chronic miasm there will be no acute miasms either. The very nature of a chronic miasm is to predispose the man to acute diseases. The acute diseases are fuel to the unquenchable flame.

Acute disease exists from specific causes, co-operating with susceptibility. Measles, scarlet fever, etc., attack sick people. Their influence might be hanging in the atmosphere - but then that is not visible. Hence, only when these diseases affect people, we are able to recognize their presence. When no child is susceptible to measles on earth, we will have no measles at all. When there is no chronic misasms, there would be no susceptibility either.

Psora is the greatest contagion topping the list. No psora, no syphilis or no sycosis! Psora is the oldest and the basic miasm for others. Let us weave our thoughts about psora a little. Basically a man is a thing of feelings. He has a very active brain and also a conscious mind. Let us go back to Adam. Adam seems to have been a very happy person - no worries - no desires, etc. Then comes along Eve, a female. Now Adam craves for company. This is a feeling. Minus the feeling (or the will or understanding) Adam would still be a happy being. It did not stop there! He went in for the forbidden fruit - Satan - may be called the miasm for our context, which entered into his mind and corrupted him stage by stage. Did it stop there? See, that is psora. Now we see the chaotic condition the man is in. Thus, psora has been the oldest and the most damaging miasm.

Unfortunately, now-a-days, psora is taken to be the itch vesicle. We will see later what Dr Hahnemann really meant by

Lecture - V

psora. Psora corresponds to the man wherein his economy is disordered to the outermost. This derangement of economy makes him susceptible to each and every surrounding influence. In a country where the central government is evil, then this evil will spread out to the states as well e.g. corruption from the centre to the state. Similarly in a man when his interior is not in order, the result of this evil will flow into his life. We talked earlier about the will and understanding. As long as there is evil inside, the life will be most definitely one of disorder only.

This disorderly condition of the economy is the underlying cause and the fundamental state of nature of psora. This ultimately ends up in body tissue changes. The man's mind is all. When the man starts consuming something not to his taste and he cheats himself into saying that he likes it and goes on consuming further the same thing (due to his belief) he becomes sick. The outermost becomes as morbid as himself.

If the interior of the man is insane, his exterior has got to be distorted. - False in the interior, false in the exterior.

Whatever we see has a cause. There is no cause except in the interior. Water flows in the path of least resistance - from a pool to outer sides - from a higher land to lower level and not vice versa. Similarly a cause cannot travel from exterior to interior. It is the natural law. Natural fixed principles and law govern homoeopathy.

Causes may be very subtle. We may not be able to see them. There is no disease the cause of which is known to man either by the sight or the microscope. Causes are so fine that any instrument cannot detect them.

Whatever we see is the representative of the cause. There is no cause except in the interior. Cause, as we saw earlier cannot flow from the exterior to the interior. It is a security lock that nature has provided.

The causes are immaterial - they ultimate in the body as tissue changes which we are able to see. These tissue changes are the results of the disease. The homoeopath has to understand this. If he does not, he will never perceive what caused the disease, what disease is, what potentiatization means or what the nature of life is. Dr. Hahnemann meant this when he spoke of the fundamental causes as existing in chronic miasms.

When a man starts to live a disorderly life, he becomes susceptible to the outside influences. The susceptibility is in proportion to the disorderly life he lives.

When the man starts thinking in a disorderly way, what happens? He pursues a disorderly life simultaneously. This ends in making him sick because of disorderly habits of thinking and living. Dr. Hahnemann stresses everywhere, in his teachings, to give the maximum attention to the mental state.

The homoeopath must begin his investigations with the signs, which represent to the mind the early stages of beginning of the sickness. This beginning will be found in the mental disorder. Signs and symptoms indicate this disorder. As it follows on, other manifestations of the disease follow. When the disease ultimate itself more in the outward form the coarser it is, and less it directs the homoeopath to the remedy.

We said earlier that the ascertainable physical constitution of the patient, etc. should be considered. This relates to the externals and outermost. The homoeopath has to take into consideration the internal as well as the external man. First consider the cause that operates in this disordered state innermost and then proceed to the ultimate. The ultimate, we repeat, constitute the outside appearance, more particularly in chronic disease. Always consider the nature of the disease and its appearance.

Some physicians will say that in the case of a tubercular patient, the bacillus of tuberculosis is responsible for his condition. But,

Lecture - V

contemplate here for a moment. If the man had not been susceptible to the bacillus, could he have become a victim of tuberculosis? As a matter of fact, the tuberculosis come first and the bacillus secondary. It has never been seen or found at any stage that it was prior to the tubercule. So, it follows that the bacillus has come as a scavenger. The cause of tuberculosis is psora. Bacillus is never the cause of disease. They come only after the disease.

The bacteria might be destroyed, but not the disease. The susceptibility will remain the same. Only those who are susceptible will become a prey to the sickness. Everything in this world has a use, so does bacteria. God has produced this world for human race to live, not to be destroyed. So there is nothing in this world to destroy human kind.

Dr. Hahnemann did not accept any such theory as bacteriology.

Soon after death, we have ptomaine poison. This is alkaloidal in character, but there are no bacteria. The poison is very much present and if a man pricks himself while dissecting that body he has to take care of the wound. If not, he may have a serious illness; and may even die. If the cadaver remained some time and becomes infected with bacteria and a dissector pricks himself, during dissection, that wound is not dangerous.

The more bacteria lesser are the poison. Let us see how bacteria controls poison. Potentize a portion of tubercular mass that is alive with the tubercular bacilli. After the optimization, after it is triturated with sugar of milk and mashed to a pulp this potentized portion will still continue to be potent as the original mass. The same symptoms will be manifested here also.

On administrating a thirtieth potency of this to a healthy man, it will establish the nature of disease in his economy and that is prior to the pthisis. Here we are able to see that we have the cause of pthisis, not in the bacteria, but in the virus. The bacteria are sent to destroy the virus. Man lives longer with the bacteria than he would without them.

The study of the disease as to fundamental cause and apparent cause is a serious and important one. We must know the government first and understand its association with the law. Here let us remember that the law directs and experience confirms.

What is law? It is nothing but an orderly state of things. In a government it operates from centre to circumference. A ship ought to have a captain - so does a government. If this aspect is missing things can only go haywire. It can be observed that order exists from top to bottom, from centre to the circumference.

A true homoeopath must always think of getting things in order. This thought must be reflected in every thought, speech and action of the homoeopath. A man cannot be an authority. Principles and law are authority. The homoeopath must constantly have the principles and law at fingertips. Then only he can see the necessity of harmony - again from centre to circumference.

It has got to be accepted; then only it will satisfy man and sustain his expectation. When you draw a circle you must establish its centre. If the centre is not established and you try to draw a circle and if you place a dot in the centre, it may not be the centre at all - or the circle may not come out as a circle and we may end up with an ellipse. Even the ellipse has to have a centre - remember the school days. Even the earthquake has its epi-centre!

Let us now look into some aphorisms and precepts from this lecture onwards.

Summary

1. This lecture deals with the fourth paragraph of Organon. The subject is discrimination as to maintaining the external causes and surgical cases.
2. The physician is a preserver of health. He must know what causes disease.

Lecture - V

3. The homoeopath must be able to discriminate. He must give a place to everything, to maintain order.
4. Individuals become sick due to bad habits. So bad habits must be shunned.
5. The man needs medicines when he becomes sick. Exterior causes are complicated with the interior man.
6. The signs and symptoms are the language of sickness.
7. All external causes that can be responsible for sickness should be removed.
8. In the fifth paragraph of Organon, we see what points guide the physician to a cure. The homoeopath must go into the constitutional make-up of the individual.
9. The disease has three periods, when acute. They are prodromal, progressing and declining periods. - Normalcy returns after the declining period.
10. Chronic miasms also have a prodromal period, period of progress, but not a declining period.
11. A chronic miasm does not progress steadily. Whenever the conditions are favorable to it, it progresses. At every arousal the condition worsens than the earlier exacerbations.
12. The very nature of chronic miasm is to predispose an individual to acute disease.
13. Acute diseases exist from specific cause co-operating with susceptibility.
14. Psora tops the miasmatic list. Psora is responsible for the other miasmatic conditions also. No psora, no syphilis or no sycosis.
15. Man is made of feelings.
16. The disorderly condition of the human economy is the underlying cause and the fundamental state of nature of psora.

17. If the interior of the individual is insane his exterior gets distorted.
18. Causes are very subtle and are not visible, either to the naked eye or through sensitive instruments.
19. Whatever we see is the representative of the causes. Causes flow from centre to circumference.
20. Causes are immaterial.
21. Disorderly life makes one susceptible. It all starts with a disorderly thought.
22. Dr. Hahnemann instructs us to give maximum attention to the mental state.
23. The ascertainable constitution of an individual relates to the external and his outermost.
24. Susceptible individuals alone become a prey to sickness.
25. Dr. Hahnemann did not adopt any theory as bacteriology.
26. Remember the law directs and experience confirms.
27. Principle and law are authority. We have to accept it as such.

Aphorisms & Precepts

1. A truth on any plane, presented to different men, is accepted or rejected by each according to the good or evil of his mind.
2. The external man is but an outward expression of the internal; so, the results of disease (symptoms) are but the outward expression of the internal sickness.
3. If you loose the attitude of the mind, which seeks the goods of the patient, you will loose your homoeopathy.
4. Those who say they have tested homoeopathy and it is a failure, have only expressed their own ignorance.

5. Every individual is susceptible to certain things; is susceptible to sickness and equally susceptible to cure.
6. Dynamic wrongs are corrected from the interior by dynamic agencies.
7. You cannot depend on lucky shots and guess work; everything depends on long study of each individual case.
8. Understand the remedy first and the keynote last.
9. The physician, who violates his conscience, destroys his ability to perceive.
10. There is nothing in this world which does not exists by something prior to itself. With the grossest materialistic ideas man can demonstrate this.
11. The sick are entitled to exact knowledge, not to guess work.
12. Throw aside all theories, and matters of belief and opinions and dwell upon the simple fact.
13. You must be able to recognize every ambassador of the internal man.
14. The signs are visible, but the *esse* is invisible.
15. Psora is the evolution of the state of man's will, the ultimate of his sin.
16. The outgrowth, which has come upon man from living a life of evil willing - is the life of psora.

Lecture - VI

The Unprejudiced Observer

Paragraph six of the Organon says:

"The unprejudiced observer — well aware of the futility of transcendal speculations which can receive no confirmation from experience - be his powers of penetration ever so great, takes note of nothing in every individual disease, except the changes in the health of the body and of the mind which can be perceived externally by means of the senses; that is to say, he notices only the deviations from the former healthy state of the now diseased individual, which are felt by the patient himself, remarked by those around and observed by the physician. All these perceptible signs represent the disease in its whole extent, that is, together they form the true and only conceivable portrait of the disease."

We shall proceed point by point. First and foremost thing is that the homoeopath must be an unprejudiced observer.

He must know who is a healthy person and his economy.

He must also know the nature of disease to the smallest detail.

He must be aware of the drugs and their manifestations. Now we come to this paragraph with the above preliminaries in our mind.

He takes note of every individual disease - the changes in the health of the body and the mind. These are what can be perceived externally by the senses. These deviations or changes from health are as felt by the patient himself. Those around the patient bring some deviations to the physician's attention. The homoeopath, an unprejudiced observer, knows and understands all these perceptible signs represent the disease, in its whole extent. All the above conjoined gives the true and only conceivable portrait of the disease in its entirety.

Well, who is an unprejudiced observer? A grand question indeed. We have seen that homoeopathy operates on law and principle. So an unprejudiced observer should stick to the law and principle. He bases all his ideas on facts. We have seen earlier that there are no opinions. Each man may have an opinion of his own. They may not agree with another, because the opinion may be an assumption not based on actualities. Facts cannot be like that. Two plus two, all over the world can only be four. Cannot be three or otherwise. An unprejudiced observer leads a plain life with good habits. The unprejudiced observer relies upon his senses to settle what is scientific and what is not. He must see the patient and the nature of the disease as an artist feels about the picture he paints. He does not depend on lucky shots or guess work. An unprejudiced observer should have conscience. If he violates the conscience he just destroys his ability to perceive. So, there is the picture of an unprejudiced observer.

Now, we shall go deeper into the study of the above paragraph of Organon. We shall see what C.A. Baldwin, M.D., has to say about this paragraph in his work *Organon of the Art of Healing - Restated.*

"The physician should understand that the observable morbid signs and symptoms represent the changes from normal in each individual disease, and that these observable signs, symptoms and sensations, taken together in their totality, represent the disease in its full extent. And the physician should understand that only with

Lecture - VI

these changes in the sensorial condition of the body and mind, discernible through the senses, should be concern himself as an observer of the individual cases of sickness.

In the examination of any particular case, the physician should not speculate or generalize and should not be biased by any previous observations. The unbiased observer - he does not speculate. He understands the facility or transcendental speculation unsupported by experience."

What does this paragraph teach?

It teaches that the sickness is represented by symptoms. These symptoms tell the intelligent homoeopath all that is there to be known about the nature of a sickness. These symptoms indicate the state of the disorder. The sickness is only a change or deviation from health. The homoeopath has only got to set this right - the disordered state.

It is a great folly for the homoeopath to look into the organs themselves for the purpose of establishing a theory to find out whether the stomach makes the man sick or whether the stomach makes the liver sick and so on.

So long as we set the mind to think about the organs and how these things are brought about there will be only confusion. This will not be the case when we meditate upon the symptoms of the sick man. We should see it as fully representing the disease's nature. These signs and symptoms must be carefully written out.

A little more about the 'unprejudiced observer' - It is very difficult to find one in the present times to suit the description. Man has fixed politics, religion, ideas of medicine, etc. When there is prejudice, reasoning is lost. Start talking to him and he will unwind his opinions and ideas; what he thinks, etc.

When men can have authority, they can get rid of their prejudices. Let us take a group of people. They all agree on how to spell some words. They make list of these words. Now all the people of that group are decided how to spell particular words and the list they prepared becomes authority. If there we have no such authority, each person of the group will spell out the same word as he likes. When I was in school, our class teacher asked each one of us to spell out pneumonia. One spell it as newmonia, another as numonia, another nuimonia (taking nui from nuisance perhaps!) Each student tried to assert his spelling loudly - ultimately chaos prevailed. The teacher tapped his table with his stick and silence prevailed. The teacher reached the black board and wrote PNEUMONIA and said 'P' was silent! After all, the teacher was the authority and we had to agree. It was settled how to spell out pneumonia. See, that is what authority means.

Once the authority is set and recognized there can be no prejudices. This is what the law and principle of homoeopathy is. It is the authority. It cannot be deviated from. It is settled from doctrine and principle. There need not be any theory at all behind this.

No organ can make the body sick. The man is prior to organs. Man will exist in spite of removal of his body parts. This sickness is from centre to circumference - but one organ cannot make another sick.

In this paragraph Dr. Hahnemann writes about the changes of state. We could observe and feel the changes that may occur in the tissues. For an intelligent observant homoeopath these tissue changes mean nothing. These are the results of the disease not the disease by itself. For the unprejudiced observer pathology does not represent the nature of sickness or disease. This is so because there are many diseases, which can bring in identical tissue changes. Wasting of the tissues, or emaciation can be brought about by numerous conditions - it is only a result.

In homoeopathy we must be an unprejudiced observer. The homoeopath must first get rid of all his prejudices. He must cast away all his whims and notions, imaginations and presumptions and his opinions. He has to stick to the law and principle given out by our doyens. These laws and principles are fixed whether you are in North or South Pole, East or West. They do not change or vary and they cannot deceive.

If the man is not open minded and if prejudiced, man will draw out his own opinions even in law. He will then misread the law and principle to suit his way of thinking. A prejudiced mind can never reason out properly. We should not draw our own conclusions - we must believe only our senses, and go for facts. Each man tries to establish his own theory. One man's food is another man's poison. But law and principle is fixed and does not vary.

The homoeopath should examine and verify the principles and doctrines of homoeopathy. All his prejudices must be cast away. The unprejudiced observer is the only true scientist.

He perceives - remember the word? - It was mentioned in Organan paragraph three and elaborated upon. A homoeopath will see and feel with his mind and sense only the changes of the state - a deviation from good health.

The changes of state as observed by the patient himself will be - when he says he is forgetful, his mind does not operate as it did earlier, he is in a state of confusion, he misses out the continuity in his thought and speech, he becomes irritable (and that he was a pleasant person to get along with earlier) there is grief in him now, there are changes in his desires and aversions, etc. Now, look at these comments of the patient with an open mind and undivided attention. These are change of state - not change of tissues. These indicate a disorderliness and disharmony. Dr. Fincke calls this a "distunement". - A most suitable word indeed. Just imagine when your radio is not tuned properly when you want to listen to your favorite programme!

Normally his friends or relatives or his wife accompanies a patient. Whatever the patient has related is noted down carefully. Now to this list, those who accompany the patient will bring out their observation - like "he is morose, now-a-days, gets upset easily" etc., etc. All these things are also noted down as precisely as told. Taking down a case will be dealt with in later pages. - (Organan paragraph 85).

The homoeopath observes as much as he can concerning the disorder. The homoeopath has another important duty to perform. He should very closely observe the patient and note down his "abnormal" actions - which he may not do when in good health. As a small example the patient may be gently massaging his foot as he is talking with the physician - This indicates pressure relieves - which the patient might not have told. Patients are awkward and they do not know it. They will do strange and peculiar things - things they would not do when in health. These are changes of state.

The homoeopath must make a note of other things also. They are 1) note down any odors - like body odor, smell of perspiration, foul smelling breath, any odor of any discharge 2) the sounds of organs - chest sounds 3) intensity of the fever, etc. This will give him an entire picture of the disease.

All these are of real value to him.

What about the tissue changes when they are present? As told earlier, the tissue always is only a result of the disease. This can, in no way point to a remedy. How do we take the presence of a tumor? Think for a moment - what is a tumor or the aspect of the tumor that can lead the homoeopath to a remedy? - Or the change in state. So such things are of minor importance - but there is something else to be perceived, i.e. how the patient acts. How he moves, how are his functions and sensations; these are manifestations of what is going on in the internal economy of the man. Nature exhibits its state in the form of signs and symptoms. These are the things to be prescribed upon, not the tissue changes, etc. They will be taken care of automatically.

Lecture - VI

Let us consider the case where no pathological changes have yet shown itself. The signs and symptoms is always a signpost to an intelligent homoeopath. It shows the nature of the disease and the change in taste. This leads one clearly, without any confusion or ambiguity to the correct remedy. When these initial signs and symptoms are ignored and set right what happens? Has the disease changed its primitive stage and ended up as tissue changes? No, the primitive stage existed all through. The tissue changes were only a result.

Bright's disease, etc. are no disease at all. It is the ultimate organic condition, which has followed the progress of the original state - a deviation or change of state from health. Under other circumstances that change of state might have affected some other organ - like his liver and lungs.

The tissue changes do not indicate the remedy, symptoms prior to morbid anatomy must gone to the very beginning. In the earlier state things were not so complicated. The homoeopathic remedy appeal to man before his state has changed into disease ultimate. The homoeopathic remedies do not change because tissue changes or morbid anatomy has set in. They apply as much after tissue changes as before it. If we cannot arrive at the beginnings how can we intelligently treat the ending? So we should dig to reach at the beginning.

No doubt a physician must know about the tissues. But his study of this must not be with the idea of curing the sick by this knowledge.

The tissue changes do indicate certain things - like how far the disease has progressed, whether it is curable or not, etc. This will help in deciding whether the course of treatment has to be curative or palliative. Study of Materia Medica is different from study of pathology.

We have been repeatedly saying signs and symptoms guide the homoeopath to select the similimum or the correct remedy. He must know to clearly distinguish the sign and symptoms, which particularly portray the state of the patient.

We have also been repeating centre to circumference. So from the signs and symptoms, if we select the most suitable remedy will the patient be cured and remain in health? We have seen the innermost disharmonies first and then it is shown in the external man. When the medicine or remedy is given to the interior, as the interior gets harmonized it follows that the exterior must also be set right.

When the vital order is restored it will end up in tissue order. Where the cure is from cause to effect, or from within out, the patient has to be cured and will remain cured.

When the disease is incurable, we can take a palliative course of treatment. It will remove the effects temporarily. The old changes will return and grow stronger. The nature of chronic disease is to increase as time goes by.

There may still be certain results of disease, which may remain with the patient even after he is cured. It is better to wait and then the remaining signs and symptoms may be removed if necessary after a cure is brought.

Remember the tissue changes are the result of the sickness - not the sickness itself.

Summary

1. In this lecture, we see that an unprejudiced observer notes only the change of state as shown by the symptoms. This is covered by paragraph six of Organon.

    (a) The Homeopath must be an unprejudiced observer.

    (b) He must know who is healthy and who is sick.

Lecture - VI

- (c) He must be well acquainted with the nature of the sickness to the smallest details.
- (d) He must be familiar with the drug manifestations.
- (e) He must be a good perceiver, and a patient attentive listener.
- (f) He must seek and stick to the facts only.

2. The signs and symptoms tell all that should be known about the sickness.
3. Sickness is only a change of state or a deviation. The homoeopath's duty is to set this correct.
4. The authority has to be recognized without any prejudices.
5. Man is prior to his organs. One organ cannot make another organ sick.
6. The tissue changes are not the disease. - It is a result of the disease.
7. Many diseases can bring in identical tissue changes.
8. Dr. Fincke terms the disorderliness or disharmony as 'distunement'.
9. A homoeopath should also carefully listen to the observations of the sick individual as told by his people or those who accompany him to the consulting room.
10. The physician must make a note of any unnatural behavior or movements, which when healthy he will not normally do like placing his hand or palm frequently to the chest, etc.
11. The homoeopath must make a note of any particular odor, nature and color of discharges if any, any peculiar sounds from the organs (wheezing while breathing), etc. All the above put together will give the complete and clear image of the disease. Every small detail counts.

12. We must investigate a case from the beginning.
13. When the vital force disorder is set right the tissue changes also will be set right and a complete cure established.
14. We better wait for all the symptoms and signs to be totally removed even after most symptoms are cleared.

Aphorisms & Precepts

1. You cannot divorce Medicine and Theology. Man exists all the way down from his innermost spiritual, in his outermost Nature.
2. The external man is but an outward expression of the internal; so the results of disease (symptoms) are but the outward expression of the internal sickness.
3. Everything is harmoniously working in the well man. Consider the man heal the sick.
4. As long as the man is capable of believing that Diabetes is disease, and that Bright's disease is a disease, he will be insane in medicine. His mind is only directed towards the results of disease.
5. A physician's attitude in performing his duty to the sick is different from that of any other person. He has a different sphere from that of the ordinary man. This is a thousand times amplified in homoeopathy. One who has entertained that peculiar "circumcision of the heart", always looking to the good of his patient, never thinking of the criticism of man, and acquires the ability to say what is right to do. He establishes a garment of righteousness.
6. Remedies operate as by contagion. He caught disease, and catches the cure.
7. The affections make the man.

Lecture - VI

8. Every ignorant man thinks that what he knows is the end of knowledge.

9. The vital force is the soul. It cannot be destroyed or weakened. It can be disordered but it is always there.

10. There is an innermost to everything, or else the outermost could not be.

11. No power known to man exists in the concrete substance; but all power exists in the Primitive Substance.

Lecture - VII

Indispositions and Removal of their Causes

Dr. Hahnemann has provided a footnote to the seventh paragraph of his Organan. It reads as under:

"It is not necessary to say that every intelligent physician would first remove this exciting or maintaining cause (causa occasionalis), where it exists; the indisposition thereupon generally ceases spontaneously."

Note the word indisposition. What is this indisposition? Disposition is orderly arrangement or harmony. So, indisposition is derangement or disharmony. We shall take a psoric individual. External causes do not inflict upon him psora. The indispositions due to external causes mimic the miasms. The group of symptoms will be an imitation of a miasmatic manifestation. The removal of the external cause possibly will restore the patient back to health.

Man is affected by many external causes. Business failure, depressing tribulations, failure in love and such are apparent causes of disease. These causes only excite the causes of indispositions. The active cause is within and the apparent cause of the sickness is without.

If the person has no psora, no deep miasmatic influence within his economy, he would be able to cast away all his business cares.

He would not be driven to insanity by his business worries. The orderly state would be maintained. From this it is seen that the homoeopath will have to discriminate between the external and internal causes; the grosser things from the true causes of disease, and also note which are from centre to circumference.

Every true sickness is referred to by Dr. Hahnemann as miasmatic disease. Here he rises the word indisposition, "Then the indisposition yields of itself," or where the psoric condition has been somewhat disturbed, order can be restored by a few doses of the homoeopathic remedy. E.g., the man has disordered his stomach - the stomach will correct itself on ceasing further abuse. Where the trouble seems prolonged a dose or two of *Nux vomica* or whatever remedy is indicated will assist the stomach in correcting itself. As long as the patient does not abuse it again and live an orderly life he will not be a victim to this indisposition again.

Strong smelling flowers, which may have a tendency to cause syncope and hysterical sufferings, must be removed from the bedside of the patient. Some nervous girls even faint when they are exposed to this odor. Some persons cannot live in the ordinary atmosphere; some people may have to be sent to the mountains; some to warm and some to cold places. By doing this, the homoeopath removes the occasioning cause - the apparent aggravating cause of the suffering.

By doing this, the apparent cause, the disturbing cause is eliminated and the patient is made a little more comfortable. But notice that the sickness is prior to this.

Organon condemns on principle the removal of external manifestations of disease by external means of any type. A psoric case has no external or traumatic cause. The patient may live an ordinary life, does not use coffee or tea at all or may be only in small quantities, very careful in diet, etc. All these will be possibly removing or reducing the external causes. Yet you will find this person sick. The signs and symptoms that are manifested are the true impress of nature. These constantly constitute the external

Lecture - VII

image of the nature of the sickness. The symptoms alone indicate the remedy most suited to relieve the disease.

Every curable disease presents itself through signs and symptoms and an intelligent homoeopath can perceive it. These symptoms alone will suffice for him to see and get the complete portrait of the sickness.

For every coin we have two sides. In homoeopathy one side is the science of homoeopathy and the other side is the art of homoeopathy. The science treats the knowledge that is related to the doctrine of cure. The knowledge of disorder in the human economy is related to the science of disease.

The symptoms of the disease indicate the disorder of human economy. We study the symptoms of the disease of the medicine that caused the disorder in economy. Studying the Materia Medica will give us the symptoms. True homoeopathic knowledge is to be well acquainted and fully understanding the nature and the quality of a remedy, it must be compared with the sickness in humans. Thus we will get a very good idea of the nature of sickness and the disease as well as that of the remedies.

The homoeopath who heals for the love of healing will practice for the purpose of verifying his knowledge and performing his use for the love of it. The love of knowledge will encourage him - first failures, then small success, then big success will have to follow. The homoeopathic knowledge has to be constantly used. This can happen only when there is love for science.

His degree of perception will help the homoeopath to see the 'outwardly reflected image'.

Many people might have memorized the Materia Medica. This memorizing will not help him unless he has a love for knowledge and the science. He has to constantly use his knowledge. He should enjoy each and every application even in the smallest details.

Dr. Hahnemann says: " In a word the totality of the symptoms must be the principal, indeed the only thing physician has to take note of in every case of disease, and to remove by means of his art, in order that it shall be cured and transformed into health."

Well, that is the essence! — From above downward, from within out and in the reverse order of the coming of the symptoms. After all this is the law and principle.

Summary

1. This lecture deals with the footnote on indispositions and removal of their cause. This is a footnote to paragraph seven of Organon.
2. Indisposition is derangement of orderliness.
3. The indispositions due to external causes mimic the miasms. The group of symptoms will be an invitation of the miasmatic manifestation. Removal of these external causes can possibly restore the patient back to health.
4. The external causes are many - like business failures, love failures, anxiety, leading a disorderly life, etc.
5. The active cause is within and the apparent cause is without. - Always from center to circumference.
6. The true sickness is miasmatic.
7. Strong odor causing hysterical sufferings or syncope must be removed from the vicinity of the patient. Those whose conditions do not suit living in plains must be sent to hilly or mountainous places. Working this way, the aggravation and suffering are minimized.
8. Every curable disease presents itself through signs and symptoms.
9. A true homoeopath will understand the nature and quality of sickness as well as the cure.

Lecture - VII

10. The homoeopathic knowledge has got to be constantly used and applied.
11. Memorizing the Materia Medica will not help.
12. The physician has to take note of the totality of the symptoms only.
13. Remember the law and apply constantly even to the smallest detail. From center to circumference, from above downward and the symptoms removed in the reverse order of their coming.

Aphorisms & Precepts

1. Memorisers have no perception; they can only remember what they see and they see only the surface.
2. Memory is not knowledge until it is comprehended and used; then goes the ability to perceive.
3. A memoriser applies the exact sentence of the proving to the exact sentence of the patient and homoeopathy never becomes alive in him.
4. Memory is a gateway to man. The outermost envelope of his *esse* is formed to be a receptacle for the will, understanding, and the memory.
5. What seems to be intuition comes from using that which is in the understanding.
6. Anything, which looks away from exactitude, is unscientific. The physician must be classical; everything must be methodical. Science ceases to be scientific when disorderly application of law is made.
7. Eternal principles themselves are authority. The law of similar is a Divine law. So soon as you have accepted the law of

similar, you have accepted Providence, which is law and order.

8. If you do not use your homoeopathy you will lose it. This is a responsibility so great that where one has gone into the truth and does not make use of his knowledge, he will become like Egypt of old.

9. Leave names out when prescribing. They are only for the foolish and for the boards of health.

10. The disease is not to be named but to be perceived; not to be classified but to be viewed, that the very nature of it may be discovered.

11. The human mind should not be burdened with technicalities. They destroy description and close the understanding.

12. Every scientific man today is trying to find something he can claim as his own. Such a man cannot understand homoeopathy. He worships himself. Has dwelt on the externals so long that it is impossible for him to think rationally.

13. Man's unbelief and opinion do not affect truth. The experience, which a homoeopath has, is experience under law and confirms the law and by this order is maintained.

14. Whenever a man settles all things by his eyes, and fingers, pseudo-science and theories, he reasons from lasts to firsts; in other words, from himself, and is insane.

15. Materia Medica never inspires perception. The physician must have the love for its use, and he becomes wise in proportion as he loves his use, and in proportion as he lives uprightly with his patients; that is desires to heal them; beautify their soul. Can the physician, who does not love his neighbor as himself, get into this position?

Lecture - VIII

On Simple Substance

In the paragraph 9 of Orgonan, Dr. Hahnemann states: —

"In the healthy condition of man, the spiritual vital force, the dynamics that animates the material body, rules with unbounded sway, and retains all parts of the organism in admirable, harmonious, vital operation, as regards, both sensations and functions, so that our dwelling reason gifted mind can freely employ this living healthy instrument for the higher purpose of our existence".

We shall break this down in parts to enable us get a better picture of this paragraph.

What happens in the healthy man?

(1) There is a spiritual vital force in every man.

(2) This is the dynamic force that animates the material body.

(3) It is the monarch.

(4) It controls and retains all the parts of the human organism with unbounded sway.

(5) The sensations and functions are controlled by this dynamics.

(6) It does this so as to enable our dwelling (the body) and the reason gifted mind to freely utilize this healthy living instrument for higher purpose of our existence.

Well, there we have the vital principle. Dr. Hahnemann could not have explained this any better. He wrote in the seventh section of the first edition of his Organan:

"There must exist in the medicine a healing principle; the understanding has a presentiment of it". As we all know Organan has gone through several editions, Dr.Hahnemann had somewhat changed. In this work, the 1883 edition, he distinctly calls a unit of action in the whole organism the vital force.

At the outlook it may appear, from some of his expressions that harmony is itself a force. We cannot consider the vital principle as harmony, nor harmony as principle. Principle is something that is prior to harmony. Harmony can be result of the principle or law.

Dr. Hahnemann was able to perceive this immaterial vital principle. He arrived at this from his own thought process. There were a few ideas at his time, i.e. ideas outside the accepted sciences. But Dr. Hahnemann applied his thought process and came out with the above expression only in the last edition. "In the healthy condition of man the immaterial vital principle animates the material body". Perhaps Dr. Hahnemann could have used the expression "immaterial vital substance". It would have been stronger and had a greater impact. It will be seen that it is a substance.

We now speak of fourth state of matter, which is immaterial substance. We now say the solids, liquids and gases and the radiant form of matter. Substance in simple form is just as positively substance as a matter in concrete form. Then you may ask, "What is this vital force? What is its character, quality or essence? Does man alone possess this vital force? Does an animal or a mineral possess it?

Lecture - VIII

For several years there has been a continuous discussion about force as force or power to construct. The idea that the force had nothing prior to it is madness. If man can think of energy as something substantial, he can, better think of something substantial having energy. If he thinks of something that has essence, has actual being, he must also think of that essence as something existing and as having something, which has ultimate.

Man should think in an orderly way, not haphazardly. He must think in a way whereby causes enter into effect and further more into a series of effects. If he does not do this, the very nature and idea of influx and continuance is destroyed.

Man should know what is continuous and must realize that there are beginning and intermediates and then ends. If he does not realize this, then he cannot think since the very foundation of thought is destroyed.

Influx - What does that mean? Let us take a chain. How is it constructed? How is the last link connected to the first link? The answer is "by the intermediate links". The last link is hooked to the previous hook - the previous hook to its previous hook and so on. Thus the last link is connected to the first link - see it? There is a continuous dependence from the last link to the first link. Whenever the chain is broken there is no longer the influx from one link to the other.

This illustration shows there must be an order and proper linking or hooking in a chain. When we speak about a few connected thoughts what do we call it? - A "chain of thoughts". See the connection? This shows that all things must be united. When it is not so the series is broken and the influxes cease to exist.

We are able to see man exists in his body. We are not able to see the finer and subtle purpose of his being.

Man becomes an irrational being when he believes he exists without a cause, his life course goes on for a while, does not exist from something prior to it, that the influx is not there constantly and continuously. Man has never been able to prove anything can exist, except it continually flows into, which holds it continuously. He assumes that energy is the first in the immaterial world. Why? We have reason, to say that energy is not energy per se, but it is a powerful substance. Man's intelligence is taken to be a substance. Energy is a powerful substance and it is endowed from intelligence.

A materialist denies the soul, denies a substantial God due to his principle. The energy, which he dwells upon so much, means nothing to him - so he has to assume God is nothing and hence He does not exist.

A rational person believes in Supreme God - He is substantial and He is a substance. This person believes that everything proceeds from Him and from the Supreme to the most ultimate matter; he also believes that everything is connected, this way. When there is a separation, there is no influx from the first to the last and then ultimate also ceases to exist.

The simple substance truly holds together the material world. When we refer to the world the two spheres that come to our mind is the thought world and the world of matter. We look at this in a different way - the immaterial world and the material world. The material world of substance is in order and harmonious. Whatever we are able to see with our eye has beginnings. The forms are harmonious. There is an order, law. Every crystal that crystallizes does so in an orderly fashion. Man's anatomy forms is in a harmonious manner. We are not able to see anything in this material world that can account for this orderliness and harmony. Yet it is so. We cannot deny it. It is obvious that this is so because of the continuous influx from the first to last. The chain is continuous and intact. Nothing can exist unless there is continuous inflow from beginning to end. Whatever man make are not permanent - they decay at one time or the other. But see things perpetuated from

Lecture - VIII

influx. Look at their order and harmony and permanence. They work according to plan and order. There is no disorder or confusion in this at all!

Simple substances have many qualities. The first thing we have to learn about *the simple substance is that it is endowed with formative intelligence*, i.e. it operates intelligently and forms the economy of the entire animal, vegetable and mineral kingdoms. Everything that has a form goes on its natural course. They assume and continue in their own private state. Man is able to detect all the elements because they are of a very orderly nature. They, themselves conduct themselves most uniformly.

The simple substance provides to everything its own type of life - gives it an identity of its own, an individuality; hence it differs from the rest and also is recognizable as such.

The crystal of the earth has its own identity, has its own association. It is endowed with a simple substance and it establishes its own particular identity - from the animal kingdom and the mineral kingdom. Why is this so? This is so because of its formative intelligence of simple substance. This is continuous from the beginning to end.

Observe frost on a glass pane of the window. It tends to manifest formative intelligence. Plants grow in fixed forms. All coconut palm leaves are identical whether in India or in Hawaii - the world over wherever it exists. They do not differ from place to place, soil-to-soil, etc. There is a universal order and harmony about it. A baby born in London is identical in its organs with that of a baby born in Australia. The structure of the framework may differ slightly - but all organs and their functions are the same the world over. There is uniformity. The gestation period does not change. The growth is gradual and controlled - come to think of this influx and orderliness. It goes according to the law of influx. All forms are subject to this —there is no exception, no compromise. We have seen that man has been gifted with a reason-minded sense. Well, when this is so, man must be rational. He is of the highest order in the creation. For all practical purposes the man is rational and so must keep himself so in continuous order so as to continue to be rational. Just see it! Is it so? Earlier we saw that a simple substance gives or provides to each, its own life. That is freedom. When this freedom is closely examined with rational lines, man is the ultimate and of the highest order and lives and leads an orderly life.

When man looses his reason and capacity to think rationally he abuses the freedom offered to him. Now what happens? Chaos! His rationality is destroyed.

This substance is subject to changes. When the orderliness and harmony is changed there is disorderliness and disharmony. From health he is pushed to sickness. Thus the man-created changes are visible and observable. Man causes this havoc.

Any simple substance may pervade the entire material substance without causing any disturbance or replacing it. Take magnetism for example. It may occupy a substance - but it does not displace it - neither does it cause derangement of its particles or crystals. Take cohesion; it is a simple substance. Cohesion does not disturb or displace the substance it occupies.

What does this prove? The first substance or the primitive substance does not exist in all distinct forms of growths of concrete forms. The material, concrete and possessing individuality is not disturbed or displaced by the simple substance, as seen above. It goes to prove that simple substance is always capable of occupying the material substance without accident to that substance itself.

Let us take the simple substance to be an active substance. *Then it controls the body it occupies.* Why? What does an active person do? He uses his force. If the force is not utilized he is not active! Force does not mean brutal - it may be passive. It is the nature of force or cause of force. It cannot be otherwise.

Lecture - VIII

When does a body move, think or act? It does so only when the interior degree of immaterial substance is separated from its characterizing simple substance and the influx ceases. Till then it has been acting upon the economy continuously in the most beautiful manner. *This energy got from the simple substance keeps everything going and in order.* This simple substance maintains all the functions in an orderly fashion - of every animal, plant and mineral.

This simple substance is responsible for all actions in this universe. It is the simple substance that keeps everything in order. It alone operates in each and every material substance. *It causes the co-operation of all things in this world.*

Observe the universe - the sun, the moon, the stars, etc. Do they interfere with each other? Each one behaves in its own orderly fashion. Whenever we turn and see we see co-operation - a co-operation that is in perfect harmony with each other. Ever gone into a forest? - For a change go and observe. The bees, birds, animals, worms, insects and the plants are all in harmony and function in the most orderly fashion. Each one does its own work - non-interfering with others. All together they maintain the serenity of the forest. The same simple substance does all this.

Look into the economy of a human. How very astonishing and wonderful! This simple life substance is responsible for all this. What happens if this simple life substance ceases to exist? Death, yes it is death. With death all the higher purpose of existence is lost. It is as simple as that. So it is the simple substance, blessed to us by the Creator, works wonders. It is able to use all creations for their highest purposes. Simple substance surpasses everything and it can be seen so.

Matter is subject to reduction: we can go on reducing continuously the matter, step by step. Matter ultimately reduces to simple substance. Note it - it is not subject to restitution. Any matter that is reduced to its primitive state cannot be returned to its ultimate form. This is the law. Man does not have the power to ultimate the simple substance. The Supreme Power holds this power in His hands. Power flows continuously from Him. It flows through all the primitive substance continuously from beginning to end; i.e. to the ultimate.

Now emerges a clear picture. A thing that does not start from the beginning with a purpose is not a thing. So it goes that everything is having its ultimate or purpose - a useful purpose. *Nothing is created without a purpose.*

When a thing does not exist in continuity from beginning to end it cannot be of any use or purpose. The end is in the first and the end is in every succeeding link to its ultimate. Then only the form can be appropriated and established for its usefulness. What a marvelous thing it is - when you establish the first link in a chain, it is the end of the next link in view - a continuous order indeed.

The simple substances may exist as simple, compound or complex state. The harmony is maintained from first to last. Thus all purposes are conserved. This compounding can be seen in chemistry, through out. We find two simple substances compounding in keeping with their own individual plan. It happens reliably and intelligently and in accordance with their affinities, for each other.

When the substances come together like that they do not disturb the simple substance of each other. There is no destruction of anything and each one retains its own identity. Now all of these enter into the human body. Every element in the human body preserves its identity throughout. Each one can be identified, wherever found. Such combination merely represents a composite state. But when these composite substance and the simple substances are brought into an additional condition, i.e., when there is a domination by something they may enter into a very complex form and in the body a life force keeps every other force in order.

Lecture - VIII

Dynamic simple substances often dominate each other in proportion to their purpose, one having a higher purpose, one having a higher purpose than another. This vital force, which is a simple substance, is again dominated by another simple substance still higher and that is the soul. Many philosophers have attempted to draw some conclusion about the soul. They all have attempted to locate it at some particular point in the body. From the above, it can be seen it is not in circumscribed location.

While considering simple substance, we cannot think of things like time, place or space. This is so because we are not dealing with something like mathematics or in the world of space and time. We are in the realm of simple substance. When you think of place and time it is finite.

Quantity cannot be predicated to simple substance. Quality alone is in degrees of fineness matter. How is this applicable in homoeopathy? We shall presently see it. We administer remedy - say *Sulphur* 50M. It is given in infrequent doses. We see that it no longer works. What do we do now? We switch on to c.m. potency and it works! What does this indicate? It clearly indicates that we have entered a new series of degrees- *dealing with quality entirely and not quantity.*

The simple substance has adaptation. If man's reasoning power interferes we are lead to false conclusions from appearances since the man has accepted the environmental theory. We should see what is it that adapts itself to the environment. Here we are not questioning whether the individual can adapt to the environment. A dead body cannot adapt itself to the environment. By careful reasoning from within we can see that it adapts its house to the surroundings. Thus the human body, under all circumstances, is kept in an orderly state - whether it be hot or cold, wet or damp. The surrounding themselves produces nothing. They are not causes, but they are only circumstances.

The soul is a simple substance. *The life substance within the body is the vice-regent of the soul. We can see that all* that there is of the soul operates and exists within every part of the human body. It is the vital force that acts and it is simple substances. The soul adapts the human body to all its purposes - the higher purposes of its being.

The simple substance keeps the body animated as long as it exists in the living human body. It keeps the body fit and moving - perfects its use. Bosses over all parts at the same time keeping the operation of mind and will in order. When there is any disturbance in the vital substance and immediately we see the non-co-ordination. Harmonious co-operation is maintained when the vital substance is continued in its normal quality.

This vital substance, when in a natural state and when in contact with the human body, is constructive. The body is continuously maintained, constructed and re-constructed. When the vital force is withdrawn from the body for any reason, havoc occurs. The forces in the body being unleashed and they become destructive. The vital force is a stern master. It is capable of keeping under control the most powerful forces in the body. But when this domination misses out for any reason, the body decays, at once.

So it is clear that the vital force is constructive and formative. Its absence spells out death and destruction.

We find from examination of the simplest form of living organism, the plasson body, we see that it possesses all the essentials of life. Everything of the highest order that life possesses. It has life properties and qualities; man and animal has - it moves, feeds, reproduces itself and it is also endowed with influx and lastly it can also be killed. Here, we have predicated much of the vital substance - from the highest to the lowest. It asserts its identity; it moves and feeds; it propagates and can be killed. It does not sustain its identity by chemical analysis since when chemical analyzed it is no longer protoplasm. Protoplasm is protoplasm, only when it lives. Chemically, all there is to be found

Lecture - VIII

of protoplasm is C, O, H, N and S, but the life substance cannot be found. Put in 54 parts of C, 21 of O, 16 of N, 7 of H, and 2 of S. What is it that you suppose will be in your hands? - Just a composite something but not the complex thing that we call or identify as protoplasm. In analyzing the protoplasm what happened to the life force? There is no difference in weight after death. Simple substance cannot be weighed. *The simple substance is just simple and it cannot be predicated of by weight, space, time etc., it does not subjugate itself to any physical law, like law of gravitation, etc.*

Let us consider this possesses power. Inert elements by nature have their own identifying simple substance. Further they have degrees of life substance varying in degrees suitable of all its uses. The innermost degrees of life substances are suitable to the will and understanding. The outermost degrees to the very coarse tissue and there is one continuity of quality, in degrees from the innermost to the outermost. Each cell has within it the innermost and the outermost because there is nothing in that which is coarse but has that which is the finest, as well. The outermost envelopes are dominated by the coarser degrees of simple substance and the innermost qualities are dominated by the innermost degrees. Each portion has an appropriate form; from the outermost to the innermost it has everything. Otherwise, the human body could not be dominated or ruled by the soul. Each tissue has, within it, its own portion of the vital substance, each having its own peculiar function.

Inert substances have their own degrees. Silica has its degrees of simple substance within it. Which can be brought out by the process of potentization, whereby it may be continuously simplified, rendered finer and finer, so that each portion which remains may, by continued potentization, be adapted to the higher degrees of simple substance of man. The thirtieth potency of silica will be sufficiently similar in form to reach, in a curative way, some of the diseases of the man viz., such as are dominating his economy in a correspondingly superficial and coarse series of the body. Silica ceases to act after a time in the thirtieth potency and it has to be further potentized in order it may be similar in quality to the inner degrees, even until it reaches the very innermost or finest degrees of the simple substance.

You take anything in this universe. It has its own aura or atmosphere. Stars and planets too have an atmosphere. The planet sun has light and heat as its atmosphere. Each human being has his own aura. So does every animal. The musk has an aura of its own? Yes, very much. It is the strong physical odor that any one can perceive. For seventeen years, a grain of musk was kept in a bottle - for experimental purposes. At the end of that period there was no loss of weight - yet giving out its perceptible aura.

Animals have extreme sense of aura, which man cannot discover. It is the instinct whereby it perceives its prey. They animal's instinct is analogous to the perception of man. The animal finds its prey by this instinct, and man is not able to discuss it. Man can smell the musk in a bottle, by his olfactory senses - it is very doubtful whether he can discover the aura by its odor. This aura becomes very useful. In the study of Homeopathy, aura finds a prominent sphere.

The consciousness between two atmospheres is that atmosphere by which one knows the other. All their affinities and repulsions are also known. They exist in two conditions - either in harmony or in antagonism. All human beings are classified as positives and negatives. There is a reason for it. Substances are extremely powerful when meeting other substances, which happen to be antagonistic in any way. They are so, also when meeting substances in a destructive way. By destruction, the formative process is brought about. Forms are destroyed so that new forms may exist. New forms are often created from simple substance.

There are two realms - one of cause and the other of ultimate. We are able to see the innermost physical world with

Lecture - VIII

the eye, touch with the finger, smell with the nose, and hear with the ear. It is the realm of results.

The realm of cause is invisible. The five senses are incapable to sense the realm of cause. It is a world of its own and *thought and understanding alone can discover that realm.* What we see around us is the world of ends - not the world of cause. Man must perceive the innermost. He should look from within upon all the things in the physical world. One cannot begin at the physical world and try to look upon the immaterial world from that platform.

Homoeopathy, as we have seen exists in law; its causes are in the realm of causes. If not existing in the world of causes, it could not exist in the world of ultimate. *In homoeopathy study we should always look in the realm of cause for primaries.*

The above is the groundwork of homoeopathy. Disease causes are in simple substance—there is no disease cause in concrete substance considered apart from simple substance. We study the simple substance to enable us arrive at the nature of the substance that causes sickness. *Potentization is sought to reach at their simple substance i.e., the nature and quality of the remedy itself.* A homoeopathic remedy has to possess the similar quality, similar action to the disease cause.

To summaries the nature of simple substance : -
1. Simple substance is endowed with formative intelligence.
2. Simple substance is subject to changes.
3. It may pervade the entire material substance without disturbing or replacing it.
4. It dominates and controls the body it occupies.
5. Matter is subject to reduction—but it is not subject to restitution.
6. It may exist as simple, compound or complex state.
7. Quality and not quantity—only degrees of fineness.
8. It can adapt.
9. It is constructive keeping the body constructed and reconstructed.

Summary

1. This lecture deals with simple substance—paragraph nine of Organon.
2. There is a spiritual vital force in every individual. This animates the human body. It is the controlling factor. It enables our dwelling (the body) and the reason-gifted mind to freely utilize the healthy living body for higher purposes of our existence.
3. Harmony is itself not a force. Harmony is the result. Harmony is what we enjoy because of good health.
4. Dr.Hahnemann says, "In the healthy condition of man the immaterial vital principle animates the material body."
5. There are three states of substances known to the man—solid, liquid and gaseous states. There is a fourth dimension - immaterial substance.
6. A dud looking seed when planted in the earth springs forth a huge tree. That is because of the power within the immaterial substance that we cannot see by naked eyes or even by sensitive scientific instruments.
7. The power within was present in the seed even before the tree—prior.
8. Causes run into effects. This can be realized by orderly thinking.
9. There is always a beginning, intermediate and end condition in thought process. Man should realize this continuous process and also contemplate on influx.
10. Think of a chain. It is made up of several links. Each link is connected to the previous and the next one. If this connection is not there or broken, you cannot call it a chain. So, one

Lecture - VIII

runs into another, from the beginning to the last. This also goes to prove that there must be orderliness.

11. One running into another is called influx. So, when the links are broken or are not connected the influx ceases.
12. Energy is a powerful substance. It is endowed from intelligence.
13. There are two worlds - the world of the immaterial and the world of material.
14. Whatever we are able to see is the material world. They have their beginnings and are harmonious.
15. But we cannot see what is responsible for this harmony. Yet it is so and there is no denial about it. It is so because of the continuous influx.
16. Whatever man produces decays and is not permanent. In due course it is gone.
17. Simple substance is endowed with a formative intelligence. It operates intelligently and forms the economy of the entire animal, vegetable and mineral kingdoms.
18. Just think of the petroleum process. How a seed grows into a plant, tree, gives out fruits and then seeds. Again they fall on the ground to propagate. Then it decays again in the earth.
19. Each crystal on the earth has its own identity, because of the simple substance in it, and its formative intelligence.
20. Uniformity and orderliness is the secret of nature.
21. Man is a rational animal and he must maintain himself so.
22. Simple substance provides to each its own life.
23. When man's rationality is destroyed only chaos can result.
24. Simple substance is subject to change. When the order is upset health is affected.

25. Simple substance may pervade the entire substance without causing any disturbance or replace it.
26. Simple substance controls the body it occupies.
27. Simple substance is always in order, and maintains harmony.
28. Matter is subject to reduction. Matter when reduced completely, step by step, is simple substance.
29. All things right from the start have a purpose. Nothing is created without a purpose.
30. Simple substance can be simple, compound or a complex state.
31. Simple substance does not disturb each other.
32. Dynamic simple substances often dominate each other in proportion to their purpose.
33. In the realm of simple substance there is no time, place or space. It is beyond these.
34. Quantity cannot be predicated to simple substance. Quality alone in degrees of fineness does matter.
35. Simple substance is adaptive to its environment.
36. Simple substance is the monarch of the body.
37. Everything in this universe has its own aura.
38. The realm of cause is invisible.
39. Homeopathy exists in law - its causes are in the realm of causes.
40. Disease causes are simple substances.
41. Potentization is sought to reach the simple substance.

Aphorisms & Precepts

1. Dynamic wrongs are corrected from the interior by dynamic agencies.

Lecture - VIII   83

2. Man cannot be made sick or be cured except by some substance as ethereal in quality as the vital Force.
3. It is unthinkable to speak of motion or force, without a simple primitive substance. Force or action of a nothing is unthinkable.
4. It is a serious matter to allow the mind to drift into thinking of anything but quality when speaking of force.
5. There is at the present time a continual discussion of force as an energy having nothing prior to it. This is confusion.
6. The simple substance is the substance of substances, and all things are from it. It is really first, in which rests all power.
7. Weight cannot be predicated of the simple substance, neither time nor space.
8. No power known to man exists in the concrete substance, but all power exists in the Primitive substance.
9. The Primitive substance, or Radiant form of matter, is just as much as matter, as matter in its aggregate form.
10. The real holding together of the things in this world is by simple substance.
11. If it were not for the simple substance, such states as antipathy, sympathy, or affinity could not be; it is the sphere of homoeopathy to deal with these things, to glean what is the real *esse* and existence.
12. There are two worlds; the world of thought, or immaterial substance and the world of matter or material substance.
13. What reason has man to say that energy or force is first. Energy is not energy *per se*, but a powerful substance. The very *esse* of God is a scientific study.
14. Bodies are not drawn together by means of their bodies, but by means of their Primitive substance.
15. The simple substance is the means of identification in nature. The mineral, the oak, the wheat, are all identified by their

Primitive Substance, and exist, only, because of their Primitive Substance, which makes them what they are.

16. Name everything that is, or moves; it is sustained from and by power of the Primitive Substance. We do not argue that it is first power, but this is first substance.

Lecture - IX

Disorder First in Vital Force

Here we shall deal with the paragraph No.10 and No.11 of Organon.

Organon paragraph No.10 reads as:

"The material organism, without the vital force, is capable of no sensation, no function, no self-preservation; it derives all sensations and performs all the functions of life solely by means of the immaterial being (the vital force), which animates the material organism in health and in disease."

Organon, paragraph No.11 reads as:

"When person falls ill it is only this spiritual, self-acting (automatic) vital force everywhere present in his organism, that is primarily deranged by the dynamic influence upon it of a morbific agent inimical to life; it is only the vital force, deranged to such an abnormal state, that can finish the organism with its disagreeable sensations and incline it to the irregular processes which we call disease; for, as a power invisible in itself, and only cognizable by the effects on the organism, its morbid derangement only makes itself known by the manifestation of disease in the sensations and functions of those parts of the organism exposed to the senses of the observer and physician; that is by morbid symptoms, and in no other way can it make itself known."

Let us go to paragraph 10 :

It says that the vital force is most essential for the functioning of our sensations, functions for self-preservation, etc.

The immaterial being along provides all the sensations and performs all the life functions. *The immaterial being is the vital force that animates the material organism, be it health or disease.*

Looking at paragraph 11, we understand: A person falls ill, what has happened? The vital force is spiritual and self-acting and automatic. It is present everywhere in the human organism. This vital force is deranged—deranged by what? Deranged by a dynamic influence upon it by a morbific agent. This morbific agent is inimical to life. When the vital force is deranged to such an abnormal state it creates disagreeable sensations. So an irregular process has now crept in, what we call as disease. *This morbific agent as a power is invisible - but it makes its presence felt by the manifestation of disease* - in the sensations and functions of those parts of the organism exposed - to the observer and physician. They are the morbid symptoms. In no other way can it make itself known, or make its presence felt.

From the above we can understand that the disorders of the activities of the internal man is a lack of harmony, a lack of balance and this lack gives forth the signs and symptoms which we recognize as disease. The disorder is expressed by the sensations and that is the language of the disorder.

The immaterial vital principle is a simple substance. It pervades the organism everywhere. In disease also this pervades everywhere - every cell and every portion of the human economy. Changes in the form of a cell are the result of disorder first. Remember the chain link analogy we dealt with earlier? It is the same here also - the derangement of the immaterial vital principle is the very beginning of the disorder. With this beginning there are changes in the sensation by which man may know this beginning. This change

Lecture - IX

occurs long before there is any visible change in the material substance of the body.

The patient can feel these changes by his sensations. These changes are inimical to life. *Life in its fullest sense is freedom.* As soon as the internal economy is deprived of its freedom in any manner, death is around the corner. Where freedom is lost, death is sure to follow. Earlier while on the subject of simple substance we saw it gives everything in its own type of life - that is freedom.

So, we see what happens when there is the influence of a simple substance, which possesses the essence of a disease. In essence, it is an evil that flows into the economy and it is a simple substance. Everything is substantial or real. Each has in itself operating and perpetuating power. The fact that it can operate and perpetuate is the evidence of power. When it has power, it results in something. Every cause of disease then has a form. Unless it is in the form of simple substance, it could not affect the form of simple substance in the natural state of economy. Moreover, it has its association from the finest forms of physical substance to the crudest - again from the beginning to the end and the inner to the outer. These changes and activities in the very crudest form are the results of disease. It is exhibited through a series of degrees coarser and coarser to the outer-most man.

Whatever we can see, and those observed with the finest instrument is nothing but the result. We have mentioned earlier that the immaterial substance is invisible. *We cannot see the immaterial substance with any faculty or instruments.* Nothing that is capable of seeing things in the world of material substance is capable of seeing through the immaterial substance.

There are instruments and instruments to see the result of disease. They can help up only in that way. They can be the most precise instruments - yet they can see the finest result of the disease only. Through these beautiful and sensitive instruments we can see the bacteria, very finest form of animal or vegetable life - but with all these precious instruments, we cannot see the immaterial substance since it is million times subtler. Nor can the human eye see it. The finest objects that are visible are the results of still finer; the cause rests within. Dr. Hahnemann refers to the morbific agents, which are extremely fine forms of simple substance - which we can call as virus. But then the viruses are gross and sometimes can be observed by the vision of man. So we should remember that within the virus is the innermost - is in itself capable of giving form to the outermost. This virus is visible and concentrated.

The coarser forms would be comparatively harmless, were it not for the interiors. The disease products are comparatively harmless but for the fact they contain an innermost. The innermost itself is the causative.

The bacteria are the result of the conditions within, evolved by the spontaneous generation. Every virus is capable of assuming forms and shapes in ultimate. The causes of ultimate are not found without - they are from the immaterial invisible centre. Whatever we are able to see, are evolved - just like the man himself who is formed from a centre and has the power of evolving. This is a blessing from the creator and operates in accordance with the fixed general laws.

Only when a disease character - which is the innermost of a virus in the form of simple substance, disturbs the vital principle - it makes its presence felt.

If there were no disturbing influence in the interior of man there can be no symptoms. Generally when we sit in a perfect state of quietude, everything is tranquil. Then we are not conscious of the eyes, limbs or other parts of the body. You have to consciously think whether you feel it or not

When all functions are in an orderly fashion, there is no consciousness of the body - meaning that we are in freedom. When freedom is not there, we say 'I feel'. This disturbance is invisible in its character, stemming out from cause and appears by

Lecture - IX

the changes in the activities of the body. There are changes of sensation, changes in functions.

An intelligent homoeopath identifies these and understands their meaning. They are warning they are for us and for purpose. Every feeling that a man has has a purpose. Remember everything in the universe has its own purpose and use. *The morbid sensation reveals to the homoeopath that disorder exists.*

The homoeopath's sole intention must be to establish freedom. *Healing the sick is placing patient in freedom - absolute physical freedom.* This is brought by removing the signs and symptoms in an orderly way - step by step - converting the disorder in such a way, they no longer have a cause. Earlier, we have seen that when economy is turned into order, signs and symptoms cease. Then we have placed our patient in freedom, both physical and mental.

Disease is the abnormal sensations that incline it to irregular actions. This is totally different from calling the result of disease, the disease. Bright's disease, cancer, palsy are all results of diseases, not disease by themselves. *Generally the conditions of human economy are called as disease - it is not correct. It is only the result of disease.* Our calling a group of symptoms a disease of one part, and another group of disease of another part is only a heresay. It leads to erroneous prescriptions and that can never be correct. Organic change is the result of disease.

Morbid disturbances can be perceived solely by the expressions of the disease in sensations and actions. Morbid sensations alone clearly indicate morbid disturbances of the invisible principle. There is nothing else to indicate this derangement. But for these indications we have no other means to restore back the freedom of a patient.

There are patients who are so sick that they cannot be put back on the road to health and freedom - they have no cure - and in these patients the internal structural changes go on slowly and the morbid symptoms are not present. These patients continuously change the doctors and climates. They recognize no one is capable of relieving them. When there is an incurable change in the vital organ, all or most of the symptoms that existed vanish; the symptoms of the disease are suppressed, as it were by the tremendous strain upon the system.

This is very true in malignant forms of the results of the disease. The symptoms that existed many years ago are no longer there. The patient may say that they did not amount to anything and he had them all his life. But those are the symptoms that would manifest to a homoeopath the nature of the remedy - they give him the true and real image of sickness.

Some doctors say that there will be remedy for cancer some day. They have in their minds only the symptoms of cancer - but then, the symptoms, which are the result of the disease, are not the symptoms of the disease itself. There is a vast difference between these two.

The doctors would not speak like this if they only knew the symptom of the result of the disease is not the symptom of the disease itself. They will think in more wholesome and proper way - they would know that to cure the patient is the cure of cancer; in order to cure the patient it is very necessary to go back in the patient's history - go to the very beginning and go to the symptoms that represent the patient in a state of disease and not the tissues in a state of the results of the disease.

In the later state, the original symptoms of the disease have vanished. They have been swallowed up. So it is when the innermost disease has acted and the whole body is full of disease results, such as dropsical conditions, or pus sacs, or hip-joint abscesses. The pains make the patient not to think about his symptoms. Here the physicians prescribe medicines for the results of the disease and they end up in failure.

Some doctors give *Silica* for hip-joint disease, *Bufo* for

Lecture - IX 91

epilepsy etc. *This is giving medicines for groups of symptoms. Well, this is not homoeopathy at all.*

A good homoeopath can listen to the signs and symptoms before morbid changes occur. If no medication has been done, the image stands out in front of him in relief and it is perfect. It is so because it has not been meddled with. It speaks with clarity and the intelligent homoeopath can learn to understand it so. Whereas the physician who is not capable of seeing that this is different from the group of pathological symptoms which represent the so called fixed diseases, he cannot make a distinction between the symptoms that represent the disease per se and the symptoms representing the result of the disease. He will never practice homoeopathy successfully.

He has to work at it till he understands it. This means application and labor till he can clearly discriminate between the organic symptoms associated with the results of disease and the pure signs given forth by nature.

Some physicians ask, "What remedy do you give for such and such a case?" Such a question can come out of an untrained person in homoeopathy, only.

You have to adjust the remedy to the patient. In homoeopathy you do not adjust the remedy to pathological conditions. The homoeopath needs symptoms, not pathological results.

Human body is capable of self-curing. If the first disorder state is removed his economy will be safe. The patient himself will restore his health, if the results of the disease cannot be removed, the morbid anatomy will undergo such changes that it will not affect his state of health. The fibrinous adhesions need not necessarily go away - a state of quiescence sets in as long as he remains well.

Do not think of a remedy for cancer- it will be just confusion. But, think of a remedy for the patient who appears to have cancer. This is orderly thinking. You will be astonished to know the wonderful changes that will take place, the conditions before cancer began. Cancer is the result of disorder. It is this disorder that has to be set right and healed.

We must consider the true morbid sensations of a healthy organism. First it is assumed that the organism is in a state of health; it is capable of performing its functions; and then the morbid sensation of this healthy organism are the symptoms, that are presented to the physician as a forerunner of death in parts; finally death of the whole.

A sick man tells the physician about the various sensations he experiences - like numbness of fingers, pricking sensation in the skin, stomach-pain, etc. These are the sensations of the parts of his body of which he is reminded. In freedom and in health he is not reminded of the parts - we have seen this earlier. When a healthy man passes urine there is no sensation - so to say. But then when it smarts or burns and tenesmus follow, immediately his attention is drawn to it - these sensations constitute symptoms.

The homoeopath can see and note down the patient's appearance - like waxy and pallid, has papules and pustules, swollen varicose veins with red face, blood-shot eyes, etc. While these are observable, there are certain things that he cannot see, certain things that the patient cannot or may not be able to tell - some things may be told by the relatives, friends who may accompany the patient to the clinic. These symptoms convey to him what is to be known about the sickness and enable him to select the remedy.

Where the strong symptoms are all gathered together, he must separate out things that were observed years ago. Those that are observed today must be listed separately. He must also note how the old symptoms have changed and why so. Sometimes they have been so changed because of drugs, so that the whole nature of the economy is speaking out a different group of symptoms.

He must note and learn all the changes along the line - from beginning to end - like what were the symptoms ten years ago and what are the symptoms now. The patient may now have a

Lecture - IX

morbid anatomy, pathological conditions in his lungs, liver and kidneys. The homoeopath, when he works upon a case in this fashion, can practically locate the morbid anatomy; he can say where it will appear, knows when and where pus is in the patient's organs and can predict for certain what can be expected to occur in the patient's economy soon.

The symptoms do not lie - they do not exist from opinions. Symptoms are facts. He, who follows this cardinal rule, will be a successful homoeopath. He must make himself conversant with the symptoms, to judge the sphere and progress of disease by means of symptomatology. Also physical examination is important. The homoeopath can make a physical examination after noting down the symptoms. The study of a sick man is the meditation of his symptoms. An able prescriber will be wise in symptoms.

There is nothing wrong in studying physical diagnosis - but then compare it carefully with the symptoms and ascertain what the different symptoms mean and indicate. The anatomy of the brain and nerves must be thoroughly known to a homoeopath. He may not be using the name of the nerves - but then he must know where it is found in the anatomy and what its functions are. This study should be continuous throughout the life. *The homoeopath must be a student forever.*

He has to be conversant with the anatomy and physiology - but by studying the symptomatology, he acquires a special knowledge of physiology. This is not possible otherwise. He has to study the operations and functions of arteries, nerves and muscles since when disturbed they call for attention. Thus he can see how the symptoms manifest themselves. Morbid pathology does not help in prescribing - but true pathology is often of greatest benefit and it helps the image of sickness to shape itself mentally.

Summary

1. The lecture deals with the paragraph ten and eleven of the Organon. The subject matter is disordered first with vital force.

2. We have seen that vital force is the most essential thing for the functioning and the sensations of the human individual.
3. The vital force when deranged by a dynamic sprit-like influence, the economy gets shattered and the individual is sick.
4. Morbific agents are inimical to life.
5. The morbific agent is invisible, but its presence is felt by the manifestation of the disease. It cannot make its presence known by any other method.
6. We see that the man is affected internally and there is a lack of harmony or lack of balance. Health is upset.
7. In disease or cure the simple substance is existent everywhere in the body and internally.
8. In disease the individual's sensations change - so does the functions.
9. Where freedom is lost, death follows.
10. Every cause of disease has a form.
11. Even the most precise and most sensitive instrument cannot aid seeing the cause of either sickness or cure.
12. Whatever we are able to see either with the naked eye or through the above instruments are only the results of the disease.
13. Coarser forms are harmless comparatively.
14. Bacteria results from the conditions within.
15. Causes of ultimate are from immaterial, invisible center.
16. Healing the sick is restoring the freedom.
17. When economy is turned into order, signs and symptoms cease.
18. The result of disease is not sickness.
19. A homoeopath must listen and perceive the signs and symptoms given out by the disease.

Lecture - IX

20. The remedy must fit the disease - it is not adjusted to the pathological changes, which are only result of disease.
21. In freedom and health an individual's attention is not drawn to his various parts.
22. The homoeopath must separate out the symptoms that were observed years back and those present now.
23. He must seek out all the facts from the beginning.
24. Symptoms never lie. They do not exist on opinions.
25. The homoeopath must study physical diagnosis for the sake of additional knowledge. He is a student forever.
26. He must study and possess knowledge of the operations and functions of arteries, nerves and muscles.

Aphorisms & Precepts

1. The signs are visible, but the *esse* is invisible.
2. The tendency of the human mind runs after things visible, that can be felt with the fingers, leads one to adopt foolish theories like bacteria doctrine and molecular theory.
3. When a physician thinks from the microscope, and his neighbor's opinion, he thinks falsely. Nothing good can come from this.
4. A time may come when Homoeopathy of the purer kind will be popular, but it is a very long time ahead.
5. The sharper the edge of the tool you fool with, the more harm you can do; so it is with high potencies in unskilled hands.
6. Technicalities are condemned in Homoeopathy. Only frame in your mind that you have seen a species of scarlet fever, a species of measles, or a species of Diabetes or Tuberculosis,

and speak of them as such; that the speech may be a true outward representation of internal thought.

7. If Homoeopathy does not cure the sick you have to despise it.

8.' A rational mind can go far beyond the idea of molecule.

9. There is nothing in the outer world but what is representative.

10. The world today accepts things perfectly incongruous and calls them science. Modern science accepts nothing which cannot be heard, felt or seen.

11. The song that is within the heart is a million times more beautiful, than can be produced by the larynx. Everything that is, or appears as real before the eyes, or to the ear in sound, is only representation of the real world, because, everything of this character is perishable.

12. All art has its Internal and External. If music is in the soul, it will give the outward reflected image of the delight, which is song.

13. The microscopists have failed to show that there is no Vital Force, no Simple Substance, no Dynamics in drugs seen, and how can we expect him to foretell when the substance cannot be seen.

14. Homoeopathy is an applied science, not a theory.

15. It is an injustice to science to practice without exact knowledge, and reasons for what you do. The whole world is but a swirl of this roundabout inheritance instead of knowledge.

Lecture - X

Materialism in Medicine

The thirteenth paragraph of Organon reads as:

"Therefore disease that does not come within the province of manual surgery, considered as it is by the allopathic, as a thing separate from the living whole from the organisms and its animating vital force, and hidden in the interior, be it of ever so subtle a character is an absurdity that could only be imagined by minds of the materialistic stamp, and has for thousands of years given to the prevailing system of medicines all those pernicious impulses that have made it a truly mischievous (non-healing) art."

Analyzing the above we see:

(1) Disease must not be considered as a separate thing from the whole living being.

(2) Not considered as a separate thing from the organism and its vital force, which animates the human organism.

(3) It could be as subtle as possible, yet not separated from disease.

Such thinking as above is absurd. Because of such thinking for thousands of years attached to the prevailing system of medicine, it has truly made the system mischievous and a non-healing art.

C.A. Baldwin uses a bit stronger vocabulary. He writes "Hence the idea that disease is a thing separate and distinct from the living whole is preposterous and unthinkable." He adds, "Disease is a condition, not a thing, a cause producing effects perceptible to the sense and discernible even by the untrained observer, but more accurately by a trained physician.

Dr. Hahnemann has expressed what existed in his time. Materialism is still on its growth upwards. Majority of men appear to have lost the sense of perception. Remember the word 'perceive' we have made a great noise about it earlier - see lecture III - Organon Sec 3.

Just for the matter of recapitulation, perception is seeing with understanding. This faculty appears to have been lost totally. A materialist refuses to believe anything that does not conform to laws of time and space. He wants everything to be measured, must be weighed, then it must occupy some space - otherwise he has no idea of that. He is convicted to fact or idea that without the above qualities it is nothing and non-existent. Anything beyond this is just poetical, dreamy or just fantasy to the material mind. Because of this notion they search in vain in the material world for a cause.

A material entity can in no way cause anything. There is no causation power, no creative influence nor propelling influence behind it. Causes are simple substances. They are in the natural state, in motion.

They cause motion in bodies they occupy. The *natural state of simple substance is that of power, mobility and activity.* The natural state of matter is rest, quietitude, silence; it has no power to move unless it is acted upon. It is like the dead man, where tissues are at rest, having no action of its own. But consider the simple substance — it dominates the matter and also animates it. The world of motion is that of power. It exists in one along with inertia. They say things go in pairs - light and darkness, heat and cold, etc. Similarly there is a world of life and a world of dead matter. Contemplate on the realm of thought and the realm of

Lecture - X

matter - they are the same as realm of cause and realm of result. Earlier we have mentioned causes are invisible - the results are visible. The actions of material substances are visible. On thinking about it we understand that what are visible in material form are only results of the existing cause in the form of simple substance; and it is invisible to the natural eye, but visible to be spiritual eye or what we call understanding.

A materialist cannot grasp this idea because he cannot think in this fashion.

You may ask, "How can you confirm it?" We have the most spectacular and grandest confirmation of these things. Just look at the remarkable action of our varying potencies in which they operate upon men - from the lowest to the highest. In course of time, you can discover that in a large number of chronic diseases our antipsorics will cause changes in economy - curative or otherwise. This is accomplished by five or seven different potencies. There, you got it - the confirmation. Note their relation to different planes in the interior of the economy.

Now we sail into Organon, fourteenth paragraph. It says:

There is, in the interior man, nothing morbid that is curable, and no invisible morbid alteration that is curable, which does not make itself known to the accurately observing physician by means of morbid signs and symptoms - an arrangement in perfect conformity with the infinite goodness of all the wise preserver of human life.

"In perfect accord with the infinite goodness of Omniscient Preserver of human kind, there is no curable, indiscernible, invisible morbidities or pathologies in the whole phenomena of disease. There can be no curable symptoms that escape the attention of the patient and an astute physician. There can be devised no rational therapeutic procedure, to meet a hypothetical morbid state, or a baseless guess concerning in the cause or nature of sickness."

Dr. C.A. Baldwin, M.D.

Let us analyze this paragraph.

(1) The homoeopath is to be accurately observing.

(2) He must observe the morbid signs and symptoms.

(3) Whatever that is morbid in the interior of man makes itself known to the physician by signs and symptoms. He has to observe accurately.

(4) This is a blessing (the indication of the signs and symptoms) given to a physician by the God Almighty, the preserver of humanity.

The above has already been mentioned earlier. The signs and symptoms can distinguish whatever that is curable. *Incurable diseases have either no symptoms or a few.* So, incurable diseases are absent in symptoms and signs. Carefully watching the patient declining gradually without any symptoms, which are the common expressions of pathological conditions, it can be understood that the case is incurable and going down to death.

Therefore all curable maladies make themselves known by signs and symptoms. This indicates the disorderly condition of the vital force or in the interior of the man. The homoeopath can understand the nature of sickness from it. The images of sickness are being formed continually. These are to be intelligently observed and properly understood. Intelligent and sincere homoeopaths can understand this well.

Dr. Hahnemann mentions about Providence. It is Divine Providence that gently guided Dr. Hahnemann to become a man and enable him perceives the law. When his little ones were pulled out of existence due to strong drugs Dr. Hahnemann thought that God had not created these little ones to die because of medicine. It appeared to him that it was inconsistent that they should have taken this miserable stuff. Those who do not recognize the Divine order will believe in false science and experimentation. They will

Lecture - X

not believe in any government of principle or in any thought of purpose or order of use.

It was Hippocrates who said first that disease might be cured either by opposites or similar. Dr. Hahnemann experimented and discovered it following strict order. Ultimately he formulated the code that is so simple and yet complete. A good homoeopath must go through Organon again and again till he is through with it. Every time you go through it there will always be some new thought that is in harmony with Dr. Hahnemann's general teaching. A continued and constant study of the Organon will most certainly bring a deeper and deeper understanding with every time reading it. It is so, because it is the truth.

We will take up the fifteenth paragraph of Organon. It is:

"The affection of the morbidity deranged, spirit-like dynamism (vital force) that animates our body in the invisible interior, and not the totality of the outwardly cognizable symptoms produced by it in the organism and representing the existing malady, constitute a whole; they are one and the same. The organism is indeed the material instrument of life, but it is not conceivable without the animation imparted to it by the instinctively perceiving and regulating vital force ('regulating dynamism' in the Sixth Edition) (just as the vital force is not conceivable without the organism), consequently the two together constitute a unity although in thought our mind separates this unity into two distinct conceptions for the sake of (easy comprehension in the sixth edition) facilitating the comprehension of it".

Dr. Kent has not reproduced the above paragraph in his lecture. But he has covered the points in paragraph fifteen of Organon.

We shall see what this paragraph conveys to the reader.

"The organism and the vital force are a unit, not a duality. They are separated into two ideas only for convenience of comprehension, or because of lack of comprehension. They stand related as produced and product. This producer, morbidly altered, producing a complex of externally perceptible symptoms, and the spirit-like dynamism animating our body in health and residing unseen in its interior, is one and the same."

Dr. C.A. Baldwin M.D.

"Vital force and the body both contribute as a single unit. The unit is inseparable."

Dr. S.G. Palsule.

Dr. Palsule has presented to us the contents of the related paragraph in a crisp and short manner.

Still for the sake of this idea getting rooted in our mind, we shall go at it, point by point.

(1) The Vital Force animates our bodies. Vita in Latin means life. In the book "Looking Within" - bringing down points from the writings and sayings of Sri Aurobindo and The Mother we see that the vital (being) is intermediate between the physical and the mental and is made up of life-energies, sensations (pleasure, pain, etc.) instincts and impulses (anger, fear, lust, etc.), desires, feelings and emotions.

(2) This spirit-like dynamism resides invisible in the interior of our body, and animates it.

(3) In a morbidly deranged body, the totality of the recognizable signs and symptoms show the nature of the malady that exists.

(4) They constitute the whole and they are not two individual or separate things. They are one. Here 'they' mean the vital force and the body.

(5) The organism is the material instrument of the life.

Lecture - X

(6) Hence, they are not two different identities. They must be taken as one.

(7) Our thoughts may separate this unity into two different components - may be for the sake of easy comprehension. (But actually it is not so!)

Presently we shall see Dr.Kent's explanation to this paragraph. Earlier we have dealt with this. Here, it is only a confirmation. Whatever that flows from the center must be considered in connection with the center. That is but natural. Man when healthy is but the result of the normal activities of a unit. So he must be considered as a single unit only. To put this in another way, his healthy vital force is the result of the action from the center.

Now, consider a man diseased. His government is deranged. Yet he is still a single unit - but now diseased - and he should be considered as such. His physiological action does not produce the morbid action. But his morbid conditions completely dominate him and he is one morbid state. We can see this illustrated again, when he is dominated by the action of a drug - wherein a drug possessed him instead of the disease process. Thus we see a morbid state. Again, he is a single unit of action only.

Three different subjects form a union. They are

(1) The study of the man in his natural state,

(2) The study of the man when in natural sickness, and

(3) The study of the man when in artificial sickness.

Each remedy must be studied first as a unit and then those units may be considered, and compared. You cannot intermingle comparative Materia Medica without a full knowledge of the units. This is found only by experience. It is better to study each remedy as a unit. Similarly, study each disease as a unit. After completely mastering one remedy or one disease, then you can compare.

Take measles as measles, whooping cough as whooping cough. In chronic diseases ascertain all the things or symptoms that have been observed in syphilis, all symptoms that have been covered in sycosis and all those that have been observed in psora. Then you are fully prepared and in a ready condition to study the Materia Medica and see the relationship of some remedies to the acute miasms and relationship of other remedies to the chronic miasms. Some remedies particularly will possess the image of measles, in some remedies the image of whooping cough and in others the image of psora, syphilis and sycosis. Once having come up thus far, we are ready for individualization. Up to now these are the generals. From here we go into comparison. This is the classical way to proceed. When this system is followed the homoeopath becomes wise and intelligent. He can apply the Materia Medica with very great precision. This is the method prescribed by Dr. Hahnemann.

Let us close this chapter with the words of Helen Keller. She said:

"The most beautiful things in this world can never be seen, it has got to be felt by the heart." This can well be applicable to simple substance too.

Summary

1. Dr. Kent deals with the paragraphs thirteenth, fourteenth and the fifteenth of Organon.
2. We should consider the disease and the living whole as one.
3. We have forgotten the art of "perceiving" - that is seeing with understanding. A true homoeopath should cultivate this habit and practice it. A materialist believes only in things that can be measured, weighed, occupies some space, etc. Otherwise, for him things are not in existence.
4. There is no causation power, no creative influence or propelling influence in a material entity.

Lecture - X

5. *A simple substance has power, mobility and activity, and that is its natural state.*
6. The natural state of matter is rest, quietitude and silence. It has no power of itself to move. It moves only when acted upon.
7. Causes are invisible but results are visible.
8. The homoeopath must observe accurately.
9. He must observe the morbid signs and symptoms.
10. All that is morbid inside the interior of the man makes itself known by signs and symptoms.
11. These signs and symptoms are God sent blessings to humanity.
12. The signs and symptoms can distinguish whatever that is curable.
13. A homoeopath must study, re-study and re-study the Organon till it becomes one with him. If he diligently pursues this path, every time he studies the Organon, he will become that much wiser about the homoeopathic principles.

The fifteenth paragraph explains:

15. The vital force and the body are not two different entities, they are but one.
16. They must be considered as such in health or in sickness.
17. We may, for the sake of comprehension consider these as separate, but then it is not correct.
18. The study of three different subjects should be considered.
    (a) Study of the man in his natural condition.
    (b) Study of the man in his natural sickness condition, and
    (c) Study of the man in an artificial sickness condition.
19. It is better to study each remedy in detail, as a unit. So, should we study each disease?

20. We must take each disease as such. In miasmatic conditions, all the things observed about each miasm must be clearly made out individually. Once all symptoms are fully covered reading up the Materia Medica can be taken up.
21. The relationship of the remedies to sickness will be distinctly clear. These will be the generals. From here, we can go into individualization. That is the classical way of doing Homoeopathy, according to Dr. Hahnemann.

Aphorisms & Precepts

1. When he questions you about homoeopathy, if you tell him what your opinion about it is, he will listen to you but when you say it is so, he looks at you in wonder and doubt.
2. The disease may not be named but to be perceived, not to be classified but to be viewed, that the very nature of it may be discovered.
3. Man's unbelief and opinion do not effect truth. The experience, which the homoeopath has, is the experience under law and confirms the law and by this order is maintained.
4. A man whose services are worth having can starve in the gutter, in order that he may do well, for the love of his neighbor; and he will acquire this power, this perception. Such a physician may realize what it is to have a duty to perform.
5. You cannot meditate on even extreme of the human race. It becomes your solemn duty to heal the good, bad and indifferent.
6. There are two worlds, the world of thought, or immaterial substance, and the world of matter, or material substance.

Lecture - X

7. In simple substance, is the means of identification in nature? The mineral, the oak, the wheat, are all identified by their Primitive Substances, which make them what they are.

8. When a man thinks from the microscope, and his opinion, he thinks falsely. Nothing good can come from this.

9. A remedy is not known simply because it has been used upon the sick. That is a confirmation only, and gives more ripened knowledge.

10. When you look at morbid anatomy from the symptomatology, you are looking at it from the interior. Morbid anatomy must not be studied as a basis for prescription making.

11. Now in a proportion as a man falsifies truth or mixes, or perverts, truth; in proportion as he mixes willing well with willing evil, so he adulterate his interiors until that state is present.

12. That changes in body correspond to wrong thinking is true. The fault of the world today, is reasoning from externals. Man elected in the early part of his history to think from lasts to firsts, and thereby lost his ability to know.

13. Man must be studied as he is, as he was, everything of man and of the human race in general, in order to understand disease.

14. Everything that is a thing has its aura or atmosphere. So as a race or class, the entire human race has its atmosphere or aura also. Each individual has his aura, or atmosphere.

Lecture - XI

Sickness and Cure on Dynamic Plane

In this lecture, Dr. Kent speaks about the sixteenth paragraph of Organon.

It reads as:

"Our vital force, as a spirit-like dynamics, cannot be attacked and infected by injurious influences on the healthy organism caused by the external inimical forces that disturb the harmonious play of life otherwise than in a spirit-like (dynamic) way, and in the like manner all such morbid derangements (diseases) cannot be removed from it by the physician in any other way than by the sprit-like (dynamic, virtual) alternative powers of the serviceable medicines acting upon our spirit-like vital force, which preserves them through the medium of sentiment faculty of the nerves everywhere present in the organism, so that it is only by their dynamic* action of the vital force that remedies are able to re-establish health and vital harmony after the changes in the health of the patient cognizable by our senses (the totality of the symptoms) have revealed the disease to the carefully observing and investigating physician as fully as was requisite in order to enable him to cure it."

"The spirit-like dynamics, when disordered, is affected only by spirit- like morbid agencies. Hence dynamic action of remedial agencies must be used for the purpose of cure. Life is the chemistry of infinitesimal, the infinitesimal only can alter its processes or correct its disorder."

Dr. C.A. Baldwin, M.D.

Let us break up the long paragraph into short connected sentences to enhance our understanding of the same. We shall go at it point by point. In our analysis in every lecture certain points will be repeated again and again. This repetition is to make the point our own from all angles - that is the purpose of this repetition.

The sixteenth paragraph, when broken up, sequentially, goes as follows:

(1) Our vital force is a spirit like dynamics.

(2) Our vital force cannot be attacked and affected by injurious influences on the healthy organism, caused by external inimical forces.

(3) These inimical forces disturb the harmonious play of life.

(4) These inimical forces will also have to be spirit-like (dynamic); otherwise it cannot affect or disturb the harmony.

(5) The physician can remove all such morbid derangements or disease from it only by means of spirit-like agents (medicines functioning plane).

(6) The platform of operation must be the same i.e., spirit-like (dynamic, virtual)

(7) Only the dynamic action of the medicines can reach the disease and fight it out.

Lecture - XI

(8) The medicines acting thus on the patient actually re-establish health and harmony.

(9) The changes in health are indicated by the totality of the symptoms. Once these changes are observed and a suitable remedy selected that can operate on spirit-like plane, meets the changes head on and re-establishes the health of the patient.

Read and re-read the above points. What does it all come down to? *The vital force is spirit-like and so are the homoeopathic Medicines.* They are dynamic in action and they alone can affect the vital force.

Now let us get into the lecture class and see what Dr. Kent has got to say in this. He is an authority. But before going into that, the reader might have observed something in the reproduction of the paragraph. Look and read it carefully and we notice an asterisk placed near the word dynamic. (See point No.6 in our analysis) What is it about - what does it denote? We refer to the footnote provided by Dr. Hahnemann. Dr. Hahnemann has given a very short footnote, in his Organon, sixth edition. It reads "Most severe diseases may be produced by sufficient disturbance of the vital force through the imagination and also cured by the same means."

We are now with Dr. Kent. This paragraph of Organon deals with three states:

(1) Of the state of health or the normal activities of the body,

(2) Of how that state is made sick or turned into disorder, and

(3) How that disordered state can be turned to health

Appears like we have heard or read this somewhere earlier and is familiar. Isn't it? Yes sir, we referred about this in lecture

10, on the subjects forming a union of study. There it was a brief touch and go. Here Dr. Kent goes into it in an elaborate fashion. Let us plod ahead.

Assume a person in a perfect state of health. We might subject him to shock, to injuries, to the actions of the cruder things around us; he would pass away without leaving upon him any disorder. The possibility is that he might be under the influence of that shock for some time. But, when reaction came, if at all it came, it would leave him free from miasm. He would not have an acute or chronic disease, therefrom.

It is only the action of immaterial substances, simple substance acting upon a plane, which is similar to the plane of his susceptibility, which can affect or infect one with sickness, the resultant action of the substance capable of operating from his innermost to his outermost. It establishes its evidence by signs and symptoms. When the outermost alone is acted upon, the vital force is temporarily disturbed, but a definite disorder is not established (not even a limited one) that can run a course with a beginning, a period of progress and decline, such as the miasms do. Remember this beginning, growth and decline - we spoke about in Lecture V.

Whatever depresses the tissues or the bodily functions of man cannot establish a true disease. Let us consider the cruder drugs, we see, used as a physic. When purgatives and emetics are given to a person, in coarser and cruder forms, he will go through the shock and return to his original state. Only after the violent and long-lasting continuous usage of liquids, a drug disease can be implanted upon him. Even this is largely superficial when compared to a natural diseased condition.

Continuous use of Bromides and Potassium will produce effects in time, but the drugs do not go to the depths. It operates upon the tissues, and produces a coarser form of disease. This is not miasmatic. Many of the coarser poisons, when taken, in crude form, manifest very little upon the vital force. The more active and virulent and condensed the poison is, the smaller the collective

Lecture - XI

symptoms. A small pox crust can be swallowed. It will be digested and very little trouble comes out of it. Whereas, the inhalation of the atmosphere containing the aura of small pox, upon an individual's corresponding plane of susceptibility will infect him. It will most certainly have a prodrome, a period of progress and then a period of decline. This shows that the foundation of the man's nature has been attacked. The immaterial substance is invisible. The disease action is on the internal man. It operates from within out. It produces ultimate in his tissues, establishing results on his skin.

Dr. Hahnemann asserts in this paragraph only a simple substance can thus implant itself upon human economy as to run its course as either an acute or chronic disease. No disease can implant upon the economy through the ultimate forms; this can happen only in its invisible form.

All diseases are in the form of simple substance. Invisible, not capable of being detected by the chemist or the microscopist and will never be detected in this natural world. The causes of disease are known from its effects only. It is beyond the natural senses and can be investigated only as to its results. Whatever that can be seen, felt or observed, or detected with a microscope is, after all, an ultimate, a result only. We can perceive the invisible disease cause only by understanding, by reasoning from beginning to end and back again.

Disease can occur only through dynamic changes and in no other way it is possible. Ultimate cannot act on the human economy, either curative or otherwise. *Vital disorder can be turned into order only by something, which is similar in quality to the vital force.* Here, remember, we are not searching for similitude in quantity, in weight or measures - but we are searching for similitude in *quality*, in power, and in plane.

We see that medicines, therefore can affect the high and interior planes of the physical economy, only when they are raised to the plane of similarity in quality.

For example, let us consider a person needing *Sulphur*, in the very highest degree. He may take sulphur to move his bowels, he may rub it on his skin, he may even wear it in his stockings, can take sulphur baths, but all these without any effect on his disease. Why is this so? It is so because the drug sulphur in that form does not correspond with his sickness. It is not able to function on the same plane in which he is sick or diseased. Hence it cannot affect the cause and flow from the cause (the centre to the circumference). This is the case with all the coarser drugs; hence they do not cure.

Sometimes, we note that crude drugs and low potency medicines temporarily remove the diseased condition. Here we see the outermost effect of diseases, diseases located in the outer planes. It is only as to the exteriors and ultimate planes. It is only as to the exteriors and ultimate that the cure is effected. It does not reach the innermost degrees and hence it is not permanent.

In acute diseases also, sometimes, crude drugs accomplish their purpose, because they affect the surface, which is the outermost. In acute disease, the tendency for the innermost is to go away of itself. If his life can survive until the disease has run its coarse, the patient will recover. In chronic miasms only their ultimate symptoms are reached; these subside temporarily or are suppressed by the action of crude or ultimate forms of medicine.

Potentized medicines would cure the sick, seemed mysterious. Lower potencies and crude drugs cured only superficial complaints. *Higher potencies operate more and more interiorly.* Chronic disease that would be relieved by moderate potencies would only improve for a matter of weeks. Administration of higher potencies continues to take up the work. Thus the patient is to be carried on from one potency to the next higher and so on. Experience of older Homeopaths says, *"Go higher"*.

It is a good policy to inform the patient not to be alarmed or astonished when such and such things happen. If not done so,

Lecture - XI

they may run after another doctor. Homoeopathy is done according to law. It has been confirmed again and again. Experience does not lead to these things, but the principles, which thereafter are confirmed by experience. Where a patient has been carried up through a series of potencies, he will often remain unaffected by that remedy in either a lower potency or in the crude state. He will be affected by the lower potency or cruder state only when he is overwhelmingly dosed by it. Then he will be poisoned.

Looking into the third proposition of this paragraph, we note the medicines will act curatively and bring the economy to order only when

(1) Potentized

(2) Potentization must correspond to the degrees in which the man is sick.

Those who are sick in a middle plane are sick from that plane to the outermost and who are sick in the interior plane are sick throughout to the outermost. When the disorder is the very depth of physical nature then it is in chronic state. In this condition all there is of the patient is only sickness and there is no tendency to recovery but a continued progress. This is the order of psora, syphilis, sycosis, and the miasms.

The nutritive plane is entirely in the outermost, which is in tissues. Assimilation goes on in the tissues. The crude things operate in the realm of tissues and ultimate. So crude things can only disturb ultimate. The inharmonious conditions are that of ultimate, the outermost plane. When the physical outermost is also affected the economy does suffer. Then the body ceases to be amenable to be operated upon by the powers within.

In a true disease having periods of prodrome, progress and decline can be implanted in the economy only by a dynamic cause. It also goes from this that only when a drug is attenuated till they are similar to the nature or the quality of disease it can cure it. The disease cause and the curing drug have to be similar in nature to produce effects. When the signs and symptoms of the disease are identical and similar with a drug that cause the same effects then it can cure, because both are similar. The causes must be similar if you want the effects also to be similar in nature and quality.

The homoeopath must always contemplate - he must constantly ask himself "Do I know a remedy that has produced symptoms like these, upon a healthy person?" The homoeopath must pass his judgment only upon the symptoms. He must look at his case as an artist, who critically views his painting - discerning the finer shades of difference and similitude.

Summary

1. This lecture deals with paragraph sixteen of Organon.
2. The inimical forces that can cause a disease have to be dynamic. Otherwise it cannot disturb the harmony.
3. The medicines can cure a malady only when it is also spirit-like.
4. The remedies selected must be attenuated to the same degree, and be capable of meeting and fighting off the disease in its own plane.
5. When dealing about dynamic cure we should remember that most severe disease might be produced by the disturbance of vital force through the imagination and also cured by the same means.
6. A homoeopath can be efficient only when:—
    (a) He has a thorough knowledge of the normal activities of the body,
    (b) He has a sound knowledge of the disease, and
    (c) He has a solid foundation of the curative nature of the

medicine.

7. The cruder things around us cannot harm a person sound in body and mind. At the most he will only be a subject to shock; that is all. When the influence of the shock wears off he becomes normal.

8. Simple substance capable of acting on the same plane as that of the person's susceptibility and it alone could affect him.

9. Many of the coarser poisons, when taken in crude form, manifest very little upon the vital force.

10. Only when an individual's plane of susceptibility is attacked on the same plane can the person be affected.

11. The immaterial substance is invisible, and operates from center to circumference.

12. We can perceive the invisible disease cause only by understanding, by reasoning from beginning to end and back again.

13. Vital disorder can be turned into order only by something that is similar in quality, similar in power and similar in plane.

14. Low potency medicines remove the diseased condition temporarily or cure only superficial complaints. The higher the potency the operation is more interior. We should go higher, step-by-step.

15. Medicines to act curatively must be potentized and the potentization must correspond to the degrees in which the man is sick. The disease cause and the curing drug should possess the similarity in potency, power and plane.

16. The homoeopath must always contemplate, meditate and must look at his case critically, discerning the fine shades of difference and similitude.

Aphorisms & Precepts

1. Materia Medica never inspires perception. The physician must have the love of its use, and he becomes wise in proportion as he loves his use, and in proportion as he lives uprightly with his patients; that is, desires to heal them, beautify their souls. Can the physician, who does not love his neighbor as himself, get into this position?

2. If it were not for the Simple Substance, such states as antipathy, sympathy, or affinity, could not be. It is the sphere of homoeopathy to deal with these things, to glean what is the real *esse* and existence.

3. Susceptibility is only a name for a state that underlies all possible sickness and all possible cures.

4. Now when a person becomes sick, he becomes susceptible to a certain remedy, which will affect him in its highest potency, while upon a healthy person it will have no effect.

5. When the dose is too large to cure, man receives it as a sickness.

6. Susceptibility exists in the Vital Force and not in the tissues.

7. The homoeopathic physician who thinks in quantities only, has such a crude mind that he cannot realize true homoeopathy.

8. The old philosophers were engaged in constant controversy here converging, there diverging. If they had only known something of simple substance, as does the homoeopath, they would have had confirmation.

9. Homoeopaths have a consciousness of what life is, what the life force is, what the nature of disease is, and can apply to all theories of the world our measure and test them. They can realize the philosophies.

Lecture - XI

10. Homoeopathy is the relation between the symptoms of the patient and the remedy, which will cure.
11. When you have discovered that this Life Force resides in a simple substance you see at once that death is not an entity. The body has no life of its own and therefore it cannot die.
12. One cannot afford to be liberal with principle.
13. When you make failures you may be sure that they are within yourself. If you think the failure is in Homoeopathy, you will begin your corrections on the wrong side of the ledger.
14. If you do not know sickness you are apt to think all things strange and unique.
15. If you love Homeopathy it will love you; such is natural charity.

Lecture - XII

Removal of Totality of Symptoms

This lecture deals with the paragraph seventeen, eighteen, nineteen and the twenty of Organon.

In paragraph Seventeen, Dr, Hahnemann says: -

Now, as in the cure effected by the removal of the whole of the perceptible signs and symptoms of the disease the internal alteration of the vital force^x, to which the disease is due - consequently the whole of the disease is at the same removed ^{1}, it follows that the physician has only to remove the whole of the symptoms in order, at the same time, to abrogate and annihilate the internal change, that is to say, the morbid derangement of the vital force - consequently the totality of disease, the disease itself. But when the disease is annihilated the health is restored, and this is the highest, and the sole aim of the physician who knows the true object of his mission, which consists not in learned - sounding prating, but in giving aid to the sick.

In this paragraph we notice an asterisk and other numbers against some words. We shall go into these after our usual analysis of the paragraph.

"A cure cancels the inner change of the invisible vital force and thus removes the entire complex of perceptible effects, removes sickness in toto."

Dr. C.A. Baldwin, M.D.

Analysis of paragraph seventeen:

(1) The disease is due to internal alteration of the vital force.

(2) The signs and symptoms indicate the presence of the disease.

(3) The cure is affected by the removal of the entire perceptible signs.

(4) Conversely, when the entire perceptible signs and symptoms are removed, the whole of the disease is also removed.

(5) So, from the above it is clear that the physician has to remove the whole of the symptoms, in order.

(6) All the symptoms to be removed at the same time.

(7) Then only the internal change can be abrogated and annihilated - the health is totally restored.

(8) The homoeopath has a life mission. He knows the true object of his mission.

(9) The homoeopath's sole aim should be to aid the sick and restore health. (Organon, 1st paragraph).

Now, we shall go to the markings.

(x) What Dr. Habnemann has mentioned here as force, he has replaced the word "force" as "principle" in the Sixth Edition of Organon.

(1) This is a footnote. The essence of it is: All the morbid signs indicative of approaching death have frequently been dissipated by an identical cause, and health re-

Lecture - XII

stored. This could have occurred only with the removal of internal and external morbid changes that threatened death.

(2) The gist of this footnote is: It is God's blessing to the humanity wherein He projects the internal malady by means of signs and symptoms. Thereby homoeopathy understands what He has to remove to restore health. Just imagine the chaos if God had not given us this blessing!

(a) In fact this is first paragraph of Organon - It says that "The physician's high and only mission is to restore the sick to health, to cure, as it is termed.

Now we will see what Dr. Kent says in his Lecture relating to this paragraph.

His very opening line is a straight punch on the nose! He says that the *removal of the totality of symptoms is actually the removal of the cause.* Causes continue into effects - i.e. *causes continue in ultimate* - may not be known. But it is true that all ultimate contain the causes of beginnings to a great extent. Cause continues into ultimate and things in ultimate shadow forth cause. Since it is so the removal of all the symptoms will have to remove the cause as well. It is but rational. From this angle let us take for example, of several symptoms manifesting themselves through a diseased ovary. Can the ovary be removed? If so, will all the problems be over? The problems may not be got over that way. By taking that route we have not removed the cause of the symptoms. Hence, it can manifest through some other part of the body that could be weak or perhaps through the other ovary.

It is a very serious matter to remove any organ through which the disease manifests itself. When there are two or more such pathological conditions established in the body and where one is removed the other immediately becomes worse.

To illustrate, if there is a structural change in the knee joint and the knee is removed, while there is a corresponding structural change in the kidney or liver, which the surgeon cannot remove, the latter worsens and breaks down as soon as the knee joint is removed.

We find this in a tuberculosis condition of the lung. It may remain in a quiet state as long as there is a fistula in ano which keeps on discharging. When this vent is closed almost immediately there is a cropping out of the disease by infiltration of the lungs resulting in the patient's early death.

The results of diseases are very necessary in many instances. Sometimes these results are tuberculosis conditions and ultimate outcome or effects due to the cause. They may contain the seeds of beginnings of a similar kind, at times. They contain the causes - but then, they are not the beginning themselves.

The disease is capable of relapse, if all the signs and symptoms are not removed from the beginning to end. Thus the disorder is changed into order - consequentially the results of the disease are completely removed. Only when the cause is completely removed the totality can be removed.

In this paragraph, Dr. Hahnemann has used words "learned - sounding practicing". What does this mean? Many people use high-sounding technical words during their course of conversation. Doctors are no exception. By this, they try to impress the world of their wisdom. Nothing but ego. But when a homoeopath sticks to his sole aim and mission in healing the sick he has no need to impress.

The doctrines of homoeopathy are simple and straight. They should not be clouded by the technicalities. Homoeopathy should be considered and talked out in the most easiest and simplest language.

When talking about Organon and its doctrines use simple

Lecture - XII

forms of speech. Technicalities are a sort of scape-goat to carry off the signs of our ignorance.

We have used the terminology "totality of symptoms" earlier in several contexts. Totality of symptoms means a lot. It is all that is essential of the disease. Whatever that is visible and represents the disease, in the natural world, visually, responding to the touch and external understanding of man, is totality of symptoms. It is this that enables the physician to individualize between disease and between remedies. The complete representation of the disease is totality of symptoms. The totality of symptoms must be able to bring to the mind of the homoeopath a clear idea of the nature of disease.

Many small symptoms can be conveniently eliminated out of the totality of the symptoms, without in any way changing the characteristics or image of the disease - i.e. it can be still individualized. These must be capable of guiding the homoeopath to the choice of the remedy.

Prescribing medicines, by perceiving the totality of the symptoms from a small portion, because of experience, is often a mistake we commit. Each case is a new case - the homoeopath must familiarize himself with the totality of symptoms to the maximum extent possible and treat every sickness as a new sickness. Where the patient is able to give out all his signs and symptoms without concealing anything the job of the homoeopath is facilitated. If the patient conceals anything or is unable to give out the signs or symptoms properly, it is hard to get at the totality of the symptoms. However difficult, the totality of symptoms ought to be arrived at for the proper prescribing, after ascertaining the nature of the sickness as well as the remedy. This is expressed in the eighteenth paragraph of Organon.

The eighteenth paragraph of the Organan states: -

"From this indubitable truth, that besides the totality of

Symptoms* nothing can by any means be discovered in diseases wherewith they could express their need of aid, it follows undeniably the sum of all the symptoms ['and conditions' in the Sixth Edition] in each individual case of disease must be the *sole indication,* the sole guide to direct us in the choice of a remedy.

* In the Sixth Edition these are added after "symptoms" (With consideration of the accompanying modalities - Para-5)

Taking consideration of the totality of the symptoms as a whole does not complete the image. Besides considering all the symptoms collectively, each individual symptom must be taken into consideration. Each symptom must be carefully examined and its relationship to the totality of symptoms must be noted down. Then only we can know its value as to whether it is a common symptom, or a particular symptom or a peculiarly characteristic symptom.

We shall now proceed to the paragraph nineteenth of Organon. It reads as:—

"Now, as *diseases* are nothing more than *alterations in the state of health of the healthy individual* which express themselves by morbid signs, and the cure is also only possible by *change to the healthy condition of the state of health of the diseased individual,* it is very evident that *medicines* could never cure diseases if they did not possess the power of altering man's state of health, which depends on sensations and functions; indeed that their curative power must be owing *solely* to this power they possess of altering man's state of health."

Let us analyze the above paragraph in our own way.

It says,

(1) When the health of a healthy individual is altered, we call him diseased.

(2) The disease expresses its presence by morbid signs.

Lecture - XII

(3) When the unhealthy condition is reversed only the cure is brought.

(4) Medicines have the power of altering the man's state of health. Hence they are able to cure.

(5) The state of health depends on his sensations and functions.

So from the above we are able to infer that the medicines must be capable of effecting changes in the human economy. Otherwise, they will not restore economy and thereby health. Where the medicine is too high to effect a disturbance in an irregularly governed economy, it follows that it will be too high to cure in that economy.

The potency of the medicine must be consistent with the patient's degree of susceptibility. Generally, susceptibility may be varied - from 30th to CM. Since the limits are very wide and broad one cannot commit an error in this. Seldom the potency is too high, but that it is higher than is necessary is often true.

A drug can act curatively only because it is capable of making changes in the human economy. It is an established fact that drugs do effect changes, by their proving. In the proving the prover takes the liberty to increase the quantity of the drug or the quality of the drug, according to his judgment.

The coarser substances do effect a few changes many times, but sometimes none at all. The higher substances make sick and this is in accordance with the state of susceptibility. Some provers are susceptible to the higher and not susceptible to lower potencies. Some patients are there who are not in the least susceptible to a single drop of tincture of coffee, but very susceptible to the higher potencies of the same drug. These patients become sick often, by large quantities of coffee. *Lycopodium* in crude form has no effect on most people. But *Lycopodium* in its higher potencies is capable of affecting almost everyone, if followed up continuously. The effect that medicines have upon the sick in restoring order can best be observed by inducing the effects upon healthy individuals. This is what we call proving.

Now we proceed to the twentieth paragraph of Organon. It reads as:

"The spirit-like power to alter man's state of health (and hence to cure diseases) which lies hidden in the inner nature of medicines ["in itself" in Sixth Edition] never be discovered by us by a mere effort of reason; it is only by experience of the phenomena it displays when acting on the state of health of man that we can become clearly cognizant of it."

Let us consider the above, point by point.

(1) A spirit-like power is required to alter the man's state of health.

(2) The power lies hidden in the inner nature of medicines. Hence they are curative.

(3) We can never discover this power just by reasoning.

(4) We are able to recognize this power only by experience. This phenomenon is exhibited by its acting in the state of health of the men.

The above details boil-down to one main theme. *The drug effects can be determined only by proving - not by any conjecture or reasoning.*

How to find out the drug effects, on the human economy? Give the same remedy to several healthy men and note down the manifestations of this drug experienced by each one. First of all we must know that drugs can make man sick and what that state of sickness is.

The homoeopath should use only drugs that have been proven thoroughly, upon healthy persons. Only by this proving can the

Lecture - XII

image of disease be brought out perfectly. We see some homoeopathic drugs in homoeopathic pharmacies are recommended for such and such a disease without any investigation as to their proprieties. Such a practice has been decried and condemned in every line of the Organon, and by every homoeopathic doctrine. This is not in line with principle; it is unscientific.

We must study in the Materia Medica the drugs that have been fully proven. The study of partially proven drugs can be done later. The "Guiding Symptoms" contain many materials, which are only partially proven. These partially proven drugs may cure, but then the cure is accidental. It is not so with drugs well proven and handed over to us by the Masters. The drugs have undergone complete trials for years. These medicines are our friends. You cannot get acquainted with a drug that is not proven properly. Pay no heed to drugs, which are referred in books as good for this and good for that. But when a book tells you that a drug has produced such and such disease symptoms study it. You will get invaluable information.

Summary

1. This lecture deals with paragraphs seventeen, eighteen, nineteen and twenty of Organon.
2. Signs and symptoms indicate the internal malady. These are the factors the homoeopath understands. They are his signposts to choose the proper remedy.
3. The totality of the symptoms gives us a clear image of the sickness or disease.
4. The removal of all the symptoms removes the causes of the disease.
5. By removing an organ through which the disease manifests itself is not a cure to the disease. The cause is not removed;

hence it can express itself through some other weak organ or elsewhere in the body. *Removal of the cause is the only way.*

6. The signs and symptoms right from the beginning have to be considered and removed, for a complete and permanent cure.

7. The doctrines of Homeopathy are simple and straight. When talking about Homeopathy and Organan it must be done so in the simplest, easy to understand words. There is no need for technicalities here.

8. The complete representation of the disease is the totality of symptoms.

9. Many small symptoms can be eliminated from the totality of the symptoms without any change to the characteristic or image of the disease.

10. It is not correct to consider a small portion of the symptoms (assuming the totality of the symptoms to be so and so) and prescribe a remedy.

11. The homoeopath must familiarize himself with every aspect of the disease.

12. Along with the totality of the symptoms, the modalities also have to be taken into account.

13. Disease is only an alteration of the state of health.

14. Medicines contain the power to affect the human economy. Hence they are curative.

15. The curative power in a medicine cannot be seen. It can only be felt by its actions.

16. The potency of the medicine must be consistent with the patient's degree of susceptibility.

17. Drug proving establishes the fact that drugs can affect the human economy.

Lecture - XII

18. The coarser drug may effect some changes many times, but sometimes none at all.
19. Higher substances make sick and this is in accordance with the state of susceptibility.
20. The capacity of a remedy to restore health can be observed from the effects it produces in a healthy individual.
21. The drug effects can be determined by its proving, only.
22. The homoeopath must use only proven drugs.
23. A well-proven drug handed over to us by the Masters is our friend.
24. Always study the proving wherein it is given that a drug will produce such and such results on introduction into a healthy individual. This will prove invaluable.

Aphorisms & Precepts

1. All art has its Internal and External. If music is in the soul it will give outward reflected image of the delight, which is song.
2. The world today accepts things perfectly incongruous and calls them all science. Modern sciences accept nothing, which cannot be heard, felt or seen.
3. The personal stamp is upon every disease and upon every proving, and the individual must be permitted to stamp himself upon the disease as well as upon the proving.
4. There are no two things alike in universe. This is so of diseases and of sick people, of thousands of crystals of the same salt. No two stars are alike. When this thought presents itself to the mind of the physician, he can see that no remedy can be substituted for another.
5. In Epilepsy, so long as Bromides suppress, nature is paying more attention to the disease of Bromides than the disease of Epilepsy.

6. A homoeopathic remedy only becomes homoeopathic when it has established its curative relation, the relation between two dynamic influences.
7. It is an injustice to Science to practice without exact knowledge and reason for what you do. The whole world is but a swirl of this roundabout inheritance instead of knowledge.
8. That changes in the body correspond to wrong thinking is true. The faith of the world today, is reasoning from externals. Man elected in the early part of his history to think from lasts to firsts and thereby lost his ability to know.
9. In proportion as man thinks against everything, his country, his God, his neighbors, he wills in favor of himself. Therefore this forms man into the nature of his affections.
10. The homoeopathic principles, when known, are plain, simple and easily comprehended. They are in harmony with all things known to be true.
11. It is not a matter of theory, or belief, or opinion; we must have something more substantial. homoeopathy must rest upon facts.
12. All quick prescribing depends upon the ability to grasp comparatively the symptoms.
13. If you do not know sickness you are apt to think all things strange and imagine.
14. True pathology is entirely unknown to the medical profession outside homoeopathy. It is morbid anatomy alone that is known.

Lecture - XIII

The Law of Similars

This lecture deals with paragraphs twenty-one to twenty-seven, both inclusive of Organon. First of all we shall reproduce the above, one by one.

"Now, as it is undeniable that the curative principle in medicines is not in itself perceptible, and as in pure experiments with medicines conducted by the most accurate observers, nothing can be observed that can constitute them medicines or remedies except that power of causing distinct alterations in the state of health of the human body, and particularly in that of the *healthy individual,* and of exciting in him various definite morbid symptoms; so it follows that when medicines act as remedies, they can only bring their curative property into play by means of power of altering man's state of health by the production of peculiar symptoms; and that, therefore, we have only to rely on the morbid phenomena which the medicines produce in the healthy body as the sole possible revelation of their in-dwelling curative power, in order to learn what disease producing power, and at the same time what disease causing power, each individual medicine possesses."

Organon - Paragraph 21

" But as nothing is to be observed in diseases that must be removed in order to change them into health besides the totality of their signs and symptoms, and likewise medicines can show nothing curative besides their tendency to produce morbid symptoms in healthy persons and to remove them in diseased persons; it follows, on the one hand, that medicines only become remedies and capable of annihilating diseases, because the medicinal substance, by exciting certain effects and symptoms that is to say, by producing a certain artificial morbid state, removes and abrogates the symptoms already present, to wit, the natural morbid state we wish to cure. On the other hand, it follows that, for the totality of the symptoms of the disease to be cured, a medicine must be sought which (according as experience shall prove whether the morbid symptoms are most readily, certainly, and permanently removed and changed into health by similar or opposite medicinal symptoms,) has a tendency * to produce similar or opposite symptoms.

(*"Proved to have greatest tendency" in the sixth edition)

Organon - Paragraph 22

"All pure experience, however, and all accurate research convince us that persistent symptoms of disease are far from being removed and annihilated by opposite symptoms of medicines (as in the antipathy, enantipathic or palliative method), that, on the contrary, after transient, apparent alleviation, they break forth again, only with increased intensity, and become manifestly aggravated (see paragraph 58-62 and 69)."

Organon - Paragraph 23

"There remains, therefore, no other mode of employing medicines in diseases that promises to be of service besides the homoeopathic, by means of which we seek, for the totality of the symptoms of the case of disease a medicine which among all medicines (whose pathogenic effects are known from having been tested in healthy individuals) has the power and the tendency to produce an artificial morbid state most similar to that of the case of disease in question."

Organon - Paragraph 24

"Now, however, in all careful trials, pure experience, in sole and infallible oracle of the healing art, teaches us that actually that medicine which in its action on the healthy human body, has demonstrated its power of producing the greatest number of symptoms *similar* to those observable in the case of disease under treatment, does also, in doses of suitable potency and attenuation, rapidly, radically and permanently remove the totality of symptoms of this morbid state, that is to say (ref. Organon 6-16) the whole disease present, and change it into health; and that all medicines cure, without exception, those diseases whose symptoms most nearly resemble their own, and leave none of them uncured."

Organon - Paragraph 25

Before proceeding to analyze the above paragraphs, let us see about the footnotes provided by Dr. Hahnemann, one by one.

Organon - Paragraph 22

(1) In allopathic medicine symptoms have no direct pathological relationship to the morbid state. Hence they are neither similar nor opposite. It is imperfect and injurious to vital force.

(X) These medicines are violent. These are chosen just on conjecture, and given in large doses. Painful operations, lead the disease to other regions.

Organon - paragraph 25

(1) The old school followed the systematic pathology and dreamed they could detect some imaginary morbific matter.

We shall now analyze the above paragraphs before going into the lecture.

Organon - paragraph 21

(1) The curative principle in medicines is not perceptible.

(2) Nothing can be observed that can constitute them as medicines - they possess only the power to cause distinct changes in the healthy state.

(3) They are capable of exciting various, but definite symptoms of morbidity.

(4) So, it follows that they can cure.

(5) We have to rely only on the morbid signs and symptoms to select the cure.

(6) Each medicine has a disease-producing and hence disease-curing power.

Organon paragraph 22 - analysis

(1) Only the totality of symptoms has to be removed to restore health.

(2) Medicines have the power to produce morbid effects in a healthy individual and power to cure a diseased person.

(3) To remove the totality of the symptoms a medicine must be sought.

(4) The selected medicine must possess a tendency to produce similar or opposite symptoms.

Organon paragraph 23 - analysis

In antipathic, enantipathic or palliative methods of treatment there might be an apparent restoration of health. The disease breaks forth, after sometime with an increased wrath. Here reference is made to later paragraph 58 - 62 and 69. We shall deal with them and correlate this paragraph when we come to them.

Lecture - XIII

Organon paragraph 24 - analysis

We should select a medicine that has the power and tendency to produce an artificial morbid state most similar to that of the case of disease in question.

Organon paragraph 25 - analysis

A medicine that has the greatest number of symptoms similar to the disease cures it rapidly, radically and permanently. It must be in doses of suitable potency and attenuation. Here, reference is made to paragraph 6-16 (Lecture VI to XI, both inclusive.)

This lecture is a summary of the earlier ones. Dr. Hahnemann gives out the conclusions. Repeating what has already been said earlier, he says and affirms that the only method of applying the medicines beneficially in disease is the homoeopathic way. We see from our daily life that antipathic or hetropathic way of treatments does not provide a permanent cure. These may be in some changes in the economy and the symptoms - but then, that is not a permanent cure. There is also a tendency to establish another disease. This disease does not eradicate the previous disease and is worse than the first.

We proceed to paragraph 26 of Organon.

It says:

"This depends on the following homoeopathic law of nature, which was sometimes, indeed vaguely surmised but not hitherto fully recognized, and to which is due every real cure that has ever taken place.

A weaker dynamic affection is permanently extinguished in the living organism by a stronger one, if the latter (whilst differing in kind) is very similar to the former in its manifestation."*

* We will now see what the footnote says:

Another similar, stronger one dominates the weaker dynamic affection, permanently.

The homoeopathic law operates when similar disease manifestations appear, simultaneously in any person, is the gist of the above paragraph.

Dr. Hahnemann definitely states that the cure depends totally on fixed law - the law of similar that governs homoeopathy. It is after studying several cases and critically analyzing them that he came to the conclusion that *the cure occurs due to similarity only and not by accident or dissimilar.* He saw that, in every case, the curative drug was capable of producing similar symptoms of the disease, which it cured. This is true in all planes, under all circumstances. All other apparent cures were nothing but suppressions and not cures.

Another extinguishes a dynamic disease, in the living economy of a man, which is more powerful than the previous one. When? When that another disease, without being of the same species, but bears a very strong resemblance to the previous disease in its way of manifesting itself.

In the above, how do we interpret the word "powerful"? Is it the intensity? On contemplating a bit on this we understand it in a different manner. Here intensity is to be understood as

(1) Having more internal qualities

(2) Higher

(3) Prior

That means from first to last. We spoke about this in an earlier lecture. We talked about quality and not of quantity. See lecture XI.

To say it more effectively *the more internal it is the more intense.* Hence it approaches the first substance in a better way. So now we understand that intensity as to cause means higher or more internal, higher in the sense of subtleness and fineness. Powerful is actually from within. *That is why we potentize, going*

Lecture - XIII

higher from one potency to a higher potency. This enables us to reach the intensity and it is in this sense that the remedy becomes more and more powerful by potentisation.

Looking at it from the material plane, or material point of view potentisation brings down the actual amount of medicine. Potentization makes the drug more powerful, from the material point of view may appear stranger, but then, that is the fact. This can only be felt. Simple substance is invisible has to be remembered.

"A dynamic disease is extinguished by another that is more powerful when the latter is similar to it." You note two points in the above statement. First is more powerful; and the second is similar. When there is more to the interior we can expect more in the exterior. Let us take sun light for comparison. It is brilliant than all lights since there is more in its interior, purer and more dynamical. In sunlight no other light outshines it. All other lights in its presence are destroyed and nothing.

The law of similar is seen in every direction we turn, in this natural world. This can be observed from man to man. How to establish this? Take the case of an insane person. This law of similar is the secret in mind cure. Many mind cures are based on this law.

A person has lost his dear one - may be any one close to him - and consequentially ill. He is depressed with grief, sobbing in solitude for the lost one and is melancholy ridden. In certain other system, the physician may say there is nothing wrong with this person - only he has to brace himself up to face the loss and get pacified. Does this work out? No. On the contrary, the person feels left out and miserable.

Consider homoeopathic treatment in this case. It is like two people having the same type or grief. May be both are jilted lovers. Now what happens? Each one sympathizes with the other. They weep it out together. A bond of sympathy is created. Sometimes a curable case of insanity can be approached this way. Is this not a mind cure? How else will you call it? Dr. Hahnemann used this method of approach in curing insanity. Where a patient would exert his or her will, but is not able to on account of the physical encumbrances, the homoeopathic remedy can step in. It will restore order.

Now let us proceed to paragraph twenty-seven of Organon.

It reads:

"The curative power of medicines, therefore, depends on their symptoms similar to the disease but superior to it in strength (see paragraph 12 to 26) so that each individual case of disease is most surely, radically, rapidly and permanently annihilated and removed only by a medicine capable of producing (in the human system) in the most similar and complete manner the totality of symptoms, which at the same time are stronger than the disease."

It is felt that no analysis for the above paragraph need be gone into. A little explanation will suffice. Just administering the drug itself, regardless of its form, for the sake of giving a drug does not suffice. The drug should be capable of meeting the disease in its own plane. So giving a drug in crude form does not work out. This requires a deep study. The attenuation also must be identical or similar to the cause of the disease. We should understand one thing - that in proving the drug could have brought forth several symptoms in one prover. But in a sick person these symptoms may not be touched at all. This is because the patient does not sustain the similar relation or susceptibility as the prover.

Dr. Hahnenann has explained the law of cure in paragraph twenty-nine. He himself states that he does not attribute much importance to it. Hence we are also omitting it

Lecture - XIII

Summary

1. This lecture deals with the law of similar.
2. Dr. Kent covers the paragraphs 21 to 27 of Organan. Paragraph 29 is not taken into consideration.
3. The gist of the above paragraphs can be given as below:

Paragraph 21: The capacity of a drug to cure sickness is determined by its capability to produce the same or similar sickness symptoms on administering it to a healthy individual.

Paragraph 22: The totality of the symptoms is clear image of the disease. So to cure, the drug must possess the ability to produce the self same symptoms in a healthy individual. A small quantity (infinitesimal) suffices to provide a cure.

Paragraph 23: Medicines, which create opposite symptoms - dissimilar symptoms - may appear to cure. It is an apparent cure. They suppress the disease instead of curing.

Paragraph 24: Homoeopathic method is the only way to cure. The drug must be similar in pathogenesis to the sickness. The drug must be able to produce the most number of symptoms in artificial disease, which is similar to the natural disease.

Paragraph 25: Experience has abundantly proved to us that a properly potentized drug will remove the totality of the symptoms. This is the Homoeopathic law of similar, similibus and curantur.

Paragraph 27: Power of the medicine depends upon its power to produce similar symptoms of the disease most certainly.

Paragraph 26: A weaker dynamic action is permanently extinguished by a stronger one - while it differs in kind - is similar to the former in its manifestations.

Aphorisms & Precepts

1. External principles themselves are authority. The Law of Similar is a Divine Law. As soon as you have accepted the Law of Similars, you accept Providence, which is nothing but law and order.

2. In chemistry one color obliterates another. This is an illustration of the outermost changes. This causes of such change lie in the primitive substance and not in the external form, so it is with cure.

3. A disease may be suppressed by a medicine as well as by a stronger dissimilar disease.

4. The physician spoils his case when he prescribes for the local symptoms and neglects the patient.

5. What is man? Is he a body? If so, we are justified in thinking of his parts, his liver, and lungs and skin, and extremities, and his body as from the life to the body.

6. The upright man, whose desires are good, wants the truth. His perceptions are intensified.

7. A prejudiced mind, decides without wisdom the way he wants to have it.

8. The outer world is the world of results. The inner world is not discoverable by the senses but by understanding.

9. It would seem as if the Old School would have asked long ago "What are the effects of drugs upon healthy people?" Their experiments on animals do not answer this.

10. "This remedy has proved useful in such and such conditions", they say. Homoeopaths say that such medicine has produced such and such effects on provers.

Lecture - XIV

Susceptibility

This lecture deals with paragraphs thirty, thirty-one, thirty-two, thirty-three and thirty-four.

First of all we shall reproduce the paragraphs in their order, and then proceed to the analysis.

Paragraph thirty of Organon reads as:

"The human body appears to admit of being much more powerfully affected in its health by medicines (partly because we have the regulation of the dose in our own power) than by natural morbid stimuli - for natural diseases are cured and overcome by suitable medicines.

Analysis: Since we have in our hands the power to regulate the doses, the human body is more easily influenced by medicines than by natural diseases. The natural diseases are cured by suitable medicines.

Paragraph thirty-one of Organon reads as:

"The inimical forces, partly physical, to which our terrestrial existence is exposed, which are termed morbific noxious agents do not possess the power of morbidly deranging the health of man unconditionally; but we are made ill by them only when our organism is sufficiently disposed and susceptible to the attack of the morbific cause that may be present and to be altered in its health, deranged and made to undergo abnormal sensations and functions - hence they do not produce disease in every one nor at all times."

Analysis of Organon paragraph thirty-one:
(1) The inimical forces, termed as morbific noxious agents, can derange the health of humans only under certain conditions, i.e., they cannot act unconditionally.
(2) These can cause sickness only when the human organism is sufficiently disposed and susceptible to the attack.
(3) So they do not make everyone sick or at all times.

You will see a footnote on this paragraph. In it, Dr. Hahnemann, goes on to say what disease is not and cannot be. They are merely spiritual dynamic derangement of the life.

Organon Paragraph thirty-two reads:

"But it is quite otherwise with the morbific agents which we term medicines. Every real medicine, namely, acts at all times under all circumstances, on every living human being, and produces in him its peculiar symptoms (distinctly perceptible, if the dose be large enough), so that evidently every living human organism is liable to be affected, and, as it were, inoculated with the medicinal disease at all times, and absolutely (unconditionally), which, as before said, is by no means the case with natural disease."

Analysis of paragraph thirty-two

(1) We term artificial morbific agents as medicines.
(2) Whenever we brand a medicine as a real one, *it will work at all times, under all circumstances, on every living human being.*
(3) It produces its own peculiar symptoms, which are clearly distinguishable, when the dose is large enough.

Lecture - XIV

(4) It works unconditionally. This is not the case with the natural disease, as said in the previous paragraph.

Paragraph thirty-three of Organon reads as:

"In accordance with this fact, it is undeniably shown by all experience* that the living human organism is much more disposed and has a greater liability to be acted on and to have its health deranged by medicinal powers, than by *morbific noxious agents and infectious miasms, or in other words that the morbific noxious agents possess a power of morbidly deranging man's health that is subordinate and conditional, often very conditional; while medicinal agents have an absolute unconditional power, greatly superior to the former.*

Analysis:

1) Medicinal powers are much more disposed towards deranging the human organism, that the natural morbific agents and infectious miasms. The medicinal agents are greatly superior to the natural morbific agents.

(2) What was said in the previous paragraph is repeated here.

Paragraph thirty-four of Organon reads as:

"The greater strength of the artificial disease producible by medicines is however, the sole cause of their power to cure the natural diseases. In order that they may effect a cure, it is before all things requisite that they should be *capable of producing in the human body an artificial disease as similar as possible to the disease to be cured,* (which with somewhat increased power, transforms to a very similar morbid state the instinctive principle, which in itself is incapable of any reflection or act of memory. It not only obscures, but extinguishes and thereby annihilates the derangement caused by the natural disease." - In the sixth edition.)

In order, by means of this similarity, conjoined with its somewhat greater strength, to substitute themselves for the natural morbid affection, and thereby deprive the latter of all influence upon the vital force. This is so true, that no previously existing disease can be cured, even by nature herself, by the accession of a new dissimilar disease, be it ever so strong, and just as little can it be cured by the medical treatment with drugs which are incapable of producing similar morbid condition in the healthy body."

Now for the analysis:

(1) The greater strength of the artificial disease produced by medicines is alone not the sole cause of their power to cure.

(2) The medicine must be capable of producing in the living human body an artificial disease as similar as possible to the disease to be cured.

(3) The greater strength in addition to the above quality it is able to cure.

(4) The accession of a new dissimilar disease cannot cure an existing one; however strong it might be.

Now to summarize the points of these paragraphs:

The drug action is always certain and positive than the action of morbific influences. The effects and symptoms produced by morbific influences depend on the individual's susceptibility. *Susceptibility is the intensified irritability of the organism.*

A healthy individual does not become infested easily. Drug action is sure, obeying the law of nature. Like causes produce like effects. Drugs act on the sensations and feelings of human organism.

We shall now see what Dr. Kent interprets as far as the above paragraphs of Organon.

These paragraphs, thirty-one and thirty-two mention about the degree of intensity (potency), depend upon the repetition of

Lecture - XIV

the dose, and upon the individual's susceptibility. A homoeopath becomes a good prescriber only when he understands and follows this principle.

We have already seen about potentisation. *In homoeopathy the quantity is not the criterion at all. It is the quality that is everything.* This has been said earlier in Lecture VIII. About potencies we have spoken in Lecture X. Earlier we learnt about the wonderful way infinitesimal material substance functions. To be effective, the remedy must be on the same plane of the disease. A homoeopath must understand why he should administer one dose and also the rationale how susceptibility is satisfied.

In contagion and also in cure one dose of medicine will suffice to cause the suspension of influx. Cause flows in the direction of least resistance. When the resistance is offered the influx stops. The cause does not flow any more.

In the beginning of the contagion there is the limit to influx. If there was no such limit established by Nature the influx will continue flowing till the individual is dead and gone! As soon as the susceptibility in the individual is satisfied the cause ceases. When the cause ceases to flow into ultimate the ultimate cease and the cause itself has already ceased.

Dr. Hahnemann states that *the drugs have more power over humans, than the disease cause. This is because man is only susceptible to natural disease on a certain plane.* We have seen disease causes are also spirit like. Only then can they attack the man. These causes flow inside the man in spite of him.

Man cannot control or resist them. They make him sick. Certain changes occur, and then man ceases to be susceptible. There is no further inflowing of the cause due to the cessation of susceptibility. Susceptibility ceases when changes occur in the human economy. It bars any further more influx.

Cure and contagion are very similar. So the principles apply to both. There is one important difference, though. In cure we have the control of potency in our own hands. This enables us to suit the varying susceptibilities of a sick man. This varying degrees of susceptibility some people are protected and some are victimized by the cause of disease. He who is made sick is susceptible to the disease cause as per his susceptibility plane he is in at the time of the contagion. The degree of disease cause fits his susceptibility at the time of attack.

Now consider the medicines. This is not the case with them. Man has, in his own hands, all the degrees of potentisation. He is like a puppeteer. He can fit the medicine to the varying susceptibility of the individual in varying qualities and degrees. So he has in his control the power of medicines and greater power in affecting the state of health of an individual when compared to the natural morbific irritation. Natural diseases are cured by suitable medicines.

When does an administered medicine cease to be Homoeopathic? - A relevant question. We are speaking about susceptibility in an individual. *Susceptibility is only a name for a state that underlies all possible sickness and in all possible cures.* The law and principle is the same. So this principle of similarity between the cure and contagion applies.

We should also remember here the Aphorism - "The homoeopathic remedy becomes homoeopathic when it has established its curative relation; the relation between the dynamic influences."

Let us take up a case of diphtheria - after studying the symptoms *Lachesis* is indicated as the similar remedy. We administer one dose of *Lachesis*. Contemplate now on the above. In this case *Lachesis* rapidly, radically and permanently cures the diphtheria. What does this mean? The totality of the symptoms of this disease is removed. Thus, the causation of the flow of the disease stops or ceases. There is no susceptibility now. We have seen that a cure can induce an artificial disease in a living human being. So, it is also capable of curing a similar disease. Once the totality of the symptoms has been removed what next. Is *Lachesis* indicated in that individual any more? No. So, as per the law and principle when there is no indication of the remedy the need for it in the individual vanishes. Then, since *Lachesis* is not indicated it ceases to act. However, if *Lachesis* is given further, it will act on a totally different plane. Not as the same one as when diphtheria was present. There it functioned in its homoeopathicity. When given at a time not indicated, it may act depressingly. We have seen earlier that the susceptibility ceases once satisfied. When the drug is in surplus, it is dangerous. In chronic diseases when *Sulphur* is clearly indicated the symptoms are gone, leaving the patient feeling better. Once the remedy ceases to be homoeopathic then further administration makes it non-homoeopathic and it is undesirable.

They say when a milligram can do good ten milligrams should do even more good. No sir, do not make this mistake. *Enough to bring in a change is all that can be homoeopathic.* Once the changes occur it will be wise for the physician to wait. Patience is a quality that a homoeopath has to develop and apply.

Administer just enough medicine to establish the order - and that happens almost instantaneously. At the most the time taken may be a few hours. As long as order continues, once it has begun, WAIT. That is how contagion takes place. In diphtheria, the disease begins and susceptibility ceases. A change takes place that protects the individual. This stops the further flow of the disease cause. Now the disease develops and it manifests itself by this symptoms.

Repetition of dose:

We just said that once when changes start occurring after the administration of the remedy "hands off". WAIT. Many wise heads go on to say, "repeat the dose". Now we shall see the wisdom in waiting. It is perfectly useless to repeat the dose without waiting.

Vigorous, robust subjects who have lightning like reaction can be administered a repetition of the dose. In this case the changes will be for the better when the remedy is not quite Homoeopathic to the cause.

Some people are injured in this way. This is because they are delicate. Here the reaction is slow; the reaction is actually prevented by the repetition of the dose. We tried to establish order, but it is prevented. *Dr. Hahnemann teaches that the human economy is more under the control of humans than under the control of diseases.* Only a disease can affect the economy, as it is susceptible to. We have seen earlier that man has in his control to vary the doses and potencies. This will help him get results. But then as already mentioned earlier, the *very susceptible individuals are damaged by the repetition of the dose.* So, now you see the wisdom in administering a single dose and waiting?

Dr. Hahnemann teaches us in the thirty-first paragraph of the Organon that disease causes have a limited effect in changing the health according to susceptibility (conditional). Dr. Hahnemann says this much - cause ceases after certain evolutions take place. A natural disease has a period of rise and decline - we talked about this at the early stages of the series of lectures. The patient will not be susceptible till there is another change of state.

Man does not go out of a state of susceptibility to a disease and in a few days get into another state of susceptibility to the same disease. A time has to elapse before an individual gets into another state of susceptibility. When we talk about the cure, instead of the contagion it would seem that a certain dose of medicine administered would last for a certain time. So, the next dose can be given only when another state of susceptibility sets in.

We now see the futility of administering the medicine again once it ceases to be homoeopathic. It will then act on the individual on an artificial susceptibility. Certain sensitive patients have a susceptibility to high potencies. Now we have to deal with two things:

Lecture - XIV

(1) Acute state, created by disease itself.

(2) Chronic state — the natural state of the patient born under miasm.

In acute cases or states the susceptibility is satisfied. (Susceptibility to the contagion). The disease cause ceases to flow and becomes inoperative. He becomes immune to any further influx. When a remedy ceases to be homoeopathic, this immunity is gone against the more power due to the possibility of variance in the hands of the homoeopath. So, where the potency goes higher than the degree of susceptibility, he may be damaged.

So, now we said in paragraph thirty-three, which has already been reproduced and analyzed earlier.

The human race has been thrown into a great disorder in its economy; all because of the improper use of medicines - i.e., drug-taking. In managing the chronic diseases, Dr. Hahnemann explicitly says the greatest difficulties inflicted in the economy of the humanity are due to continuous taking of the drugs. A life-long disorder is developed. The disorder sometimes is so heavy that it literally takes years of very careful prescribing, to restore the economy to order.

From here, we proceed to paragraph thirty-four of Organon. It says that in order to cure:

(1) The medicines must be capable of producing in healthy living individual symptoms that are similar to the disease it is expected to cure.

(2) The artificial disease created by the medicine must be of a greater degree of intensity. We have spoken about this intensity earlier - it must be something higher, more internal, something superior or prior.

The intensity of power is proportionate to the degree of approximation towards primitive substance. There is no other way to think about this.

The cause of disease as well as cure exists within the primitive substance, and not in ultimate material form. But remember that the immaterial cause of disease continues in the disease ultimate. Causes are continued into ultimate. The bacteria may contain cause as causes continue into ultimate, but the primitive cause is not in the bacteria; the bacteria themselves have a cause.

Summary

1. This lecture deals with susceptibility - the related paragraphs of Organon are thirty, thirty-one, thirty-two, thirty-three and thirty-four.
2. The human body is more easily influenced by medicines than by natural disease.
3. Natural diseases are cured by suitable medicines.
4. The effects and symptoms produced by a morbific influence depend on the individual's susceptibility. This depends on the constitution and disposition determined largely by living regemen.
5. Bacteria or morbific potencies are of secondary importance in infection.
6. The morbific agents can affect the humans only under certain conducive conditions. The individual must be sufficiently disposed and susceptible to the attack.
7. From the above it can be understood that all can be made sick at all times.
8. Disease is merely a spiritual dynamic derangement of the life.
9. The medicines are also morbific agents. They induce an artificial disease in healthy living human beings.
10. A remedy works at all times, under all circumstances, on every human being.

11. A remedy produces its own peculiar symptoms, when the dose is large enough. These symptoms are clearly distinguishable.
12. The natural disease can affect only conditionally. The medicines work unconditionally.
13. The drug action is never failing — always characteristic - in accordance with the law. Like causes produces like effects.
14. The medicinal agents are superior to the natural morbific agents and the miasms. They are much more disposed towards deranging human organisms.
15. Medicines have greater strength. This alone is not responsible to make it curative. The medicine must be able to produce similar symptoms as the disease.
16. The entering of a new dissimilar disease cannot cure an existing disease.
17. A healthy individual does not get infected easily.
18. The cure is accomplished by nature by super imposing similar symptoms.
19. In Homoeopathy, quantity is no criterion; it is the quality that counts.
20. A remedy can be effected only when it can operate on the same plane of the disease.
21. A properly selected remedy with sufficient intensity and power will meet the degree of susceptibility on its own plane and wipe it out.
22. An influx cannot continue forever - if enabled so, it may flow till the individual is dead. The influx stops after a limited flow - i.e. when the susceptibility is satisfied.
23. Drugs have more power over humans than the disease causes.

24. Susceptibility ceases when changes occur in the human economy.
25. Cure and contagion are similar. The law is the same for both.
26. We have two things that can be controlled, in our hands. They are 1) the potency and 2) the dosage.
27. Drugs being superior to natural disease cause the additional two things mentioned above is a big boon to us, when properly used.
28. Susceptibility is only the name for a state that underlies in all possible sickness and in all possible cures.
29. On administering a dose of medicine, wait, to see the changes. Do not rush to repeat the medicine.
30. Administer just enough medicine to establish the order - it happens almost instantaneously or at the most in a few hours.
31. Repetition of the dose without waiting may prevent the reaction.
32. Very susceptible individuals are damaged by the repetition of the doses.
33. Man does not go out of a state of susceptibility and in a few days get into another state of susceptibility to the same disease.
34. Drug taking, when continuous creates a great disorder in the human economy. A life-long disorder is created. Then, only very careful prescribing will restore order.
35. The artificial disease by the medicine must be of a greater intensity — something higher, more internal and something superior or prior.
36. The immaterial cause of disease continues into the disease ultimate.

Lecture - XIV

37. Very high potencies seldom require repetition if clearly indicated, to produce a long curative action in chronic cases.

Aphorisms & Precepts

1. If there were no Idiosyncracy there would be no Homoeopathy. Every individual is susceptible to certain things; is susceptible to sickness and equally susceptible to cure.
2. Cure rests in the degree of susceptibility.
3. Remedies operate as by contagion. He caught the disease, and catches the cure.
4. Dynamic wrongs are corrected from the interior by dynamic agencies.
5. Principle teaches you to avoid suppression. A homoepath cannot temporize. Those suffering are necessary sometimes to show forth sickness in order that a remedy may be found.
6. Man cannot be made sick or be cured except by some substance as ethereal in quality as the vital force.
7. Susceptibility is only a name for a state that underlies all possible sickness and all possible cures.
8. Now when a person becomes sick, he becomes susceptible to a certain remedy, which will affect him in its highest potency, while upon a healthy person it will have no effect.
9. Susceptibility exists in the Vital Force and not in the tissues.
10. Measles and Smallpox are not on the outside. Man is protected on the outside, and is attacked from the inside, when there is susceptibility.
11. There are degrees of susceptibility. The old school calls a certain kind of susceptibility "Idiosyncracy", though they have failed to find out what it is.

12. Think how susceptible a man is to a sickness, when the Rhus vine will poison him when he is on the windward side, half a mile away.
13. An individual may be susceptible to nothing else; gross, coarse, vigorous in constitutions yet there is one thing he is susceptible to, and that is what he needs.
14. The sharper the edge of the tool you fool with, the more harm you can do; so it is with high potencies in unskilled hands.
15. While we conceive that innumerable causes may give rise to the same pathological condition, we see that the pathological condition in itself, cannot furnish us with the slightest idea of the remedy.
16. Under homoeopathy treatment progress of chronic disease the highest degree of susceptibility must be present, until a cure sometimes becomes possible.
17. Man is more susceptible to drugs than to disease, because their action may be forced upon the economy. In disease the highest degree of susceptibility must be present.
18. Man is susceptible to all things capable of producing similar symptoms to those, which he already has.
19. The law of sickness is the law of sickness whether produced by drug or disease. It is the law of influx.
20. It is inconsistent and irrational to think there are several active diseases in the body at the same time.
21. Contagion does not come by quantity but by quality.
22. The quality of contagion is similar in its nature of the cure.
23. The symptoms, themselves, point to the thing, which the individual is sensitive to, and every one is susceptible in just this way to the remedy that will cure. That which he most

Lecture - XIV

wants, is that which nature has provided him with the means of reaching out after by the symptoms.

24. A crude drug may poison a patient, when the substance potentized would have cured him. The individual comes in contact with too much of something he is sensitive to and gets sick.

25. If a man were in perfect health he would not be susceptible.

26. The same susceptibility is necessary to prove a drug, as to take a disease. That is Homoeopathic relation. Hence we see what contagion is.

27. All prescriptions that change the image of a case cause suppression.

28. The limit of drug action is symptomatology.

29. If we were to undertake the study with the microscope what susceptibility is or what affinity is, we would not succeed.

Lecture - XVI

Oversensitive Patients

This lecture deals with Organon paragraph forty-four onwards. Drug poisoning was dealt with in Lecture XV. It is not always due to prescribing of the crude drugs. When we associate ourselves for long with sensitive patients we will realize that there are patients who have been actually poisoned by the inappropriate administration of potentized medicines as well. Such patients are over-sensitive patients. These people would have received repeated doses of medicine. We have seen that medicine can be homoeopathic only in appropriate dose and potency. So, when this limitation is overlooked and doses are repeated carelessly the medicine acts otherwise. Hence this drug poisoning. Let us go into this in a detailed manner.

For any disease to get cured the most appropriate medicine has to be chosen. This medicine can be called homoeopathic only when administered in proper doses and potency. A time also has got to be allowed for the medicine to act and produce results. Where this is not so and the medicine is repeated or continued, what happens? In some such cases the drug establishes a miasm. Now, the miasm imitates one of chronic diseases or one of the acute miasms as per its capability. There has been examples of a patient suffering for seven or eight years due to the ill effects of

Three methods are available. They are:

(1) When two dissimilar natural diseases meet together in one person;

(2) The result of the ordinary medical treatment of diseases with unsuitable allopathic drugs not capable of creating an artificial morbid condition identical to the disease to be cured.

(3) It may be stronger then the stronger one has its sway over the body.

Epidemic — think of it. In an epidemic several people are affected. Yet we see that some people are not at all affected by it. Now, we have a question to answer here. Why is it some people escape the wrath of the epidemic? Our natural assumption here will be that those who escaped had better immunity, they were unusually strong, more vigorous and of very good order. But is it true?

Among those who escaped we notice that they were anything but strong, some were invalids, some had consumption, some were diabetic, etc. So the above assumption was found to be wrong. *These people did not suffer in the least due to their non-susceptibility to the influences of the epidemic.* That is the fact and the reason why they escaped the epidemic.

We are able to see here that these individuals were sick. In spite of their sickness the epidemic had no influence on them. It is clear here that it is impossible for the epidemic to suppress their sickness. This epidemic was dissimilar to the disease they had and it could not suppress it due to its virulence.

Supposing they had a milder form of chronic disease, such as severe attack of dysentery, it will cause that to disappear temporarily. Then the epidemical disease would have taken over and would have run its course. When the epidemic attack subsides

Lecture - XV

his old symptom would be back again as though nothing had disrupted it. Here this is a case of dissimilar and goes to prove the message in the Organon to be correct - *i.e. dissimilar cannot cure, but they can only suppress.*

Let us see what happens when the chronic disease is stronger than the epidemic disease - i.e., if it has an organic hold upon the body and that it cannot be suppressed. This is mainly the relation of the acute dissimilar disease to the chronic disease of severity.

There are some differences though between the relationships of chronic dissimilar diseases. We shall take an example of a case of Bright's disease in earlier state. Let the symptoms be clear enough to make a disease. This individual takes syphilis and almost at once the kidney disease is held in abeyance. The albumin in the urine almost vanishes. Waxy appearance also makes a disappearance.

This individual is now treated for syphilis. What happens? For about a year's careful medication, the syphilis state is gone. Now the albumin in the urine is present again, dropsy returns and the individual expires of an ordinary attack of Bright's disease.

It is observed in some cases that two chronic diseases seems to alternate with each other - i.e. one seems to be subdued for some time and the other chronic disease prevails. In this case, when one chronic disease A is treated homoeopathically and cured or reduced in its activity the other chronic disease B exhibits its presence. Normally this condition is met within an individual who is syphilitic as well as psoric. The psoric manifestation of skin eruption in one or various other forms, takes syphilis. Now all the psoric manifestations like the nightly itching of the soltrheum just vanishes and the syphilis eruption will appear in their place.

On treating individual for syphilis now, after some time the syphilitic manifestation is subdued. Now the psoric manifestation will show its countenance to the proportion of the subdued syphilitic condition. The syphilitic state, which was not completely cured, is still present. The psoric manifestation will keep the syphylitic residue in abeyance. Now we will have to abandon the syphilitic correction and go on with anti-psoric treatment. The apparent order of the economy will be restored. The vicious cycle starts again - now it will be the turn of the anti-syphilitic treatment since the syphilitic manifestations have appeared. Thus the vicious circle is set up. **In syphilitic eruption there will be no itching - but in psoric manifestation there will be itching present.**

Under the above circumstance, a proper treatment cycle is to be followed. Any haphazard or careless treatment may lead to complexity. It will not be a good proposition. As told in the previous Paragraph, there will be syphilitic eruption (without itching) and psoric itching. Under these conditions Mercury must be considered. When we seek a proper homoeopathic treatment there is a separation, whereas inappropriate treatment complicates the issue very much.

We shall take another case. A chronic malarial diathesis, which has existed for several years and it is complicated with psora. In this case, once the quinine is antidoted the malarial manifestations like the chill and fever return in their original form. We know that the trend of homoeopathy is to separate. The malarial manifestation is treated. It cannot be cured when complicated since the remedy will not be similar to cure. The first prescription antidotes the drug and liberates the individual from the drug disease. Then the most acute or the last appeared natural disease makes its appearance now. Remember the law of homoeopathy. This return is in accordance with the fixed law. The sickness symptoms appear in the reverse order i.e., the last miasmatic symptom, which was removed, will now return first, and go away, never to return.

In the paragraph thirty-six of Organon we find another thought coming up. It is when two dissimilar diseases meet; the stronger one has its sway, in the body.

Lecture - XV

A non-violent homoeopathic treatment leaves the chronic disease unaltered. For suppression violence must be present upon the body. One must bring into the body an enormous amount of violence to the economy by heavy dosing, tremendous physic, much sweating and even blood-letting, etc., was practiced in those olden days. Their tactics may subdue or suppress the disease for the time being. The symptoms jump back and stage a come back. Now it will be in a more agitated and turbulent state than before. The more violent the drug disease upon the body, the greater the change in the chronic disease.

Violent treatment alters the nature of the chronic disease. A new disease, that is more intense, suspends a prior dissimilar one existing in the body. As long as the effect of quinine continues, it will suppress and hold in abeyance to the disease to which it is dissimilar. Homeopathic drugs can induce an artificial disease in the human individual. So, quinine also inflicts an artificial disease upon the human economy and continues for years till it is antidoted by a suitable medicine. Remember what was said earlier - when quinine is antidoted the malarial manifestations will now pop up.

The malarial manifestations were kept under control by quinine, since it was capable of creating similar disease symptoms, and it was more violent than the malaria present. Arsenicum is also capable of inducing upon the human economy serious conditions.

In some cases where there is a lot of complexity, treatment is difficult. We have to treat one layer and go to the next. Here the last group of symptoms that was removed will be the first to reappear. When this happens it is the sign of proper way of treatment and it indicates we are on the right path. We go to the next layer and so on. The disappearance of the symptoms should in the reverse order of their coming - just like one layer piled upon the other.

When we stack bags of cement, we go on putting or placing one bag on the other. When we want the cement how do we take it? The topmost bag first. We take it in the reverse order of stacking. Similarly the last group of symptoms to go will be the first to reappear.

We have now seen how two different diseases occupy, so, to say, two different corners of the same economy. *Here while one pervades, the other lies low.* We also saw how it will be in complexity. In the first instance they stay apart from each other. In the second instance they become complex. We also saw how such conditions are to be treated. It is difficult to know whether each of the drugs had introduced an artificial disease.

Every administered drug may be capable of establishing an artificial disease. Where the symptoms are only partially developed and the drug that caused the symptoms is known, it is better to include the anti-dotal relation to the drug with the rest of the symptoms. *To put it in another way always select a drug that has a well-known anti-dotal relation to the drug that caused the suppression. We should also see to it that the drug so selected is also the most similar of all drugs to the few symptoms that are present.* So we make the maximum use of similarity. The similar remedy is most likely of all others to antidote their drug. Remember the principle of similars. That is the most important thing.

Paragraph forty-three of Organon reads as:

"Totally different, however, is the result when two similar diseases meet together in the organism, that is to say, when to the disease already present a stronger similar one is added. In such cases we see how a cure can be effected by the operations of nature and we get a lesson as to how man ought to cure."

A real union takes place between two similar diseases. These results in the vanishing of old things, new things come into existence in a state of order. So, when two similar diseases meet in the same human organism the result is totally a different one. Here nature

Lecture - XV

accomplishes the cure. So, nature shows the way as to how this is achieved.

Summary

1. This lecture deals with the paragraphs thirty-five onwards to forty-three of the Organon. It deals with protection from sickness.

    The method of cure comes under this topic. This covers:
    - (a) When two dissimilar natural diseases meet together in one individual.
    - (b) The result of ordinary medical treatment with disease with unsuitable allopathic drugs.
    - (c) When two diseases meet in a human individual the stronger one has its sway over the body.

2. An epidemic has been taken as an example. Here, we see many people are affected by it. Yet some escape. Those who escape are not completely healthy individuals either. How is it that they escaped — what gave them the immunity? It was their non-susceptibility to the epidemic.

3. The epidemic was dissimilar to the already existing disease and it could not suppress it due to its virulence.

4. Supposing they had a minor chronic disease the epidemic would have overtaken it and suppressed it temporarily. As the epidemic attack subsided the earlier chronic disease would have returned in all its glory. So we see that dissimilar diseases cannot cure. They will suppress.

5. When there is a chronic disease present and it is stronger than the epidemic, it cannot be suppressed. This is due to

the relationship of acute dissimilar disease to the chronic disease.

6. In chronic dissimilar diseases when one disease is cured, the other one, which was kept in abeyance, will come out. When this is treated, again the older manifestations will appear. The cycle will be repeated.

7. When old symptoms reappear, they should come in the reverse order — i.e., the last symptom removed must be the first one to re-appear. In that case, we are in the proper direction.

8. Only when violence is present suppression can be there. So, in the violent ways of a case like heavy dosing or bloodletting, etc., there will be suppression - an apparent cure. But this will only be temporary.

9. Violent treatment alters the nature of disease.

10. In complex cases treatment has to be very careful. We should remove the symptoms one by one, layer by layer as a pile.

11. It is a good policy to select a drug that has a well-known anti-dotal relation to the drug that caused the suppression. This will be the most similar drug also.

12. Where two similar diseases meet together in the same human individual a real union takes place. Old symptoms vanish and new things come into existence creating a state of order. This is the way nature acts and we have to learn this from nature.

Aphorisms & Precepts

1. The old philosophers were engaged in constant controversy, here converging, there diverging. If they had only known

Lecture - XV

something of simple substance, as does the homoeopath, they would have had confirmation.

2. When you have discovered that this Life Force resides to a simple substance you see at once that death is not an entity. The body has no life of its own and therefore it cannot die.

3. When the old symptoms return there is hope. That is the road to cure and there is none other.

4. The outer world is the world of results. The inner world not discoverable by the senses, but by the understanding.

5. Irregular action expressed in signs and symptoms is the disease. The disturbance in the vital substance has no other means by which it can make itself known to the intelligent physician. This is in accordance with law. This leaves the morbid anatomy out of the question.

6. Unit of action, in health, unit of action in sickness, unit of action in cure, all are one.

7. Individualization is blocked by this inability to distinguish between the finer features of sickness, and of medicines.

8. Take the simplest form of substance known to have life. If we subject it to physical and chemical forces it is killed: it no longer moves, feeds, propagates or can be killed. There is then something that can be withdrawn by physical force. Can we not perceive that it is a something added to these forces that make it alive? It is not merely a motion of this substance, for move, as you will, it is dead. Something is withdrawn, which can only come within the perception of understanding.

9. We now see that we have something substantial; that something is disturbed by something as invisible and substantial, as itself. These two, coming together, disturb each other under fixed laws relating to Primitive Substance.

10. It is just as dangerous to suppress symptoms by drugs, as it is to remove them with the knife.
11. It is better to do nothing at all than do something useless; it is better to watch and wait than do wrong.
12. The diseases themselves cannot be suppressed, but symptoms can. The totality of the symptoms must disappear in an orderly manner in order to constitute a cure.
13. All physicians recognize that suppressing an acute rash is dangerous, but all are not far-sighted enough to see that such is the case with chronic eruptions, excepting that the resulting symptoms come more slowly.
14. Only a few drugs will be similar enough to cure, and there will be only one similimum.

Lecture - XV

Protection from Sickness

This lecture deals with paragraph thirty-five onwards and forty-three of Organon.

Paragraph thirty-five reads as:

"In order to illustrate this, we shall consider in three different cases, as well what happens in nature when two dissimilar natural diseases meet together in one person as also the result of the ordinary medical treatment of diseases with unsuitable allopathic drugs, which are incapable of producing an artificial morbid condition similar to the disease to be cured, whereby it will appear that even nature herself is unable to remove a dissimilar disease already present by one that is unhomoeopathic, even though it be stronger, and just as little is the unhomoeopathic employment of even the strongest medicine ever capable of curing any disease whatsoever."

Analysis of the above paragraph:

This paragraph starts as "To illustrate this"—

To illustrate what? What does "this" refer to? "This" stands for methods of cure by super-imposing similar symptoms. With this illustration in mind let us view the above paragraph.

Lachesis; there have been patients suffering from the ill effects of deep acting remedies like *Sulphur* due to many repetition of the medicine. This has been observed in diseases where such medicines were truly indicated and otherwise. These are all sensitive patients. The suffering from repeated doses emerge years after the abuse. A close observation confirms the drug poisoning by the periodical outbursts typical to that drug.

The crude condition of a drug could be perfectly harmless. But it may be poisonous when in a dynamic plane and could hurt an oversensitive patient. A person may drink a glass of milk and absorb all its nourishing qualities. But the same person will be greatly affected by a drop of highly potentized milk when repeated beyond its homoeopathicity. This will establish a miasm that can affect the person for years.

A lady who was oversensitive was a prover of *Lac caninum*. She had a periodic return of the symptoms. Since she proved the medicine indiscriminately she suffered from its poisonous effects. If only this had been administered in a prudent manner the disease would have established itself as an acute miasm, running its own course and ultimately disappeared. We learn a lesson from this incidence. *Never choose an oversensitive person to be prover.*

In another case a single dose of very high potency of *Lachesis* was administered to an oversensitive patient. This patient ran a course of *Lachesis*. In about two months time the symptoms vanished, never to return. When *Lachesis* had taken hold, during its period of action the patient's symptoms were suppressed. But, after *Lachiesis* had run its course and disappeared her chronic symptoms appeared. This is in accordance with the doctrines. The patient was over-sensitive and when the dissimilar disease of *Lachesis* was in full swing her chronic disease was suppressed.

There are examples where a patient is homoeopathic to a remedy, and when enough medicine has been administered cure has been effected; but when the remedy is repeated beyond this,

Lecture - XVI

the remedy stops functioning homoeopathically and acts through the general susceptibility creating a miasm in the extremely oversensitive patient.

From the above, we must learn that for hypersensitive patients we should not administer CM potencies, or other high potencies. This will make the patient sick. In such cases it is wise to use 30th and 200th potencies. Wherever the remedy is a truly indicated one such potencies will work quickly.

We now proceed to paragraph forty-four to forty-eight, both inclusive. They are given below serially.

Paragraph 44 — Two dissimilar diseases repel, suspend or complicate each other.

Paragraph 45 — Where two diseases differing in kind, similar in symptoms while appearing on the same individual, the stronger one will overcome the weaker.

Paragraph 46 — Gives several examples and also says that two similar diseases cannot exist in one individual at the same time.

Paragraph 47 — Nature teaches us that curative process can be accomplished only by art. We must choose a remedy that matches the disease and select a potency considering the intensity of the disease.

Paragraph 48 — The cure is brought in by the state of the art. The correct remedy in a potency that can produce similar symptoms is to be administered. This will be superior in strength to combat the disease producing influence, which causes the disease.

We now proceed to paragraph forty-nine of the Organon. It goes like this:

We should have been able to meet with many more real natural homoeopathic cures of this kind, if, on one hand, the attention of observers had been more directed to them.

We now retrace our step to paragraph forty-six. It is full of several examples of these natural cures. These cures are not that common, now patients suffering from phthisis re-locate themselves to places where the climate suits them better. They return cured. Some go to places where the climate is wholesome. But, they are not cured. Let us analyze this situation. People who ran to damp climates got cured. This is because the evils of these places were similar to the evils of the patient's economy. This similitude is antidotal to their condition and is curative to them. This similitude brings back into order the suffering economy. We can see clearly that this is in perfect accordance with the eternal law, which governs the law of similar.

We saw two similar diseases cannot, like two dissimilar diseases repel each other, suspend each other or complicate each other. On the contrary let us assume that a particular individual is affected by two different kinds of diseases, but similar in their symptoms. Now what happens? We saw that the stronger of the two diseases overwhelms the weaker one. This can be put in other words - the Vital Force of the body which was thrown out of harmony by the earlier disease is pushed to the back-stage and the stronger one takes over the Vital Force. So, here the weaker disease is wiped out. Let us verify this principle. A successful vaccination with pure cowpox will offer resistance to smallpox even though it is most similar to cowpox.

Dr. Hahnemann has offered several examples illustrating this phenomenon. He has quoted diseases that are dissimilar in kind but similar in their manifestations.

(1) Smallpox produced ophthalmia. Inoculation of smallpox cured ophthalmia.

(2) Blindness of two years caused by suppressed eruption cured completely when the patient had an attack of smallpox.

Lecture - XVI

(3) Deafness and dyspnoea cured when the patient suffered from smallpox.

(4) Smallpox has cured swelling of the testicles.

(5) Dysentry caused by smallpox was cured by an attack of smallpox.

(6) Cowpox vaccination is a recognized preventive of smallpox.

(7) Cowpox often cured itching eruptions.

(8) Measles has cured skin eruptions.

(9) Dr. Hunter has observed cowpox cured intermittent fever. The two fevers similar in nature could not exist in the same body at the same time.

At this point I like to bring to your attention that Homoeopathy does not recommend vaccination. For the benefit of the readers, reproduced below is a quote from Stuart Close's work:

"Homeopathy is opposed to the methods of vaccine and serum therapy, although it is claimed by many that these methods are based upon the homoeopathic principle. It grants that this may be true so far as the underlying principle is concerned, but opposes the method of applying the principle as being a violation of sound, natural principles of medication and productive of serious injury to the living organism."

It has been proven experimentally and clinically that such methods are unnecessary, and the results claimed by their advocates can be attained more safely, more rapidly and more thoroughly by the administration of the homoeopathically indicated medicines in sub-physiological doses, through the natural channels of the body, than by introducing it forcibly by means of the hypodermic needle or in any other way."

In the earlier days of homoeopathy there were only very few medicines at the command of a homoeopath who had to face a great array of diseases. He was worried to find similar remedies to meet all his cases. But today this is not the case. *When and where a homoeopath proceeds in a systematic manner armed with the Material Medica can often meet all the diseases he comes across.* Any reliable and good Material Medica gives the symptoms, which are not most scientifically and sufficiently proved. A sound knowledge of each disease and its symptoms as well as the symptoms of the remedy will go a long way.

Every Homoeopath has got to be an eternal student throughout his life. He must take up the task of studying (not reading) his Materia Medica thoroughly. He must take up this practice day in and day out. Every repeated study of each medicine will provide him many insights. He will be able to know each medicine completely.

The physician of the present day can have no excuse in not studying the Materia Medica. There are very good and reliable Materia Medica books that are mostly used by the physicians the world over. A physician cannot say the proper details of the remedies were not available. All these Materia Medica are very scientifically and systematically brought out. Each medicine has been proved.

The present day physician must not divert his attention towards traditional ways. These lanes are dark and treacherous. Remember that the physician's first and foremost mission of his life is to cure the patient reliably, rapidly and permanently, with minimum or no discomfort. For achieving this there are no short cuts. The physician has to proceed scientifically and systematically.

A physician cannot take things for granted and do anything with his patients. A scientific approach according to the laws of doctrines of Homoeopathy is the only way. There is no other way.

Lecture - XVI

If a physician ignores this cardinal rule, God save him. He will then be a total failure. His patient may be a total wreck.

Some physicians calling themselves homoeopaths administer remedies that palliates and relieves the patient's suffering. They go to any length to justify their doings. They do not listen to the patient's suffering. An honest and sincere homoeopath will turn every stone in his path to find the most suitable remedy for his patient's suffering. He should find out every symptom of the patient to get at the proper remedy. The physician must exercise every care and most scientifically and systematically arrive at the appropriate remedy using the homoeopathic laws and principles. Only then can he be successful and the patient will also derive the cure.

Some physicians cannot grasp the homoeopathic doctrines fully and properly. Such persons fall into interpolation, taking a bite of homoeopathy and allopathy. Under these circumstances, an allopath is better and to be preferred to one who calls himself a homoeopath, who does not know enough homoeopathy to practice the art.

Some physicians provide a local application of a crude medicine and also administer a remedy to the patient. Let us take a typical example - crude medicine is applied on a diphtheritic membrane. In addition a remedy is also administered. Think on this. Now what happens? The crude medicine will spoil the appearance of the throat. The physician cannot observe what and how his remedy has worked out. Such dual medicine administration can damage the case. So, what is the purpose? Why not stick to the remedy alone? There is no point in such a treatment.

In an association meeting, a doctor recommended the use of Hydrogen Peroxide to clean pus cavities. He said it was harmless, and it did no damage. Here the question is does this application of Hydrogen Peroxide do anything at all? If it does anything, the changes it effects will injure the case. The virginity of the case is lost. Understand this principle well. *Make it a principle not to use anything in addition to your remedy that can effect any change.*

The physician will be eager to know what his remedy has done for his patient. When should he come back for a review? This is based upon the nearest homoeopathic remedy that the physician has chosen to administer. Each and every change must be carefully watched. This is an absolute necessity for only this observation will be able to guide the physician as what to do next. Sometimes the patient listens to his friends and upon their suggestion he could take some medicine. Under such circumstances there will be some changes. Then there is utter confusion at the physician's end! In case if no changes have occurred after his remedy the physician is the master of the ceremony and he knows, for sure, his next step. There will be no confusion and the physician will not falter.

A patient comes in howling with pain. With him his relatives and friends also come. They do not know what to do and in their dismay they crowd around the patient. The patient is yelling with pain. These people in their anxiety ask "Doctor, please do something for his pain. Kindly give him some medicine to relieve him of his pain quickly." The doctor is now in a fix. He has to silence those around the patient and also relieve the victim of his suffering. Due to the pressure, the doctor does not thinks twice. The doctor quickly gives a dose of Opium. Why has the physician taken this drastic step knowing fully well that he is injuring the patient and his action is against his best judgment? He has taken this rash step to silence those people who brought in the patient. But the physician knows fully well that he has damaged the case and also he has let slip the beautiful opportunity to cure the patient homoeopathically. The above is typical occurrence everyday in every clinic, unless where the physician is wiser.

Lecture - XVI

Stop to think here. The patient may suffer, what if? Can we ever pardon a doctor destroying his own power to heal the patient? Can we accept the physician justify his action by saying "I had to give a dose of Opium, otherwise these people would criticize me". Can this argument be sustainable? If you are a member of the jury will you accept this explanation? What lesson does this type of occurrence teach the physician?

A genuine homoeopath must have honesty, sincerity and immense will power to proceed in accordance to the homoeopathic principles and doctrines. He must have the character and grit to face any criticism, from any quarters. Under all circumstances he should and must only consider and do only the right thing in every case. He must learn to ignore the rattling of the people who bring in the patient. He must take full responsibility for the patient.

In case the patient dies due to the negligence of the physician, will the law pardon it? Is it not a violation of the law? Has not the physician violated his conscience? Is this not equivalent to suicide on the part of the physician? Criminal, isn't it?

People will trust and respect the doctor who sticks to the laws and principles of homoeopathy, through any type of crisis. Such a doctor will ignore the yelling of the people or critics who comment that the doctor is ignorant or incapable.

A doctor, who has no respect for the laws and doctrines of homoeopathy, will flout them; will bend down at every threat; will violate his conscience. Such a doctor can be bought, hired or do anything, will abandon his color in an emergency. He will not command any respect of his community or the society. No one will stand by him in his tribulations. Public's attitude must not decide what a doctor has to do.

A good homoeopath has to study the patient and his symptoms, very carefully. He cannot afford to miss or ignore any symptom, however insignificant it may look. As mentioned earlier the homoeopath is on a fact-finding mission. By this, whatever is right is protected and anything that is wrong is degraded. By the fact finding mission and doing the right thing on a scientific and in accordance with the laws and doctrines of homoeopathy, in assuming full responsibility of the patient, the physician has acted courageously and in the proper manner as he is expected to act. When the physician has acted in the interest of the patient he can look squarely in the face of the patient's relatives and friends, even if the patient dies. Of course, this does not put a brake on the wagging tongue of the people and their criticism splashed against the doctor. In this case the doctor has not violated his conscience or the law. We proceed to the actions of the medicines from here.

There are two actions of each drug. They are primary and secondary actions. These are dealt with in the paragraphs sixty-three and sixty-four of the Organon. The primary and the secondary action of a drug is simply the one action of that drug. It does not matter what ails the patient from the primary action or the secondary action of the remedy, because that drug will cure all the same. The symptoms due to the action of the remedy oppose the symptoms already existing.

Let us take an example. In an earlier stage sleeplessness is indicated and in later stages sleepiness is the symptom. One state will be more prominent than the other. We find from the proving of *Opium* that some of the provers experienced sleeplessness first and sleepiness later. The cause was a small dose of *Opium*. So, we understand that where *Opium* is indicated, it can cure sleeplessness as well as sleepiness. From this we can draw the conclusion that there is no need to see whether *Opium* produces in one place one state and its opposite state in another place. In some provers *Opium* produced diarrhea in the beginning and constipation in others. We can consider the case of alcohol. In one drunkard we observe an effect and the same alcohol produces an exactly opposite effect. These examples clearly indicate the dual action of a remedy about which we are currently talking.

Now, we come to the constitutional states. These states affect the patients in a particular fashion. These states are observed as leftovers after proving or in cases where the patient has been poisoned by a drug. Remember we talked about drug abuse earlier in this lecture. These symptoms will alternate and tend to confuse the physician. Once the physician knows the patient's constitutional state things will become obvious. So it is very very important to know the constitutional state of a patient. Only knowing this will help us choose a proper remedy. In acute diseases the symptoms are so blatant, which helps the physician choose an appropriate acute remedy. In such a case there is no need to consider any constitutional state. All the acute symptoms can be established in any patient.

As an example of this, a *Calcarea* patient will need an acute cognate of *Calcarea* where his sickness symptoms are acute. Here the acute symptoms fit into those established and formed by his constitutional condition. Hence, we should remember that the constitutional remedy plays a very important and vital role in a sick person.

Summary

1. This lecture covers the aspects discussed in paragraphs forty-four onwards.
2. Drug poisoning can occur in homeopathy by:
    (a) Administering crude drugs
    (b) Administering inappropriate remedies.
    (c) Administering inappropriate potencies of the remedy.
3. The people who are most prone to drug poisoning are the over-sensitive patients.
4. Each dose of medicine must be allowed some time to act.

5. Where the due time for the action of the drug is not allowed and repetition of the dosages are made it is drug abuse. In such cases, the remedy establishes a miasm. The miasm initiates a chronic disease or an acute disease.
6. Where the dosages of the remedy is carelessly repeated, years later the drug poisoning rears its head. The outbursts are typical of that remedy.
7. The crude condition of a drug may be harmless but will be poisonous on potentisation, when repeated beyond its homoeopathicity. It will establish a miasm that can affect the patient for years.
8. We should not give CM potencies to hypersensitive patients. It is better to use 30th and 200th potencies in such cases.
9. Two dissimilar diseases repel, suspend or complicate each other. Several examples are given in Paragraph 46 of Organon.
10. Two different diseases with similar symptoms when appearing in a single person at the same time, the stronger disease will prevail over the weaker disease.
11. Similar diseases cannot exist in one individual at the same time.
12. Homoeopathy is a science and an art. The administering of the appropriate remedy in the appropriate potency, repeated after the drug action of the previous dose has stopped is an art. Such administration results in complete cure.
13. Homoeopathy is opposed to any vaccination. Where sub-physiological administration of homoeopathically indicated remedy is given the patient obtains the benefits similar to the vaccination. Vaccine is introduced forcibly into the body by hypodermic needles. It does not go into the body by natural channels.

Lecture - XVI

14. A homoeopath has several medicines to deal with any disease now.
15. Every homoeopath has to be an eternal student.
16. A homeopath cannot afford to be negligent at any time.
17. There are many reliable and valuable Materia Medicas at the disposal of a homoeopath, today. Repeated studies of the Materia Medica provide him with a lot of insight.
18. A homoeopath should not divert his attention to the traditional ways.
19. Patients must not be taken for granted.
20. A homoeopath can be successful only when he sticks to the laws and doctrine of his science.
21. A homoeopath should do what is right according to his doctrines, under any circumstance. He cannot afford to be negligent.
22. In cases of dual application of remedies - one externally and another internally - external application can infuse the case and cause confusion to the physician. So give only what is necessary. By administering a single drug the physician can observe its effect on the patient. This will surely and certainly guide the next step to be taken, for the physician.
23. A genuine homoeopath has to be honest and true to his conscience. People will trust such a physician and respect him.
24. All symptoms, major or minor, have to be considered before prescribing a remedy. No symptom can be ignored.
25. Each drug has a primary and secondary action.
26. The patient's constitutional drug or remedy is a very important one and is not to be ignored.

Aphorisms & Precepts

1. If you love homoeopathy, it will love you; such is natural charity.
2. It is an entirely different business to comfort from what it is to cure.
3. The will is expressed in the face; hence the countenance of the people. Have murderers and evildoers a placid face?
4. What a man wills to do is his life and character.
5. Proceeding from the will is man's understanding. If the will is good to obey the commandments, he selects his very education in accordance with it.
6. The upright man whose desires are good wants the truth. His perceptions are intensified.
7. The outer world is the world of results. The inner world is not discoverable by the senses but by understanding.
8. One, who is not acute in observation, goes through life, seeing only indifferent similarity. Most men only know the toxic power of a drug.
9. No two remedies are absolutely equal in their similitude.
10. We cannot educate a patient until after he is cured. We have to let him think in his own way. But steal in and cure him. Do him good. That is the all-important thing.
11. The questions of palliation will annoy you, especially in early years. You will be pressed upon all sides by women who wring their hands and by men who hear the cries of women. But what authority have you to hush the cries of the patient, if by palliating you do away with the ability to heal him.
12. The more violence you see, and the more necessity for haste, and the more severe and the greater suffering of the patient, the more harm you can do by a false and foolish prescription.

Lecture - XVII

The Science and the Art

In the previous sixteen lectures, we learnt the principles of the knowledge of Homoeopathy. In this lecture we are to learn about their application by means of three steps.

(1) What are the means for the physician to arrive at the necessary information, relating to a disease, which direct him towards the cure?

(2) The second step is to discover the disease creating nature or power of the drug. We also know that each drug is capable of creating an artificial disease, with its own characteristic symptoms, in a healthy individual. Homoeopathy is based on facts, not on opinions. Materia Medica is based on facts. The facts are the proving and recorded facts.

(3) How and what are the most effective ways that the physician has in his hands to apply this knowledge of the morbific influence of the drug for a rapid, gentle and permanent cure. Here he needs to be totally discriminative and selective.

We have seen that the above relates to the disease in general and the patient in particular. Here, we recall paragraph three of the Organon. It says:

The physician should understand,

(a) What is curable in disease in general and in each patient in particular.

(b) What is curative in drugs in general and in each drug in particular.

(c) How we must apply with clear and precise reasoning what is curative in drug to what is curable in disease.

To put it in other words:

(i) How to match the proper remedy to the disease,

(ii) How to administer properly the correct dosage of medicine,

(iii) How to repeat the dose,

And finally

(d) How to recognize the blocks in the way of cure and how to remove these obstacles out of the way.

From here on, Homoeopathy, which was taken as a science so far, takes the form of the ART OF HEALING.

In allopathy there is a name for every disease. So, the allopath prescribes a medicine for the disease known by a name. By keeping a record or perusing such a record we will know nothing more about the disease, or its nature. Hence this falls under a general classification. Whether the patient be A or B or C — when the affliction is classified and identified by a name, the treatment or the prescription is always the same. In Homoeopathy, it is not so.

Dr. Hahnemann classified the diseases. The two classes on a broad scale must be known. They are 1) Acute and 2) Chronic.

We have already dealt with these briefly in our earlier lecture. An acute miasm has a prodromal period, progress and finally a

Lecture - XVII

period of decline naturally. A chart also illustrated this. After the decline of the acute miasm there is recovery.

In the case of a chronic disease, this also has a prodormal period, period of progress. But the chronic disease has NO period of decline. The process is continuous. Whenever the proper conditions of the body permit its progress the disease progresses. When the physical or mental conditions are not favorable to its progress, it lies dormant. A chart also illustrated this.

Acute diseases are short-lived. They die a natural death sooner or later after it runs its course. So, this class requires lesser study than the chronic disease. Acute miasms are contagious or infectious. They run a definite course.

We have a patient who has a stomach disorder and vomiting. This patient has no trouble from these problems after that. This is only an indisposition. When these troubles are due to external causes, like eating foods that disagreed with him, it is not miasmatic, just indisposition. Here the problem was due to food, which caused a disturbance. A similar condition could arise at a later date when the patient again makes the mistake of taking such food. Till then he is healthy.

The pure diseases shall be considered now. They are not like the above. We have already seen that a Government governs the human economy. Its seat is in the brain at the top. It has also been brought to our attention that the disease whether acquired or inherited, flows from the inner most to the outermost, while making a man sick. We have also studied about influx. This influx of simple substance causes sickness in humans and they run a fixed course. As mentioned earlier each one has a prodormal period, its own period of progress. The traditional school has fixed defined and made out particular symptoms for each. It is called the pathognomonic symptoms of that disease. Knowledge of these symptoms will be useful for the purpose of association.

When we think of a child having measles, the homoeopath may not think of measles. He will be able to visualize the character of the sickness and will imagine the sufferings of that child. A homoeopath understands the sickness from the symptoms and not from the name attributed to the disease. That is why we have been repeatedly hammering that the homoeopath must be well familiar with the disease picture.

This is not to discredit the diagnosis aspect. It is not useful for the purpose of writing out the prescription.

Earlier we said that a homoeopath must be able to discriminate. In cases like measles in the earlier stages things may confuse to be like a scarlet fever or *vice versa*. He must analyze calmly and properly and decide the nature of fever. In case of measles he will choose *Pulsatilla* and in case of scarlet fever he will choose *Belladonna*.

The idea of saving the patient must be on the top most of the homoeopath's mind. So he must choose the remedy that the patient needs. Hence he need not worry about the classification. However, he can have an idea of the classification, in a general way.

The next step is choosing the correct remedy to administer the medicine and what are the steps necessary to be taken to protect the people when there is a contagious disease.

A homoeopath must be after facts. So he must know the nature of diseases in full. He must explain it to the family for their protection sake. They may appear simple - but nevertheless important in the interests of the community.

Sometimes, chronic diseases closely resemble acute diseases. E.g., those mimicking acute attacks that comes regularly as periodical headaches. When you consider a single attack it will look like an acute miasm. *But when taken as a whole the tendency to progress and not to recovery clearly indicates that this headache belongs to the chronic class.* The disorders

Lecture - XVII

that result from debauchery, drinking and over eating, from immediate circumstances that are periodical are due to the latent psoric conditions present. They are momentary sickness, and man suffers from chronic miasms. Hence he has all these diseases. These attacks form a sickness and appear like an acute disease because of the miasms. *All these small recurring attacks are due to chronic miasms in the human body.* When carefully observed we notice that those do not have a prodromal period, progressive period and a period of decline. They may progress and decline but do not have a prodrome.

Here, we have to read a portion of Organon, paragraph 71. The relevant portion reads as follows:

"How is the physician to ascertain what is necessary to be known in order to cure the disease?"

The question is straightforward and understandable. So no further explanation or analysis is necessary. What answer does Dr. Hahnemann offer as a reply to this query?

Paragraph 72 answers this question. It reads as under:

"With respect to this point, the following will serve as a general preliminary view. The disease to which man is liable are either rapid morbid process of the abnormally deranged vital force, which have a tendency to finish their course more or less quickly, but always in a moderate time - these are termed acute diseases; - or they are diseases of such a character that, with small, often imperceptible beginnings, dynamically derange the living organism, each in its own peculiar manner, and cause it gradually to deviate from the healthy condition, in such a way that the automatic life energy, called vital force, whose office is to preserve the health, only opposes to them at the commencement and during their progress imperfect, unsuitable, useless resistance, but is unable of itself to extinguish them, but must helplessly suffer (them to spread and) itself to be ever more and more abnormally deranged, until at length the organism is destroyed; these are termed chronic diseases. They are caused by infection with a chronic miasm."

Analysis:

Diseases that affect the human organism are of two types; the first one is rapid, the morbid process is caused by abnormal states and derangement of the vital forces. These run a course within a brief period. These are called as acute diseases.

The second category is one that develops from imperceptible beginnings. They advance to such a condition that they dynamically derange the living organism. The health is undermined progressively and ends up in death - destroying the organism. These are called chronic diseases.

To make the above brief:

Acute diseases always tend to recovery. Chronic disease has a tendency to progressively mature and continue to damage the human organism.

While we are on acute disease we can as well peruse Organon paragraph seventy-three. This paragraph is reproduced below:

"As regards acute diseases, they are either of such a kind as attack human beings individually, the *existing cause* being injurious influences to which they were particularly exposed. Excess in food, or an insufficient supply of it, severe physical impressions, chills, over-heating, dissipation, strains etc., or physical irritations, mental emotions, and the like, are exciting causes of such acute febrile affections; in reality, however, they are generally only a transient explosion of latent psora, which spontaneously returns to its dormant state if the acute diseases were not of too violent a character and were soon quelled. Or they are of such a kind as attack several persons at the same time, here and there (*sporadically*) by means of meteoric or telluric influences and injurious agents, the susceptibility for being morbidly affected by which is possessed by only a few persons at one time. Allied to

Lecture - XVII

these are those diseases in which many persons are attacked with similar sufferings from the same cause (epidemically); these are diseases generally become infectious (contagious) when they prevail among thickly congregated masses of human beings. Thence arise fevers, in each instance of peculiar nature, and because the cases of disease have an identical origin, they set up in all those they affect an identical morbid process, which when left to self terminates in a moderate period of time to death or recovery. The calamities of war, inundations and famine are not infrequently their exciting causes and producers - sometimes they are peculiar acute miasms which recur in the same manner (hence know by some traditional name), which either attack persons but once in a life time, as the small-pox, measles, whooping cough, the ancient smooth, bright red scarlet fever of Syndenham, the mumps etc., or such as recur frequently in pretty much the same manner, the plague of the Levant, the yellow fever of the sea-coast, the Asiatic cholera, etc.

Foot note: The homeopathic physician, who does not entertain the foregone conclusions devised by ordinary school (who fixed upon a few names of such fevers, besides which mighty nature dare not produce any others so as to admit their treating these diseases according to some fixed method) does not acknowledge the names goal fever, bilious fever, typhus fever, putrid fever, but treats them each according to their several peculiarities."

A brief analysis of the above paragraph:

Acute diseases are separated into further classes or categories. There are two major headings under which they are classified.

(1) Artificial acute sickness, due to

    (a) Over exertion

    (b) Injury

    (c) Over-indulgence

(d) Drugging

(e) Exposure

(f) Un-hygienic living

(g) Un-hygienic surroundings

(2) Natural acute sickness due to natural causes

(a) Epidemic

(b) Endemic

(c) Sporadic

(d) Contagious

(e) Infectious

When the living human organism is exposed to the above injurious influences and also to excess of food, insufficient food supply, physical impressions, chills, over-heating, strains, dissipation, physical irritations, mental emotions, etc., it suffers from febrile affections that are acute. These affections are short living over bursts of the latent psora inside. This is dormant within the human organism.

Sporadic: Several persons are affected at the same time in a spread out manner. People who are susceptible get affected.

Epidemic: Many persons are affected with identical sufferings. The cause for this is the same. Epidemic diseases become contagious when it spread in thickly populated areas.

Then, there are fevers, etc. of peculiar nature of identical origin. They all possess the same morbid processes. They terminate in recovery or death. The causes for these are the calamities due to war, severe floods, and famines.

There is also another group of peculiar acute miasms. They recur in the same manner. These are all known by some traditional

Lecture - XVII

names. They attack people once in a lifetime. E.g. Measles, whooping cough, smallpox, scarlet fever, yellow fever of the seacoast, plague of Levant and Asian-cholera, etc.

Dr. Hahnemann classified the diseases in a very pertinent manner. The classification is provided here for the reader's benefit. Dr. Hahnemann has said there are three miasms, which are chronic and torments the living human organism. They are psora, syphilis and sycosis.

The worst cases are those where all the three chronic miasms or some part of the three are complicated by the administration of drugs. Once we are able to nullify the effects of the drug, we can study the pure miasms. But in the present the miasms are so complicated in most men. Whenever we are confronted with a chronic disease we notice chronic drugging there. Remember this has a devastating effect on the vital force.

Dr. Kent feels that this drugging has bombarded the human race in a most violent manner. The human race was not torn to pieces so miserably when they resorted to treatments like bloodletting, administering emetics and sweating which was adopted earlier. The huge doses of jalap and calomel rushed through the intestines flushing out the patient. The result was the patient felt better after this treatment. He did not carry any after effects to his grave. He did not suffer for his lifetime due to the internal results of the powerful emetics and sudorifics. But presently we note that small doses of very concentrated drugs are being administered. These have a great damaging effect on the patient affecting gradually his economy and building up of chronic symptoms step by step. A very slow suicide indeed!

There is a statutory warning now-a-days printed on cigarette packets. It is "Cigarette smoking is injurious to health". I feel that there must be a similar warning printed out on the colorful and attractive boxes containing medicines too!

Continuous taking of alkaloids, etc. creates most dreadful condition in the history of medicine. The aim is to get small doses, to get insidious effect. The milder preparations like the medicine Sulphanol take a long time to develop their chronic effects. They are the most tenacious and troublesome drugs. These drugs are mild and appear to produce a mild primary effect. Then, what we forget is the devastating severe after-effects, which creep in silently and gradually. Even in Dr. Hahnemann's time, he has said, the most troublesome chronic diseases were those that were complicated by drugging. It is even worse now. *The headache medicines, catarrh cures, etc. which are so commonly dispensed and consumed appear so simple and innocent, in their first effects. But contemplate on this - visualize the after-effects, which is so spine chilling.*

Simultaneously, give a thought to the Homoeopathic medicines. *They are so natural and effective. They do not possess that lingering silent killing nature.*

Before closing this lecture, I would like to bring to attention of the readers what Dr. Stuart Close, M.D., has said in his work "The Genius of Homoeopathy".

"Homoeopathy as set forth by Hahnemann, while not perfect, is complete in all essentials as a system. It is supreme within its legitimate sphere because it is the only method of therapeutic medication which is based upon a fixed and definite law of nature."

We started this lecture, as homoeopathy is both a science and an art of healing. Let us end this lecture with the same idea in Dr. Stuart Close's words: —

> *"Homeopathy, the science and art of therapeutics of medication, has a two fold existence - as an institution and in the personnel of its loyal, indivividual representatives."*

Lecture - XVII

CLASSIFICATION OF DISEASE

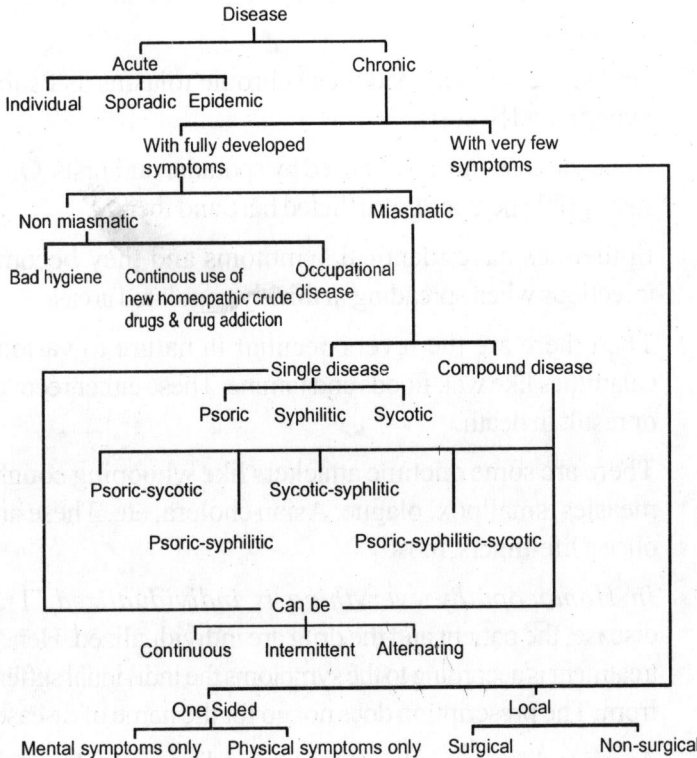

Summary

1. Homeopathy is a science and an art of healing. In this lecture we learn about the application of the scientific principles, we have so far seen.

2. There are many acute diseases that torment the human race. These are caused due to exposure to injurious influences such as excess of food, insufficiency of food, physical impressions, chills, over-heating, strains, dissipation, physical

irritation, mental emotions, acute febrile affections, etc. This is due to the latent, dormant lying psora miasm in each individual.

3. Dr. Hahnemann named these chronic miasms as Psora, Syphilis and Sycosis.
4. Acute diseases are also caused by sporadic outbursts. Only susceptible persons get afflicted here and there.
5. Epidemics have identical symptoms and they become infectious when spreading in thickly populated areas.
6. Then there are the fevers peculiar in nature to various calamities like war, floods and famine. These either recover or result in death.
7. There are some onetime attackers like whooping cough, measles, smallpox, plague, Asian cholera, etc. These are once a life-timers, mostly.
8. *In Homoeopathy everything is individualized.* The disease, the patient and the drug are individualized. Hence treatment is according to the symptoms the individual suffers from. The prescription does not go for the name of disease.
9. An acute disease is only a short-term indisposition. It cannot be called a disease. Acute diseases have a prodrome period, progressive period and a declining period.
10. However knowing the disease by the traditional name is useful for the purpose of comparison or association. This knowledge does not help in making out a homoeopathic prescription. The homoeopath understands the language of the disease by the symptoms given out. It is nature's way of expressing the malady.
11. Patient's need and his suffering must be the top-most in a homoeopath's mind.

12. Sometimes chronic diseases may closely resemble acute one. A headache that keeps on coming again and again when considered, as a single attack appears to be acute. But when there is no recovery and viewed from a holistic angle we understand that these outbursts are due to latent miasms.
13. Acute diseases after running their course recovery. The chronic ones develop slowly and terminate in death.
14. It is better to know the classification of diseases as given out by Dr. Hahnemann.
15. Dr. Hahnemann christened the miasms as *Psora, Syphilis* and *Sycosis*.
16. Cases become complicated where the three chronic miasms are continuously improperly medicated.
17. The small non-homoeopathic pill that looks so innocent may apparently provide a short-term relief. But its after-effects are devastating. It is a slow killer.
18. Homoeopathy as given to us by Dr. Hahnemann is complete in every way. *It is the only method of therapeutic medication, which is based upon a fixed and definite law of nature.*
19. *Homoeopathy is a scientific system and healing by homoeopathic method is an art.*

Aphorisms & Precepts

1. The value of service is nothing, your use is first, and so long as you have this in your mind, you will grow.
2. The idea that you must relieve a patient of his chills at all hazards, that you must give him Quinine, and Arsenic afterwards, if that does not work, is all wrong. You will be

tempted to do these things, unless you have grown up within yourself a new conscience, and realize that it is criminal.

3. The physician who ceases to study a case before he sees what the patient needs, neglecting that case. He falls into a habit and it becomes second nature to prescribe without reflection.

4. You see homoeopathy in a superficial way only when you see the similarity of the symptoms to the remedy, the mere outward manifestation. You must see that the interiors are related to each other.

5. When the Materia Medica is fully learned you see at a glance the image of the remedy. It looms up before you. You know it as a physician of experience knows measles or scarlet fever.

Lecture - XVIII

Chronic Diseases - Psora

For anything there should always be a beginning. *For all physical sickness Psora is the beginning.* Psora is the basic miasm and from this the other two miasms blossom out. But for Psora acute diseases would have been impossibility. Psora is the base or the foundation of all human diseases. Psora came first and all other sicknesses followed suit.

Psora is primitive. It is the underlying cause of all disorders of the human race. Like any other condition of sickness, Psora also disharmonizes the human economy. Many chronic manifestations, affecting the human race is due to Psora. Had the human race remained in perfect order, Psora could not have existed.

The susceptibility to psora is by itself a very vast subject. It is very extensive since it is the most primitive one its roots go to a great depth - in fact to the first wrongs of the human race.

Dr. Hahnemann says psora is the common wellspring of many chronic diseases. They seem to differ in essence but ultimately are one and the same.

For thousands of years it has disfigured and tormented the human race.

"If illness is an imbalance of the vital force, an imbalance which issues from thought and transcends the whole being, this anomalous thought must necessarily and inevitably issue from a mind and will which are already defective. We are of-course, talking about an illness of miasmatic origin, while we leave aside for later discussion the origin of this initial miasmatic illness, merely pointing out that man's liberty permits him to commit this transgression and leads him to the imbalance which is the initial illness."

Dr. Hahnemann

Further Dr. Hahnemann in his book *Chronic Diseases* says that Psora is that most ancient, most universal, most destructive, and yet most misapprehended chronic miasmatic disease — and during the last centuries has become the mother of all the thousands of incredibly various acute and chronic (non-venereal) diseases, by which the whole civilized human race on the inhabited globe is being more and more inflicted. *Psora is the oldest miasmatic disease known to us and this is most hydra-headed of all the chronic miasmatic diseases.*

Dr. Allen in his book, "The Chronic Miasms", says about Psora that it is like an octopus, taking in everything, both physical and the mental, and in many cases largely influencing the spiritual. There is no life process free from it.

Dr. Hahnemann found records of psora among ancient Greeks, Romans, Arabians and the Israelites.

So, from the above we see that Psora is also a spiritual sickness and the human race developed a susceptibility to psora year by year and from generation to generation. It developed in leaps and bounds.

We all have seen a Banyan tree. It is so huge and keeps on growing. It shoots out roots from its branches. They in turn go into the earth and nourishes the tree and helps it grow bigger and bigger. Just think of it. How is this tree propagated? It springs out of a seed (by germination) that is so small. This is quoted to show that all huge things have a very small seed or small and simple beginning.

Lecture - XVIII

Psora also has spread out similarly from a very small beginning. In the earlier days, it was itch that affected the skin. Then it had a surprising growth and spread out into its underlying states and manifested itself in large portions of the chronic case, which torments the human race.

Let us now see what diseases are covered by psora. Epilepsy, insanity, the malignant diseases, tumors, ulcers, catarrhs, and a great portion of the eruptions are due to Psora. Psora's progress from very simple state to a highly complex condition is not always alone by itself. We said earlier that Psora confined to the skin at the earlier stages. By drugging from generation to generation it has grown to gigantic proportions and complexity due to the drug poisoning—like a Banyan tree.

This is due to the physicians endeavor to eradicate the external affection. By their eagerness to drive this away the external affection was pushed in deeper and deeper into the body. *It did vanish (?) from the external - but now by virtue of its delving deeper and deeper internally it became more dense and also as invisible enemy within.* The human race is almost threatened with extinction.

It makes one shudder to see infants die and the little ones having no efficient vitality to live. This is largely due to the outcome of psora. Think of the growing congenital debility, marasmus, and many chronic diseases, which pluck the children away from us. The underlying cause is psora, then syphilis and then sycosis.

Dr. Hahnemann toiled for twelve long years to collect proof and evidence to reach this conclusion. How did he accomplish this great conclusion? Dr. Hahnemann took pains to note down many details whenever any patient, who manifested chronic disease in any way, came to him. He noted down all the symptoms of the patient, from the beginning to end. He also took down the medical history of his parents. Armed with these details he was able to collect all details of many diseases and was able to draw out the full and complete picture of psora, in all its forms.

Till Dr. Hahnemann brought out the theory of miasms, the medical world looked upon each of these varying diseases distinct by itself. For example, all the striking features of affection was collected together and labeled as a disease - say, epilepsy. But that school of thought was ignorant of that epilepsy is the result of the disease and never appeared twice alike.

It is to be noted that whether it is epilepsy, diabetes, cancer, Bright's disease or any other so-called disease, had a beginning - one beginning. They are not distinct as it was thought. It operated in each person in accordance to that individual. *This tells us why homoeopathy is a science of individualization.*

Dr. Hahnemann was struck with wonder about certain short-action remedies before he started collecting details in the aforementioned manner. Certain short-acting medicines like *Nux vomica* and *Ignatia* cured only a single manifestation, a group of symptoms, or the relief would be for a short duration. The disease returned back after a short time in spite of Dr. Hahnemann's best efforts to cure it. He observed that there was a constant progress of the disease though he had relieved his patient of the suffering well many times.

The above phenomenon was due to psoric doctrine. *Short acting remedies contain the counterparts of acute psoric manifestation. So the acute remedies will palliate the suffering from time to time.* On carefully observing the record of such cases, it could be seen that the case has been steadily progressing. This shows that the underlying cause has not been eradicated and that something is at the root, which prevails, encouraging the disease to steadily grow worse.

Dr. Hahnemann was a master of acute disease and acute remedies. He was hounded by the thought of the disease relapsing and steadily growing worse. Remedies like *Belladona, Aconite,*

Lecture - XVIII

Bryonia, Arnica, China, Nux vomica had been well proved by this time as antipsorics, and were found perfectly suitable for acute psoric manifestations and other acute miasms. Dr. Hahnemann was yet to stumble on the fact that acute miasms were strictly acute miasms. Hence he could not compare them with chronic miasms or *vice-versa*. He had not seen them yet as miasms.

We must first understand clearly the acute miasms. Only then will we be able to compare them with chronic miasms. They go hand in hand and manifest wonderfully. *The acute miasms can be violent enough to cause death or with lesser violence there is a period of progress and thereby a tendency to recover.* Since they cannot prolong in the patient, they have to subside. Acute miasms are not governed by any fixed time - they have a prodromol period, period of progress and a period of decline. This was explained in an earlier lecture and also with a chart. They have their own lifetime. Similarly there is no time after the lapse of which the chronic miasm is labeled as such.

The old school divided acute diseases into three categories: 1) acute, 2) sub-acute and 3) chronic. Sub-acute meant sickness with duration of more than six weeks and sickness that ran indefinitely was chronic. *Hence we have to understand that a chronic miasm is chronic right from its beginning; so was the acute miasm.* We should study its nature, its capabilities and from what it will do to the human race and name it accordingly.

Dr. Hahnemann confesses that he was astonished to note no progress after a period of treatment in chronic diseases. The symptoms followed a particular pattern appearing with their own regularity. *At every appearance it was stronger than the previous one, clearly indicating the disease was progressing.*

Dr. Hahnemann now had on his hands a project that was difficult to study. He also faced all sorts of difficulties. To surmount this it took a minimum of twelve long years. He discovered that in all the chronic cases there was an underlying chronic miasm. It had a tendency to progress and ended with the life of the patient. Then he worked on the proving of the remedies to discover in them a total likeness to the chronic miasms. Only these conclusions assisted him to notice such things.

How did Dr. Hahnemann accomplish this difficult task? He brought all the symptoms in one grand collective view. Then he began to observe and reflect as to what was the first, the second, and later appreances in the line of progress in the deep-seated chronic miasm. By this reflection he was able to reach back the origin or the first symptoms of the disease. As an example, in cases dying with phthisis he was able to go back to the sufferings of the patients in their younger days. The patients had suffered vesicular disease between the fingers and upon the body. Some ointment had suppressed this, which was in vogue in those days. What has this amounted to? It amounts to the suppression of the vesicular disease.

Now, accepting the above as suppression, does this suppression have a part in the later development of the pthisis. Dr. Hahnemann has written about how he solved such a puzzle in his book "Chronic Diseases". There he has provided in many pages his experience and observations. By the use of appropriate remedies and application of the principle to the progress of the disease we can see the truth of Dr. Hahnemann's conclusion. Application of this principle will also lead to the curative effects of many diseases.

The remedy's appropriateness can be seen from the fact that the latest symptoms will be the first to vanish. The older symptoms will appear and disappear in the reverse order in which they appeared. So, the old symptoms come back in the form of eruptions, old chills that have been suppressed, come back and many other chronic manifestations appear, in a sort, successively. When we observe these things we can conclude that we have driven these earliest and deepest troubles back to their original

Lecture - XVIII

manifestations - like a vesicular eruption. Where we see nothing simpler than the eruption what is that can be a natural inference? Do you not see it written in big red letters? Yes, *the suppression of the eruption was the beginning of the disease!* Obvious, is it not?

A good and successful homoeopath will observe these details. Many patients are very badly off because this is never observed. This results in the disease progressing onwards. In such a case the patient declines instead of the disease declining. *When the patient is only better symptoms-wise and the old symptoms not coming back goes to prove that the remedy has acted palliatively. So, this is not a cure.*

It is better to apprise the patient of his condition and also what the remedy would do for the patient. Otherwise, the patient takes too much courage and such a person will not be able to take any discouragement when the reverse occurs. So, be careful. When a patient comes after treatment and profusely thank for having relieved him/her and as a good, successful homoeopath, no backward progress has been observed it is always good to inform the patient that if any eruption, etc. crop up at a later date do not meddle with it and suppress it. As a good policy it is wise to check back the records when the patient comes in with a wonderful progress. The patient has to be warned not to do anything in case any earlier symptoms return. He ought to be instructed to report the fact to the physician. The physician must also tell the patient that such and such symptoms can re-appear. This, of course, is possible only when a proper history of the disease is maintained, and checked out correctly.

How does this point help the physician and the patient? When the patient is instructed not to take any medicine or apply any external remedies for such a re-appearance of the earlier symptoms and should contact the doctor immediately, the physician knows for certain that he has taken the proper course in treating the disease.

This will help him to throw out the cause of the disease. The patient benefits by the sure cure he will thus obtain.

On the return of any earlier symptom the patient must not take any drugs; keep his life simple and pure as far as possible, try to keep the physical forces untrammeled by violence of any sort. Then, under such conditions, the physician is able to observe the re-appearance of the old or earlier symptoms, which were suppressed for long time.

The patient may come back long after the cessation of the treatment, for a symptom that has re-appeared. Checking up of the old records will confirm that psora existed from the childhood and that it was suppressed.

Cases such as above are simplest of psora since these can be collectively seen in one person. *Complicated cases of psora are those that are inherited.*

In simple cases of psora, the eruptions come and disappear, and then catarrhal troubles crop up. They vary in their manifestations. Prescription for all these symptoms brings back eruptions that appeared in childhood. We do not get the patient to the original form of psora, as the parent was afflicted with psora and the child gets a complex form from those which were present when the patient came to the physician. We rarely come across the vesicular form or simple form brought back since these can be seen only in persons who have had the simple form. But then, if the vital energy of the economy is being turned into order forms approximating the simple form will return.

Since this is the natural form of economy we are able to notice our moving backwards. We are moving towards the beginning of psora or its earlier forms. Let us take up a case of vicious form of scaly eruptions, dry, hard horney scales. Under accurate prescribing the scaly formations disappear. When the vital force has sufficiently become stronger, the vesicular eruptions develop. How is this?

Lecture - XVIII

The original disease was having vicious squamous form. As the vital force developed, the appropriate remedy helps the vicious form to become milder. Different types of skin diseases were called by different name. Skin disease is skin disease - that is all. So, what is in a name? A rose is a rose by whatever name we may call it.

The different forms of eruptions change into varying forms. But we know that they all spring out of one cause. When proper homoeopathic treatment is afforded they come back in their successive stages. This goes to prove that psora begins with the simple isolated vesicular form of eruption.

In more advanced and complicated forms of psora, there could be organic changes. In such a condition and where the patient undergoes homoeopathic treatment for some time it comes to a standstill, and looks as if it is doing nothing. But in course of time vicious and ugly eruptions spring out on the body. *This is an excellent sign because now the disease manifests upon the skin or in catarrhal discharges; the internal organs are safe.* In case these external manifestations are stopped or suppressed the disease travels inside and affects the internal parts. See how logical the homoeopathic law 'cure takes place from inside to outside' is? - From a more important organ to a less important organ. Hence suppression of any externally appearing disease will prove disastrous. It may not be so immediate, but in the course of time it will be extremely dangerous.

A good and successful homoeopath knows the chaos that could be created by suppression by external applications. In allopathy today there are several ointments, which are applied locally. Can the homoeopath accept this principle of so-called cure? Think of it. What a great damage and injustice is done in these cases? What a tremendous shock to the patient's internal economy! What has this kind of suppression done to psora? Psora has been made worse, made more complex year by year, generation by generation to such a glory that it is the fundamental disease of the human economy and the basis of all troubles in man.

In any particular case, we can learn more about psora by watching it in its backward progress than by watching its onward progress. Psora is the cause of chronic manifestations of diseases that are not syphilitic or sycotic. We are able to gather all the vicious constitutional states named as organic disease as the result of psora. Remember that any disease of the human body is the result of upsetting of the economy. That is why Dr. Hahnemann gave us the rule 'Treat the person and not the disease'. Once again we are able to see that the name has little or no value.

Bright's disease is categorized in five forms. According to what we learnt above, these five forms of Bright's disease are not diseases. They are the results of the psora being active and present. It operates on the economy and attacks the kidneys. What do you then say of the common chronic diseases of the liver? It is not a disease of the liver, but due to the localization of psora in the liver. Similarly lung, heart and brain diseases are not diseases. They all have a common denominator and one single origin. When we follow their progress and study and reflect on them and analyze them from their beginnings to ends, from causes to ultimate, we get a clear picture of their internal cause and beginnings.

We shall discuss psora further in the next lecture.

Summary

1. Psora is the basis of all human sufferings.
2. From psora, syphilis and sycosis spring out.
3. Psora is ancient and primitive.
4. Psora is the wellspring of many chronic diseases. Though

Lecture - XVIII

they differ in essence they are all one and the same, ultimately.
5. Psora has disfigured and tortured the human race for thousands of years.
6. Illness is an imbalance of the vital force.
7. The imbalance coming out of thought transcends the whole being. This is the initial illness.
8. Psora is most universal, most destructive and the most misapprehended chronic miasmatic disease.
9. Psora is the mother of all various non-venereal diseases. Psora is like a gigantic octopus spreading its vicious tentacles, taking in everything, both physical and mental. It largely influences the spiritual being as well.
10. Psora existed among the ancient Greeks, Romans, Arabians and Israelites. From that time onwards the human race has developed susceptibility for psora.
11. Psora starts with a small beginning and at the end manifests itself into chronic disease.
12. Psora is hydra-headed and is at the base of all chronic and acute diseases.
13. When external affections are eliminated by outer applications the disease is driven inwards and the internal organs suffer.
14. Congenital debility, marasmus and children born with very low vitality are caused by psora.
15. It took twelve long years for Dr. Hahnemann to discover that miasms were the cause of chronic diseases.
16. The disease could be labeled under any name, say diabetes, epilepsy, Bright's disease, etc., but they are of one origin, psora. These are only different manifestations. Each form of manifestation affects the individual in a particular manner according to the individual.

17. Acute miasms are acute miasms and chronic miasms are chronic miasms. They must be accepted as such.
18. The nature of acute miasms must be well mastered to enable compare it with chronic miasms. They go together in devastating the human economy.
19. They have no fixed time. Acute miasms have a prodromal, progressive and declining period.
20. The earlier symptoms may reappear after the disappearance of the symptoms for which homoeopathic treatment was afforded. This is a good sign.
21. It is always the last manifestation that goes first. Then the earlier symptoms go successively one by one in the reverse order under proper homoeopathic treatment.
22. The reappearance of earlier symptom may take some time. When such reappearance takes place the patient has to be instructed to get in touch with the physician. The patient must not meddle with the reappearance.
23. The reappearance could be an eruption or catarrhal discharge.
24. In complex cases organic changes could be there.
25. Remember the law of cure takes place from inside out. So any external manifestation indicates a cure, in the proper direction.
26. We have to treat the person, not the disease.
27. Lung disease, brain disease, heart disease etc., etc., indicate psora being localized in those organs.
28. To know the miasm properly and fully, we should study the case from the beginning to end step by step. So we will know when suppression meddled with the picture of the disease.

Lecture - XVIII

Aphorisms & Precepts

1. There is nothing in the world, which does not exist by something prior to itself. With the grossest materialistic ideas man can demonstrate this.
2. You must be able to recognize every ambassador of the internal man.
3. Susceptibility is only a name for a state that underlies all possible sickness and all possible cures.
4. Susceptibility exists in the vital force, and not in the tissues.
5. The signs are visible, but the *esse* is invisible.
6. Homoeopaths have a consciousness of what life is, what the life force is, what the nature of disease is, and can apply to all theories of the world our measure and test them. They can realize the philosophies.
7. That changes in the body correspond to wrong thinking is true.
8. Man must be studied as he is, as he was, everything of the human race in general, in order to understand disease.
9. Psora is the evolution of the state of man's will, the ultimate of his sin.
10. This outgrowth, which has come upon man from living a life of evil willing, is Psora - is the life of Psora.
11. When psora had become complete ultimation of causes, it became contagious.
12. Thinking, willing, and doing are the three things in life from which finally proceed the chronic miasms.
13. The whole miasm in a chronic disease does not come out in an individual, but in the human race.
14. When old symptoms return, there is hope. That is the road to cure and there is none other.

Lecture - XIX

Chronic Diseases - Psora (Contd.)

We are recalling Dr.Hahnemann's words here. It was given in the earlier lecture. He says, "Psora is the oldest, most universal and most pernicious chronic miasmatic diseases, yet it has been misapprehended more than any other. The oldest history of the oldest nation does not reach its origin. Psora is as tedious as syphilis and sycosis, and is moreover, hydra-headed. Unless it is thoroughly cured, it lasts until the last breath of the longest life. Not even the most robust constitution, by its own unaided efforts, is able to annihilate and extinguish psora."

All the three miasms, psora, syphilis and sycosis are all contagious. In each of these, there is something prior to the manifestation. We call this disease. We speak of the signs and symptoms of a disease; speak of the out-cropping of the symptoms. When we speak of these in relation to, say syphilis. Remember there should have existed a particular amenable state to syphilis. Otherwise conditions relating to syphilis could not have broken out.

At this stage the following aphorisms and precepts are recalled.

1. There is nothing in the world, which does not exist by something prior to itself.
2. Susceptibility is only a name for a state that underlies all possible sickness and all possible cures.
3. Man is susceptible to all things capable of producing similar symptoms to those, which he already has.
4. Susceptibility is prior to all contagion.
5. If a man has no chronic miasm he would not have acute disease. It is because he is susceptible to these outside influences.
6. Never look for a cause within the thing itself. It must be prior, or within the organism.

We can go on with many more aphorisms, but at this stage, this is sufficient to prove the point in question. *So, we do see that, in this case of syphilis, or in the case of any other miasmatic problems, it could not descend upon the man except where a suitable environment for its development is there. Hence this environment is prior to the disease!* To extend this a little further the miasmatic disease could exist only in a body wherein suitable condition for its development exists.

Earlier, we have mentioned psora as being the first while syphilis and sycosis followed. It is now proper to deal with psora first. We shall see about its development. First of all, there must have been a state or condition of the human race, which ought to permit psora to develop. We cannot expect psoric affection to depend on a perfectly healthy race since it would not be welcome there and allowed to flourish further. The condition would be adverse. So, this is ruled out in a healthy race. Then, the question arises how psora could have developed. There must have been some sickness prior to this state, which is recognized as the chronic miasm. It could be some state of disorder, some state that it would be perfectly rational and proper for man to solve as to its cause, as to its history and as to its very nature.

Lecture - XIX 213

Earlier we have said thinking, willing and doing, are three things in life from which finally proceeds the chronic miasms. Think for a few minutes or reflect upon this. A man thinks of adultery. This thought leads him to a prostitute or a misguided woman. Even now it is not too late for he can run away from the scene - chicken out of the situation as we say. But his will says, "come on man, go ahead!" He succumbs to the adage the best way to avoid a temptation is not to resist it. Now what happens? The woman has syphilis. Our hero also gets his share of that. The scene comes to THE END! From the above it is all due to the man's act. Now it is the result of his action. This is not THE END, but the starting of his troubles.

Syphilis is due to impure coition - man going places where syphilis is and contacting with those who have it already. This is by means of an action, but that is not the case with psora. In case of psora man does not seek it, he does not go where it exists, he does not necessarily associate with those who have it.

Syphilis is due to the action of a contact, although after once ultimated may be perpetuated by accident. Recall what was said in the earlier paragraph about his thought and willing. The man thought about going to a woman. Then he willed to go to the woman. Up to here, nothing has gone amiss. He could have realized his folly even at this stage and run away from the scene. He did not do it. He favored the contact with the woman and went into action. What do we understand from this scenario?

There is always a state and condition that existed prior to the man's action. So syphilis corresponds to a man's action. Prior to that was a diseased condition. That diseased condition was thinking and willing.

Let us elaborate a little more about thinking and willing. What is the man's original way of thinking? As man grows in years, his way of thinking changes from his original condition to a corrupted way of thinking. Then, how do we get to the bottom of man's original thinking? Where do we obtain a sample of the original human being? A baby or a child is the specimen. The child's thoughts are virgin and uncorrupted. From observing the child, we understand that the man's original way of thinking was true and honest, good to the neighbor, upright and just. So, as long as the man remained in this natural condition, he remained free from susceptibility to disease, because that was the state in which he was created. Till man maintained to that state preserving his integrity, he was not susceptible to disease. There is an aura surrounding every body. This aura gets corrupted when one falls sick. So, till the man maintains the original condition he was created in, he does not exhibit an aura that could become contagious.

When man wills things due to his false thinking he stepped into a state of a corrupt interior. The external man is what he wills and his understanding. Man leads his life as he wills. So is the body of man. The life and the body of the man make one in this world. So, when there is the original state maintained the aura is undisturbed. When the man goes astray, this aura is disturbed. The disturbance of the aura is in proportion to his viciousness of his departure from virtue and justice into evils.

Natural calamities and destruction is a great tragedy. But then every cloud has a silver lining. They say that these natural calamities come to destroy, but it cleanses. Cleanses what? It cleanses the evils on the earth. It is said that prior to Noah's floods leprosy was wide spread. This was due to the frightful profanity that existed in that period. Of course, natural calamities do not carry off only the evil. Chances of some good are also wiped out. But then that is a risk taken for granted. Luckily the natural disorder of the human race is a much milder form of psora upon a different race of people.

In natural catastrophes human race is destroyed and new races appear due to the catastrophe. If the human race of Noah's flood period had survived the floods we could have been of the same

Lecture - XIX

race of people. So then leprosy could have been wide spread here now also. But then due to the disconnected human race, we today suffer from milder forms of psora. In ancient times leprosy was referred to as an internal itch.

From all the above we understand that this state of human mind and the human body is a state of susceptibility to disease. This is due to willing evils, from false thinking making the life into a continuous heredity of false things and so this disease psora. This leads us to the fact that these outward manifestation psora is prior to man.

Psora differs from syphilis or sycosis. The later two are due to or the result of the man's action. But psora is due to an influx from a state or condition. It progressed and established itself upon the earth, and we see it as manifestation outwardly of man's very nature.

Today's human race is a little better than a moral leper. That is the state of human mind today. In other words, every one is psoric. We have been seen earlier that the present human race is a victim of a much milder form of psora. A new contagion comes with every child. We also saw that psora progressed from generation to generation. *What does this mean? It means that the susceptibility to psora is also increasing from generation to generation.* If this is true for psora it must be true of every miasm and so true of every drug.

We find that when Mercury drugs a person he becomes more and more susceptible to Mercury, and is more easily poisoned by it. People poisoned by it that they couldn't go near it. Similarly persons poisoned by psora in their early stages of psora become very sensitive to it. A slight whiff of it from their schoolmates would bring on a crop of vesicles between the fingers attended with acarus.

Allopaths have a term. It is "Idiosyncrasy". They say where there is no idiosyncrasy there would be no disease. In a future lecture we would be dealing with idiosyncrasy. This word has its origin in Greek language. Idios in Greek means one's own. Syn means together and trasis mean a mixing. So, coining it together we get the word Idiosyncrasy meaning a peculiarity of temperament or constitution, any characteristic of a person? This is what we call susceptibility in homoeopathy. This is a state that is disposed to admit. So, now we know for certain what the term susceptibility in our context means.

Now we return to what we were dealing with. What is acarus? Acarus is an order of the class "Arachorida". Ticks and mites belong to this. Some people may argue that acarus is prior to the eruption. A healthy person will not be affected by acarus. Why? The miasm is simply evolved out of a state. The result of this state is acarus, which is the ultimate. It is clear that the state is prior favoring the development of the itch-bug allowing it to be active. When there is no activity, it is death. The itch-bug cannot thrive in a healthy body; they will be thrown out and not allowed to be active since a healthy condition remains.

We have seen that the penetration of the miasm increases from year to year and from generation to generation. What does this indicate? It shows that the human race becomes more and more sensitive, generation-to-generation to this internal state and the miasm keeps on ploughing deeper and deeper, internally. We had taken up syphilis for consideration. So, this syphilitic miasm is the under-lying cause that predisposes the man to syphilis. We saw syphilis was due to contact or impure coition. This damaging thinking and willing for practical purpose is psora - now it is clear then if psora was not present in him, he would not have contracted syphilis. There would have been no ground in his economy for syphilis to thrive and develop. Again we prove that psora is the cause of many miseries to the human kind.

The will and the understanding are the reasons for man's action. When there is no thinking and no willing, no action could happen.

Lecture - XIX

So willing and understanding is prior to action and this is fundamental. Man does not act until he wills. He wills what he carries out. Only a robot would do something that it did not will. It has no thinking power. It does what has been programmed. This programming and giving commands can come only from a thought and will power source, the human being.

A man wills to go to a house of ill fame. He wills to copulate with a woman there. She is affected by syphilis. Now she transmits this disease to all those who copulate with her. Now, this is due to sex. Hence now-a-days we call the veneral diseases as sexually transmitted disease or STD for short. Our hero in this story also is donated with his share of the syphilitic miasm, with pleasure. What does this correspond to? The will the act and this disease corresponds to the man. Now, we are caught in a vicious circle! See how it is so?

The man was in a good stead. He thought of the pleasure of copulation. His will tells him that loose-character women were available for the act in any house of ill fame. So, he wills to go there and his will makes him act. So that action of reaching the brothel is accomplished. Even now no damage has occurred to his healthy state. So far so good! Finally the action of taking the woman came in. That was the climax. But the anti-climax was his contracting a S.T.D. miasm. This is quoted only as an example. Contemplate on the trio, i.e. thinking, willing and acting. Does this not hold good for every action of the man? In the above case, the miasm, which succeeded psora, was only an outward representation of the action and this is the result of his thinking and willing.

Psora, we have seen is the most ancient of the diseases that torment the human race. From this vital beginning and the next state correspond to action. Thinking, willing and acting are the three things that relate to the life of human beings. Man thinks, wills and acts - it is basic. The aura that is given out from the human race at any given period corresponds to the state in which it is. The children inherit it from their parents and when they become parents their children inherit it. This process is continuous. We have seen that the internal corresponds to the external and they cannot be different from one another.

Thus we see that the internal state of the man is prior to his surroundings. So the environment is not the cause. The environment only reacts upon and reflects the internal. One that is pre-existent or prior internally is the same as that follows externally. So the internal state flows externally in the form of symptoms to the external. It affects the skin, works on the organs and upon the body of the man. The abundant accession or the influx always has the tendency to take the direction of least or no resistance, that is, in the direction of man's affections and his loves. Things flow in the direction in which he wants them to flow.

The diseases correspond to man's affection. Based on this, the diseases that torture today's human race represent his interiors. The diseases are only the outward expression. Today, man flouts all the laws of nature and causes his own misery. He hates his neighbors, violates every commandment and so forth. This is his internal state. This internal state is exhibited by the diseases he suffer from. All diseases on this earth, acute or chronic represent his interior state. Only when this is so, he can be susceptible. We repeat again that only his interior image comes out as disease.

Man has been corrupted stage by stage, from generation to generation. Today he lives a life of hypocrisy. Anger, greed, lust and ego govern today's human race. Man thinks only of himself. He has become an introvert - he does not socialize and if at all he socializes he does so to gain something for himself. Today's man lives in apartments with many floors where there are several other families. He does not know the person living next doors. That is miserable condition. His interior condition has not deteriorated to this extent overnight. Today "man eats man". The human race has

Lecture - XIX

gone to this level only in stages, deteriorating year by year. Each generation got into this state by inheriting it from its earlier generation and then added a bit more poison from its own "ingenuity" and false thinking. This is the cause for the present day terrorism. What was simple psora initially gave birth to syphilis and sycosis. This state of affair has now assumed gigantic proportion and has corrupted the mankind totally. The human race has become very susceptible to acute affections. Every small thing or every little epidemic of influenza brings the man down with an acute attack. The cause of this complication is due to what the man has driven himself into. As told earlier this has not occurred over night. It has accumulated till now and will go on till we have a history of man. If man had lived righteously free from guilt and sin, generation to generation, we would not be facing the great misery and torture today. Then man would not have been sick. Some call man as an animal. Had not these states been allowed to pollute the man, be would have been a perfect natural animal free from diseases.

Look around and see the plants, birds, etc. See how perfect they are. Man alone, in God's creation has entered a state of evil thinking and by his false willing carved for himself a niche of misery and disease. Man has lost his freedom, his internal order. He alone is undergoing changes, which the vegetable and animal kingdom of his period did not take on.

Man has not been affected by the miasms alone. The burden and torture that he experiences are complicated further by an external source. The thousand-fold complications that add to man's misery is the allopathic treatment.

As a matter of fact, every external manifestation of the miasm is the natural course for correcting the mankind. But the human race is violently damaged; diseases are being complicated because the external expressions are forcibly attempted to disappear by the administration of some violent or stimulating drug. People rarely admit they had itch in their childhood. They could have totally forgotten their early affection. When we question some one elder in the family, like the mother, uncle, etc. they confirm that as a child he had itch.

Itch is looked down as a doormat. Something that is disgraceful; so is every thing that has a similar correspondence. It is because itch by itself corresponds to adultery. Adultery is internal and the itching external. One succeeds the other. This is true with all miasms.

We have great miasms to treat. They are full in their complications. Where a true sycotic affection, gonorrhorrhoea appears as second hand, it is in its suppressed form. The suppressed form is a thousand times worse than the original form. All external manifestations have been made to disappear. This is true with psora also. The vesicular and squamous eruptions and all the outgrowths and out-cropping belong to psora. As said earlier, all the methods conceivable, however novel and effective it looks, destroys the original manifestations. Then the disease grows to gigantic levels. No one can predict its outcome. The cancerous affections, organic diseases of the heart and lungs, pthisis and the general destruction are all due to the suppression of psora. This devastating and miserable condition will prevail till Homoeopathy spreads out and it establishes upon the earth its doctrines. Then sick people could be headed under its principles and this threatening state will diminish.

Look around you. How many allopathic clinics and hospitals have sprung out? Compare their numbers to what existed in your childhood. Every year the medical colleges are turning out thousands of fresh doctors. Already there are so many allopaths. The tribe increases in thousand folds every year- thanks to the numerous medical colleges already in existence and many more that come into existence every year. What does this mean? Does it not mean that the sick people are on the increase - otherwise so

Lecture - XIX

many clinics and hospitals and the army of allopaths cannot flourish?

The allopathy system has violent drugs and there are also after effects. The allopaths are doing what they have been doing from the beginning - only now this is in a larger scale due to the greater number of allopaths being turned out.

Homeopathy can be the savior. Homoeopathy deals with the persons and not the disease. Here the disease refers to the name that has been allotted in allopathy. *Homoeopathy does not have specific medicines for any particular ailment. The medicines are for the individual's symptoms.* For the same ailment in two persons one same medicine will not prove effective even though the ailment is called by the same name. May be for the sake of conveying the suffering in a particular region in a particular organ a name is used commonly. But homoeopathy does not go by these names.

Psora has developed to be the most contagious of diseases. Our children become more susceptible to its beginnings as psora becomes more and more complicated, and its contagion adds to the disease. When psora affects the children, they become increasingly more sensitive to the other miasms, as well. The present day human race is intensely susceptible to psora, to syphilis and sycosis. Dr. Hahnemann has said, "Psora becomes, therefore, mother of man's common diseases. *It can be said that at least seven-eights of the chronic maladies existing at the present day are due to psora.*"

We have seen what is a proper cure. By the administration of appropriate remedy or remedies the cure is brought in steps. In the process the last symptom that appeared goes first, the next one, second and so forth. So in the case of psora we come to the simple form of skin eruptions as the last step since that was the beginning of psora. When this condition is reached the external body will not be nice to look, but then the interior is saved and is in a much better stead. Sometimes the vesicular eruptions may be something dreadful to look upon, hurts the vanity of the patient but this has to be tolerated and the economy is set right. Hereditary states are also involved in these manifestations. As mentioned above, internal evils flow into external manifestations with the help of homoeopathy. It is still driven further out affording the economy a comparative freedom.

Often we notice that itch does not yield to the homoeopathic treatment readily. This is because the remedy is routing the hereditary state within, causing it to flow out more exteriorly into manifestations without. Ignorance of this fact makes one lose his heart, when his remedies do not clear the eruptions immediately.

When a child is sick due to psoric manifestations and treated properly by homoeopathic methods the sickness will flow out in the form of eruptions on the skin. Now, here the process of curing is taking place. In homoeopathy, the cure is from within to outward. Finally after much tribulation this skin eruption also will disappear, carrying away with it the internal trouble as well. So we should not get dejected or disappointed if the skin eruptions are not immediately wiped out by the administration of the remedy, homoeopathically. Under such circumstances the external applications like Sulphur or Zinc ointments should not be resorted to. This is a violation of the law, capable of injuring the patient.

Dr. Hahnenmann has provided a long list of cases authoritatively with quotations and references in this connection. This list must be carefully studied. He has also elaborated it with the numerous ones he collected in the course of his investigations. These collective symptoms have presented us with a wonderful picture of psora. The observations helped him to the selection and using of Sulphur. Many remedies bear close similarity to the psoric symptoms; all-deep acting remedies have more or less something resembling psora.

More About Psora

"Disease is the totality of the effects, by which we recognize or perceive the action of a peculiar order of subversive forces upon an organism which has been exceptionally or specially adapted to, or prepared for their reception."

Hemple

The subversive force is the miasmatic affection. To know how it can progress we must have a sound knowledge of the miasms; their mysterious, but persistent, progressions, pauses rest, advancement, retrogression and attacks along unfamiliar lines and their modus operandi. Will it be possible to fight with an unseen enemy about whom we are ignorant? So, it is imperative to know every thing about the miasm.

The skin never produced an eruption upon itself except in traumatic or chemical causes. So, eruptions can occur only when there is an internal cause for it.

An eruptive disease, as a rule, causes the disappearance of the whole of the original trouble.

Suppression, by external applications or by strong internal drug, will result in the secondary manifestations of the chronic affection, soon or later.

Today psora is the parent of a multitude of functional and pathological changes that affect the human organism.

The Israelites of Christ's period led a pure life. They were comparatively free from psora. They lived a simple life, had good habits, did not over - indulge in liquor, meats or rich food. The Greeks also involved themselves in the physical culture and physical training thereby these two sectors of the human race were comparatively free from psora. In them, psora was largely confirmed to the surface of the body. This was the observation of Dr. Hahnemann.

Psora originally came as a form of itch and was highly contagious. So contagious was it that even a touch of an affected person or a handshake with him could pass it on to the other. Syphilis and sycosis are not so.

The unscientific and suppressive methods of treatment resulted in psora assuming a diversity of character and such huge proportions.

Due to suppression, where psora was complicated with either or both of the other miasms, the conditions and the situation are worsened. Under such a state psora very easily inter-twines with syphilis. Appears like "Made for each other".

Summary

1. Psora is the oldest, most universal and most pernicious chronic disease. Yet it is the most misapprehended.
2. Psora is equally serious as are syphilis and sycosis. The most robust constitution can annihilate and extinguish psora, unaidedly.
3. Psora, Syphilis and Sycosis, all the three miasms are contagious.
4. In every disease there is something prior to it. There must be 'a something', a state that permits the disease to take hold in a body.
5. Man is susceptible to all things only when he has a state corresponding to those particular disease symptoms.
6. Man is susceptible to the outward influences.
7. Chronic diseases could thrive, flourish or develop in a body wherein suitable condition exists in the body.
8. Thinking, willing and acting are the three fundamentals in a living body. The chronic diseases start from here.

Lecture - XIX

9. Psora corresponds to false thinking, guilt and wrong acting. From this stems out the venereal diseases Syphilis and Sycosis.
10. In the case of psora, the man does not seek and go after it. Neither does he have to come into contact with the persons who have it. Here we are speaking of virgin psora, without any complications.
11. Man's original state is purity in thought, will and act. Unfortunately this state has been very corrupted in today's human race. This deterioration has been slow, but steady, step-by-step, over the years, from generation to generation.
12. In his original state he could not have contracted any disease of miasmatic origin. But in today's corrupted state, he has become the victim of numerous simple and complicated diseases.
13. The body and the mind constitute a single unit. They are not different from each other.
14. In today's human race every one is sick in one form or the other.
15. The itch-bug cannot thrive and develop in a healthy body.
16. The internal man is prior to his surroundings. That which is prior internally is the same that follows externally. It cannot be otherwise.
17. The abundant influx always takes the path of least resistance. The man's affections and loves are the paths of least resistance.
18. Man's misery is due to his own thinking.
19. Every manifestation of the miasm is the natural course for correcting the mankind.
20. External manifestations are the result corresponding internal state. Unfortunately the external manifestations are forcibly

made to disappear by the external application or some violent drug. The external manifestations disappear by going inward, deeper and deeper.

21. Adultery is internal and the itch is external. One succeeds the other.

22. The cancerous affections, organic disease of the heart and lungs, pthisis and general destruction are all due to the suppression of psora.

23. Psora is the mother of man's common diseases.

24. Seven eighths of the man's chronic maladies today are due to psora.

25. In proper path of the cure, the last manifestation disappears first; the other manifestations go in succession in the reverse order.

26. Psora's affection in children makes them become more and more complicated and its contagion adds to the disease. The children become increasingly sensitive to other miasms.

27. Heredity psora also creates complications.

28. Itch may not readily disappear by the medications. In homoeopathy, we have to wait since the appearance of the external manifestations indicates our proper course of treatment. This is due to the Heredity State within that prevents the immediate cure of the skin eruptions.

29. Homoeopathy cure is always from within outward.

30. The external applications of ointment or an internal strong drug will cause the disappearance of the skin manifestation. But this will drive the manifestation deep inside and cause a great havoc and damage to the internal organs.

31. The deep-acting homoeopathic remedies have something resembling psora in them.

Lecture - XIX

Aphorisms & Precepts

1. You cannot divorce Medicine and Theology. Man exists all the way down from his innermost Spiritual, to his outermost Natural.
2. The external man is but an outward expression of the internal; so the results of disease (symptoms) are but the outward expression of the internal sickness.
3. Everything is harmoniously working in the well man. Consider the man healing the sick.
4. If there were no Idiosyncracy there would be no homoeopathy. Every individual is susceptible to certain things, susceptible to sickness and equally susceptible to cure.
5. Cure rests in the degree of susceptibility.
6. Principle teaches you to avoid suppression. A homoeopath cannot temporize. These sufferings are necessary sometimes to show forth sickness in order that a remedy may be found.
7. When the dose is too large to cure, the man receives it as a sickness.
8. Evils must take place, and changes, which are the ultimate of his internal thought, will take place in the body.
9. One sick man is to be treated not the disease.
10. Thus a man is what he wills. As his love is, so is his life. When man thinks about the neighbor, he wills one of the two things - he wills good to his neighbor or the opposite.
11. Everything that is a thing has its aura or atmosphere. So as a race or class, the entire human race has its atmosphere or aura also. Each individual has his aura or atmosphere.
12. This aura becomes intensified with the growth of evil in the interior of man.

13. The human race exists as a changed *esse*.
14. If you do not know sickness you are apt to think all things strange and unique.
15. Sharp prescribing is attended with immediate results. If you do sharp work you will see frequent aggravations of the remedy. When you do poor work you never see them.
16. The physician spoils his case when he prescribes for the local symptoms and neglects the patient.
17. What is man? Is he a body? If so, we are justified in thinking of his parts, his liver and lungs and skin, and extremities, and his body as a whole. But we are to consider man as from the life to the body.
18. Susceptibility is prior to all contagion. If an individual is not susceptible to Smallpox he cannot take it, and will not receive it though he goes near the worst cases, or eats a Smallpox crust.

Lecture - XX

Chronic Diseases - Syphilis

Under homoeopathic treatment there are some generals related to syphilis. We shall see what the dictionaries define as syphilis:

(1) Twentieth-century Chambers Dictionary: Syphilis — A hereditary or markedly infective disease, propagated by direct contagion or by the transmission of the virus through some vessel or medium, which has recently been contaminated — most commonly caused by impure sexual intercourse.

(2) Stedman's Pocket Medical Dictionary: An acute and chronic infectious venereal disease caused by Treponema pallidum (spirochaeta pallida) and transmitted by direct contact though sexual intercourse.

(3) Gould's pocket Pronouncing Medical Dictionary: A chronic, infectious, venereal disease, which may also be hereditary, inducing contagious and other lessions; it is due to Treponema pallidum.

From the above we understand that syphilis is a sexually transmitted disease. It is disease caused by Treponema pallidum. Syphilis is an eruptive disease, basically. There are different syphilitic eruptions in all their manifestations as to the time and color. The prodromal period is usually twelve to fifteen days. Sometimes it could be even fifty to sixty days. The reason for this delay could be some acute miasm or bad cold which prevents the syphilitic manifestation and prolong the prodromal period. It could also be due to a drug disturbing the economy. Without any interruption, the prodromal period is usually twelve to fifteen days. The prodromal period increases with the contagion of the various stages. This is not elaborated in any books, but can be observed and verified in homoeopathic practice. The books give the primary contagion as the only contagion in connection with the syphilitic miasm.

Let us assume that the syphilitic miasm is disease that will run for a definite time. A patient with syphilitic disease approaches the physician. He has gone through with the primary manifestation. The physician tells him he can safely marry. His wife becomes an invalid. She does not experience the primary manifestation of the lesion and roseola. The wife gets the syphiloderma or a syphilitic skin disease, with symptoms belonging to the later stage of the disease. Where or how was this infection contracted? Naturally, she got it from her husband who was treated for the syphilitic primary manifestation. *The wife took up the infection from the husband at a level in which it was operating on the husband. From here on it progresses.*

The above situation is equally true for psora and sycosis. Similar things do not happen in the acute miasm. All the three miasms have contagion in the form in which they exist at that time. The state that is transferred in the advanced state of psora to the patient's wife is the level of psora he has at that time. The wife takes it up at that level and the psoric miasm progresses in her also from thence on. To this condition is added her own and it progresses in full swing with the peculiarities.

There is law of protection by dissimilar about which we have seen earlier. That law enters the scene at this stage and shields the wife's system from taking up a new infection; be it psora, syphilis

Lecture - XX

or sycosis. The disorders that are already present in her economy may be so wholly dissimilar which keeps her safe and sound, and away from the contagion.

From the above we understand that a woman might copulate with a man affected by sycosis in the form of gleet. But she would have been protected by her own system and not be affected by sycosis. Similarly in case of man who had a chancre might have copulated with her and she may not be infected by it. She may be his wife and even have a child by him. That child would get the syphilitic miasm and be born black while the mother does not have it. The reason is that the mother is the land and the father's sperm the seed. *The seed possessed the syphilitic contents from the father. The mother has only provided the groundwork.*

The above has been demonstrated time and again. Several children have been born black with syphilis, but the mother had no indication of the syphilitic infection. The primary stage of syphilis condition cannot be disguised. In its secondary or tertiary stages the progress is insidious and hence there is no way of detecting it immediately. Where the husband has the primary sore, the primary stage will manifest in the wife, whereas if he passes on the infection in a tertiary stage, wherein all the manifestations were suppressed on passed by we cannot know whether the wife has taken up the disease or not. This leads us back to the principle we learnt earlier. Two dissimilar diseases repel one another. So, where the wife has some chronic disease and her economy disturbed, say from a phthisical condition, the lady remains protected. *A disease overwhelms the body already and that condition protects her.* Remember the law "dissimilar always repel each other and similar cure each other." Where there is psoric manifestation is of a milder variety and can be substituted by the contagion a syphilitic condition sets in. It is necessary to know the action of disease upon each other. There we can see the principles of cure in how one disease affects another.

Anti syphilitic homoeopathic remedies give a lot of details about syphilitic miasm. When the prodromal period ends chancre appears as the external manifestation. About six weeks later we can expect the roseola and other eruptions. Succeeding these, throat ulcers and falling of the hair occurs. These are all associated and succeed each other rapidly. These are the most common external manifestations of the earlier period of the secondary stage of syphilis. Weak persons affected with this stage are affected feebly. Where the constitution is robust and vigorous the manifestations are also vigorous. In other words the manifestations are in proportion to the stage of the constitution.

Here we should understand one thing. It does not matter whether the constitution is weak or robust and how feeble or how strong the manifestation happens to be. The main point to be considered is the miasm is internally active. This is a very dangerous proposition. The internally active maism tends to attack the important organs like the brain, the kidneys, the spleen, the heart, the lungs, the tissues and bones. After all, these are the interiors of man.

As the syphilitic miasm commences to overwhelm the interior tissues, the periosteum, the bone and the brain are the main targets. Psora attacks more frequently the blood vessels and the liver and this causes deposits beneath the skin forming suppurations and boils. The syphilitic boil is not a true boil. It is a multiple tubercular mass most vicious in character.

If we carefully back track the progress of the syphilis miasms we will be able to go back to it's beginning, presuming they had been suppressed. We know that homoeopathy in the earlier stage of the disease attacks the root of the evil. Thereby it becomes latent bringing things into order. A painful chancre becomes painless and continues as a mild and harmless sore. The bubo will be hastened to suppurate. Mucus patches will be checked. Sore throat will be greatly relieved. The patient becomes more and

Lecture - XX

more comfortable. In this earlier stage the backward stage in the form of ulcers, etc. is not seen. The homoeopathic remedy quickens and subdues the manifestations and takes a deep and permanent hold of the affected economy and then the manifestations gradually subside. This is one good reason for us to wait for the remedial action to take place.

So far we have seen the action of the homoeopathic remedies upon the earlier manifestations. When we see or examine the very latest manifestations, we can observe the opposite state. We shall now see a case of ten or fifteen years standing. The patient might have undergone all sorts of vicious treatment. The patient experiences awful bi-perietal head pains, becoming weaker in mind, getting the tertiary manifestations in general, the tendency to gummatious formations and deep seated ulcerations and breaking down in his health. How is he to be brought back to good health or how can his economy be restored? The solution here can only be had in a constitutional remedy. This constitutional remedy will bring out the external manifestation somewhere upon his body. The primary sore may not appear immediately. It may not appear at all. But the constitutional remedy will bring back an ulcerated sore throat resulting in the destruction of the soft tissues in view, including the soft palate. When this ulceration appears the pain in the bones, which threatened to become necrosed, will stop. The periostitis will subside. Iritis is likely to become a troublesome symptom and may come with secondary symptoms or appear several years later mingled with tertiary symptoms. The appropriate homoeopathic remedy will promptly relieve this last appeared symptom. The patient may complain that he had not had this throat trouble for a long time. On examination the physician can observe a membrane sacrificed by the administration of Nitric acid and other caustics. The membrane will be indurated, hard, gristly like tissues that are infiltered with gummatous deposits. Now that patient will have to undergo much trouble. Under appropriate homoeopathic treatment the suppressed manifestations will come back. These will come back by the appropriate treatment only.

Summary

1. Syphilis is a sexually transmitted disease.
2. Basically syphilis is an eruptive disease. Its prodromal period is twelve to fifteen days, normally. But when an acute miasm is active in the body it takes anywhere upto sixty days. This could also be due to a drug disturbing the body's economy.
3. When the patient is treated for the primary stage still it is not safe. He can transmit the disease to his wife. She will take up the disease in the same platform in which her husband is at that time. It will progress from there.
4. The law of protection of dissimilar protects the wife's system. This is true of syphilis, sycosis and psora.
5. But a child born of wedlock in the above case will be affected by syphilitic miasm, even though there is no trace of infection in the woman. This is because the father's sperm is infected.
6. Primary stage of syphilitic condition cannot be disguised. But the secondary or the tertiary stages will progress insidiously.
7. Dissimilar diseases repel each other. Similar diseases cure each other.
8. The most common manifestations of the secondary stage of Syphilis are throat disorders, hair loss in that order, in the earlier stages.
9. These manifestations are weak in weaker constitution and strong in a robust and vigorous constitution.
10. Whether weak or strong, the miasm is active internally. The miasm has a tendency to attack the more important organs like the brain, the kidneys, the spleen, the heart, the tissue and bones.
11. The main targets for a syphilitic attack of the internal organs

Lecture - XX

are the periosteum and the brain. Psora's main targets are the liver and blood vessels, and due to it deposits under the skin forming suppuration and boils. The syphilitic boil cannot be called a true boil.

12. With the help of homoeopathy if we carefully study the pattern of the disease backing out or the backward process, we can lay hands on the beginning. When we have reached that condition, the ulcer becomes painless and is mild, harmless sore. The bubo will also suppurate. Mucous patches will be relieved and throat problems much milder. Periostitis becomes milder. Totally the patient becomes relieved.
13. Wait and see the action of the remedy, is a good policy.
14. To treat a case of long standing the one and only solution is to give the constitutional remedy that matches the patient's constitution. This will bring out the external manifestation. Sometimes the secondary stage and tertiary state can manifest together. An appropriate homoeopathic remedy will relieve the last appeared symptom first. By suitable further remedies in succession we can relieve the patient further.

More Information on Syphilis

1. We shall see here how syphilis develops.
2. It appears in the form of a small pustule. Then it changes into an impure ulcer with raised borders and stinging pains. If this is not cured it remains in the same place during the man's lifetime. In the years it is active internally.
3. The infection started at the moment of contact and only when the internal malady developed further in a period of twelve to fifteen days does the external manifestation, the

chancre, is thrown out. So the whole living body received the miasma's presence. Any amount of cleaning, wiping off or washing, even immediately after the coition will not help. The damage is already done.

4. The best anti-syphilitic remedy is pure semi-oxide of Mercury.

5. Syphilic chancre, when not complicated with psora can be cured easily.

6. When syphilis is complicated with psora it reaches the tertiary state. The latent psora is awakened violently. This is sometimes referred to as masked or spurious syphilis.

7. The rude awakening of psora affects the patient by undermining the general health and breaks out as a chronic suffering.

Lecture - XXI

Chronic Diseases - Sycosis

There are two types of gonorrhoea. One is the chronic gonorrhoea, which has no disposition to recovery. It continues indefinitely. It involves the whole constitution in varying forms of symptoms. The other type of gonorrhoea is the acute one. The acute gonorrhoea can be cured in a few weeks or months. Both the forms are contagious.

We shall now see how the dictionaries define gonorrhoea.

(1) Chamber's Dictionary: A specific contagious inflammatory discharge from the urethra or vagina.

(2) Steadman's Pocket Medical Dictionary: A contagious catarrhal inflammation of the genital mucous membrane transmitted chiefly by coitus and due to Neisseria gonorrhoea. May involve the lower or upper genital tract especially the uterine tubes or spread the peritonium and other structures by the blood stream.

(3) Gould's Pocket Pronouncing Medical Dictionary: A contagious inflammation with a purulent discharge from the genitals.

The term is of Greek origin, "gone" meaning seed and "rhoia" meaning a flow. The muco purulent discharge is known as gleet.

There are simple forms of inflammations of the urethra accompanied by discharges and they are not contagious. We have simple inflammations of the urethra and also specific inflammations of the urethra. Of the specific variety, we have chronic and acute. The majority of the cases in this group of acute conditions have the regular three periods - namely prodromal, progressive and the period of decline. The books deal with gonorrhoea only on its beginning state - the discharge.

The acute can be really referred to as gonorrhoea, since of this there is only discharge. In acute condition, if a suppressive treatment is resorted to, the system throws off the after-effect in most cases. The suppression cannot bring on the constitutional symptoms called sycosis. Fig warts or the constitutional states such as anaemia cannot follow it. This is in the case of acute conditions. In the case of suppression of chronic miasm, these will follow, and become very serious. Most of the cases, which come to the physician, have been suppressed. These cases are very much more grievous compared to their primary state.

The prodromal period for acute and chronic state is same for both - from eight to twelve days. There is discharge in both and there is no essential difference between the discharges. The chronic condition discharge is a muco-purulent discharge. It may have all the appearances of any acute discharge taken up by the urethra. The constitutional sycotic gonorrhoea can be cured and the health restored by any simple anti-sycotic remedy, which conforms to the nature of the discharge. There will not be any necessity in earlier stage. But, after the disease has progressed for a few weeks a distinction has to be made. In that stage, an appropriate remedy, which conformed to the more acute symptoms matching a fully developed sycotic condition, would be required. The process of selecting the appropriate remedy for sycosis is the same as that for any other miasmatic disease, viz., tracing the past history of disease i.e., by making an anamnesis.

Lecture - XXI

An anamnesis of all the sycotic cases will provide us the pathway to the constitutional state of sycosis. This is exactly how Dr. Hahnemann ascertained the nature of psora. He selected the similar remedies for psora by ascertaining its nature and action. *We call medicines as anti-sycotic, which not only conform to the nature and action of sycotic, but also those remedies which are able to reproduce the earlier sycotic manifestations. The discharge will reappear when the remedy confirms to sycotic nature and action; it tends to drive the disease backwards.* Remedies, which conform only to a particular portion of the disease cannot establish return of the earlier symptoms. This is because that remedy is not fully similar enough to the disease conditions and hence cannot act deep enough. Such remedies cannot be considered as truly anti-sycotic ones.

At this juncture it is not necessary to describe the acute form of gonorrhoea. We shall concentrate on sycosis as a chronic miasm, the beginning being a urethral discharge. We have already said that the pure and simple sycosis case is not found often as the number of cases of acute gonorrhoea. This disease appears to be on the increase.

We see a good many cases among the women and children. Gonorrheal cases that are suppressed by injections are considered cured by the old school. The doctor advises wedlock. The complete cure has not been effected - it has only been suppressed. The patient better delays his marriage. The proper condition is that the discharge has to be brought back by appropriate homeopathic treatment. Injection only suppresses. Treatment must be afforded properly by an anti-psoric remedy, homoeopathically. Only after that the patient may be counseled to marry a healthy woman, and bring forth into this world healthy children.

It is common for a wife to breakdown in a year or about in eighteen months to come with ovarian diseases or abdominal troubles complicated with all sorts troubles peculiar to females. Here it is imperative to trace out this history of the husband's affliction. You will discover that he had two or three attacks of gonorrhoea that were treated with silver nitrate, by injections, which stopped these discharges. It will also be seen that young man was never healthy after the disappearance of the gonorrheal discharge. *This suppression in the man followed the contagion in the woman.* This type of study surely is interesting.

Sometimes the severity is great, and the trouble comes very soon after the suppression. The young husband himself will realize that this present sufferings are due to the suppression of that discharge. Sometimes they are latent and their progress is gradual. The blood is affected, gradually the increasing anemia sets in, the patient becomes pallid and waxy.

Earlier we said that the disease is transmitted to another person by the infected person. The level of the infection that is transmitted to the other person corresponds to the donor's level. Can we call him a donor here? This is true for all the miasmatic affections. Here the recipient's peculiarities also join hands with the contagion.

We saw that the discharge was stopped by medication. Yes, the discharge had stopped for certain, but was that a complete cure? We will presently see. This young husband was also advised that he could marry. But his wife who has been healthy till the marriage suddenly becomes ill after the marriage. The nature of disease that the young man had gone through was a sexually transmitted disease. In this case a discharge. When this was apparently stopped, suppression has taken place. So the disease was not completely cured and the wife took up the contagion obviously. Hence she became another victim. This can only be seen and understood by a homoeopath.

Now, we will take up a man who had the sycotic trouble for ten to fifteen years. You find him waxy, body full of verucae. His lips are pale, ears almost transparent; he is declining in his health

Lecture - XXI

and various kinds of manifestations are observed. We are able to collect several symptoms in this case. Now the homoeopath has to do his homework. He should study and carefully consider the case. If his perception corresponds to some long acting, deep acting remedy and he administers it then the patient is bound to progress in health and improve. The homoeopath must remember that the disease gets well in the reverse order of its progress.

Let us assume that the troubles have manifested itself in other mucous membranes of the body, the waxiness, the pallidness disappear. This is because the conditions become busy in other regions. The catarrhal manifestations may be the catarrhal conditions of the eyes, but generally it is the catarrh of the nose. It is common for the nasal catarrh to be sycotic. Further it appears when gonorrhoea is suppressed, the catarrh settles in the nose and posterior nares with thick copious discharge. With local treatment it does not get suppressed. In a vigorous enough constitution the discharge will be maintained in spite of administration of different specifics. In feeble constitution the diseases are driven to the center and the outermost of man left unaffected. *Calcarea* is an antisycotic remedy, deep in its action. When this is administered in a patient who has yellowish green nasal discharge, his old discharge will reappear. The young man would not possibly have contracted this because he was chaste now. In his earlier life he must have had gonorrhoea, the nature of which was sycotic. Unless it possessed a specific nature and character the human economy would not have been affected, resulting in the affection of the nose in its own way. *Here the nasal discharge has been transferred from its nasal location to a new site bringing in the original discharge back.* The first and the original manifestation have appeared. An appropriate remedy can achieve this, homoeopathically. This must be explained to the patient. He must also be informed that he will get well soon, getting rid of the catarrh. He must also be warned that he must not tamper or meddle with the penis discharge. That will make him irrecoverable. This observation has been repeatedly experienced and there is no doubt about this.

Gonorrhoea manifests itself on the surface in its earlier stage. Hence, soon after suppression, the catarrh emerges in vigorous constitutions. It gets located in the nose. Where the catarrh does not appear soon, the constitution is feeble and hence represents the disease in the deeper tissues. In these cases this disease will represent itself on deeper tissues. Bright's disease, breaking down of the lungs, liver and rheumatic disease of worst forms may appear and finally kill the patient. It becomes catarrhal only in the earlier stages. The young man whose wife was infected may feel that he has escaped the outward manifestations of the disease due to his feeble constitution. But see what happens. He may think he is cured. As we said earlier, in feeble cases where it is not thrown out as catarrh the disease is represented on deeper tissues. What does this mean? The disease goes on to an advanced stage and attacks the blood. The man becomes anaemic.

Let us look at a case where the man is a bachelor. In the above apparently cured condition he marries. The wife does not roll in to the catarrhal state. The contagion is contracted in the bladder trouble, but she gets the anaemia stage. Some may call this a secondary state, but it really a more interior form of the disease. From the anaemia condition it spreads into all the functions of the body.

Let us see why the woman did not come into a catarrhal state. If you recall our earlier statements, it can be obvious. The writing will be on the wall! The husband skipped the catarrhal condition due to his feeble constitution. The disease appeared to be cured - but it was represented in deeper tissues. The principle behind the woman not getting into that state was 'she got the contagion in the same level of that of the man, when she contracted the disease'.

At this level, since she had circumvented the catarrhal stage, what are the sufferings we could expect? She gets the fibrinous state, inflammation of the uterus and soft tissues or low-grade changes in the kidneys. The constitutional diseases peculiar to the female community of today may also be present. *Coming to think of it, it s a bit strange that only the soft tissues are affected and the bones are left out. Syphilis targets the soft tissues and bones. Psora affects the whole economy, leaving nothing to escape causing a general breakdown.*

In a man sometime the catarrhal stage is not seen, instead inflammation of the testes or inflammation of the rectum may be there. Where a man has used strong injections for the purpose of suppression of the gonorrheal discharge you will find him writhing in pain. He will be twisting and tossing with pain. Only continual motion will give him relief. The pains experienced by him will be tremendous, tearing from head to foot. If he can get up from the bed he will keep on walking day and night. This is rheumatism without swelling; it appears to be along sheath of the nerves. It could be relieved only by motion.

The first remedy that may strike you in this case will be *Rhus* - since pain relieved by motion is its characteristic. In the above case *Rhus* will be of least or no value at all. This is because *Rhus* is not an anti-sycotic remedy. *Rhus* will not relieve his distress and anxiety. The pains will only continue and attack him violently, his tendons will begin contracting, they will shorten and calf muscles will become sore. The thigh muscles will become so sore that they cannot be touched or handled. In some cases, the infiltration of the muscles and their hardness will create a severe soreness, which will extend to the bottom of the feet making it impossible for the patient to walk. He is forced to sit in his bed or lie in his bed or crawl on his kness and hands. These cases are violent ones. These cases will go on for years. In apllopathy they may suggest to apply some oil, this could be used for years but there will be no use.

A homoeopathically selected appropriate remedy will bring back the patient to health. *The remedy must cover the whole nature of sycosis and the remedy must be an antipsoric one.*

This will relieve the soreness of the foot and in turn the discharge will appear. Whenever the old symptoms return, the patient is on the recovery path and the physician has taken the proper path to deal with the disease. When the discharge appears the above said horrible symptoms are relieved. *Under sycosis, only when the discharge does appear we are heading towards the cure.*

Now we will take up the case of a woman - we are aware of the fact that the woman took up the contagion at the same level as her husband was in that particular time of infection. Let us assume she has the fibrinous inflammation, very worst condition of anaemia and the skin patchy, sallow and waxy, and the withering and organic condition. A carefully selected homoeopathic remedy that is truly anti-sycotic and administered to her will help her. But in this case we need not look for the discharge. Here the condition of her husband at the time of infection plays its part. Even without the reappearance of the discharge she will get alright. Here in her case, the reverse order of reappearance of the symptom is only the reverse order of those she had. She may not have had the primary, but all that her husband had will be seen in her case too - stage-by-stage and symptom-by-symptom.

The innocent woman is the grievous sufferer. You see a woman in anemic condition with rheumatic state and an anemic condition of the blood. It takes hold of the blood first and conforms to the subjects who have advanced in deep-seated troubles subject to epithalamia. Such subjects are especially victims of Bright's disease and to acute phthisis. If they had pneumonia, it is likely to end in a breakdown of some sort in the lungs. In cases where any acute disease, prolonged in nature like typhoid, etc. always the recovery will be slow.

It is always a good proposition to know the history of the patient and his peculiarities of the life. *It is very important to find out whether the patient is syphilitic or sycotic. We are aware that everyone is psoric.* Persons who have lived a healthy

Lecture - XXI

and proper life escape the two contagious diseases, which the man acquires by his own seeking. When a lingering disease like typhoid etc. has ended we can understand that the patient is psoric but when the physician is aware that the patient is also syphilitic or sycotic, the patient's recovery can be hastened, see how a closer knowledge of the patient helps! When this knowledge about the patient is not got, things will be puzzling to the physician.

A sycotic patient, at the end of a typhoid fever will slide into a state of do nothing and decline; convalescence will not be established; she will lie with an aversion of food; she does not react, she does not repair; there is no tissue making; no assimilation; there is no vitality; she lies in a sort of semi-quiescent state; she is sinking in her health day by day. The physician should suspect this disease, as the culprit. He should not allow this to go without a suitable investigation. He must call her husband and must find out whether the husband had experienced any of the specific diseases in his younger days. He should do it in utter confidence. If you were the family physician this must be done.

The husband will confess he had these troubles earlier. His earlier doctor had said that he was cured and he could marry, no trouble would ensue. In all innocence he entered wedlock. His previous doctor also confirmed the wife will not be affected. This drove the young man into marriage. Under this situation the homoeopath should also watch the children born to them. *They will be few since sycosis makes a woman sterile.* If she has more children there will be a strong tendency towards marasmus in the first year or a strong tendency to consumption in the first or second year or they will appear withering and old in appearance of face. Anyone of these three miasms will pre-dispose the children to this state. But if you find the children anemic and waxy, and is accustomed to lienteric stools, having no digestion, when every hot spell bring on complaints that appear like cholera infantum, *it does not grow, does not thrive it has to be suspected as a sycotic case.* In all these ailments sycosis is the most frequent cause.

This disease manifests itself in the form of warty growths. It does not manifest itself by eruption similar to syphilis and psora. *If the physician knows that the patient is sycotic, the patient must be administered an anti-sycotic remedy.* Then he will rally. *In case he is a syphilitic patient, he should be given an appropriate anti-syphilitic remedy. Where neither of the above miasmatic conditions is present an anti-psoric remedy that corresponds to his condition and state will cause him to rally.* The nature of these three miasmatic conditions must be constantly kept in view. It must also be remembered that these chronic miasms are present in the economy and often after an acute illness, will have to be fought. If the physician is ignorant of this, the patient will gradually sink and die for apparent want of vitality to convalesce.

In case of a sycotic infant a truly suitable anti-sycotic remedy will bring back the same stage, which the infant began with. Hence the discharge will not come to the infant. Such affected infants, in their grown-up stage will be sensitive to sycosis. They are already prepared to receive the sycotic gonorrhoea whenever the first exposure occurs. Here the parents lay the susceptibility to psora and the parents also lay the susceptibility to syphilis.

Man can have only one attack in his natural lifetime, of any of the three chronic miasms. *Neither psora nor syphilis nor sycosis attacks a person more once.* When a person is asked how many times he has had gonorrheal discharge many say about half a dozen times. Out of these, only one must have been sycotic. The sycotic constitution cannot be taken a second time. One attack gives immunity to that person forever. The offspring becomes more susceptible to all the miasms the more they become developed in the human race. The more they become complicated with each other the susceptibility to acute and epidemic diseases in the human race also increases. This goes to show how the human race increase in susceptibility to the chronic miasms from generation to generation.

Summary

1. There are two types of gonorrhoea, the acute and the chronic. Acute can be cured in a few weeks. The chronic progresses involving the entire constitution and there is no recovery. Both varieties are contagious.
2. Gonorrhoea is a contagious inflammation with a purulent discharge from the genitals.
3. We have simple and specific forms of inflammations of the urethra. Specific forms can be broken down as acute and specific varieties.
4. In the acute there is only discharge. Suppression of this discharge cannot bring the constitutional symptom called sycosis.
5. If the chronic miasmatic discharge is suppressed the constitutional symptoms fig warts, anemia etc., can follow.
6. There is no need to make any distinction of the earlier discharge. But after the progress of the disease for a few weeks the distinction is necessary.
7. Any remedy conforming to the nature of the discharge can cure it in the very early stages. In a progressed stage, which is a few weeks old, anti-sycotic remedy will be needed.
8. Analyzing the history will lead us to the beginning of the sycosis and its progress.
9. The anti-sycotic remedy properly chosen will enable the discharge re-appear. This remedy drives the disease backwards. Remedies that may conform to only particular

portions cannot establish the return of the earlier symptoms. Such remedies are not truly anti-sycotic.

10. The old school suppresses the discharge and calls it a cure. Only when treated homoeopathically by appropriate medicines a complete internal cure can result.

11. When a woman comes in for treatment of this miasm, the physician should not stop his investigations with her. He should call in the husband and go into his history as well.

12. The wife receives the disease at the same level as her husband has it at the time of infection.

13. When a woman who was perfectly healthy before marriage gets sick after marriage having sycotic symptoms, the husband must also be investigated.

14. When a man has carried on with the disease for ten or fifteen years he will have warts and his skin waxy, lips pale, ears almost transparent, his health declining. Where the troubles have manifested in other mucous membranes of the body he will not be pallid or his skin waxy.

15. In feeble constitutions, the disease is able to penetrate deeper and progresses towards the center and the man's outermost is left out.

16. When the discharge does reappear, it should not be trampled with. If meddled the patient may become irrecoverable.

17. In feeble constitutions after medication, if the catarrh does not appear soon it affects the deeper tissues. Bright's disease, breaking down of the lungs, liver, worst forms of rheumatic disease may result in the death of the patient. In the advanced stages, the disease may attack the blood and the patient becomes anemic. From the anemic condition it spreads into all the functions of the body.

18. The constitutional diseases peculiar to the female community is also roped in along with the attack on the soft tissues.

19. Strange it may seem the bones are not attacked. Syphilis attacks the soft tissues and bones. Psora affects the whole economy, causing a break down.
20. Where a man has used strong injections to suppress the discharge he will writhe and twist in pain. It is because the nerval sheaths are involved. The rheumatic non-swelling pain is relieved by constant motion. Hence he writhes and twists or even keeps walking day and night. His tendons will contract violently and become sore. He cannot walk. He will crawl on all the four.
21. A proper homoeopathic remedy will correct or relieve the patient from the above sufferings and will bring back the discharge. He will be in his path to recovery.
22. When a woman is treated the proper homoeopathic remedy will drive out the disease in the reverse order of what all she had to the condition in which she received the infection. So here we may not see the discharge condition or the catarrhal condition.
23. In a sycotic patient who is also attacked by an acute disease like typhoid, etc., the recovery is slow.
24. In all these causes the physician must find out whether the patient is psoric or syphilitic. Sycosis and syphilis are the two chronic miasms affecting the human race by their own seeking.
25. A sycotic patient may become sterile. Where she has one or two children they will be affected by marasmus in the first year, a strong tendency towards consumption in the first or second year. They will appear withered and old in face. Any one of the three miasmas will predispose the children to this condition.
26. The nature of the three miasmatic diseases must be well understood and known.

27. Children take up the disease as a hereditary disease due to their susceptibility. The parents lay this.
28. The miasmatic condition can attack the man but once, in his life-time.
29. The children become more susceptible to all the miasms the more they become developed in the human race. The human race becomes more and more susceptible to acute and epidemic diseases, from generation to generation.

How Sycosis Develops

1. Sycosis is a sexually transmitted disease caused by impure coition. On infection, it overwhelms the human organism first. After developing completely, internally, it manifests itself externally in the form of excrescence.
2. The incubation period is normally twelve to fifteen days. Sometimes the external appearance may take several weeks. They are dry and soft, similar to warts. There is also a fetid discharge. They bleed easily, look more like cauliflower or coxcomb. In males they appear on the glans or under the prepuce. In females it appears around the genital organs. The pudenda are swollen.
3. Dr. J.C. Brunett made a study of sycosis and observed vaccination is another carrier for sycosis. He gave it the name vaccinosis.
4. Secondary and tertiary stages result from suppression. The various methods of suppression may look like cures. But, in fact, by this way the disease is driven deeper and deeper.
5. In the first stage mild form of cystic condition is present. When local treatment is sought the result is abscesses about the neck of the bladder or urethra.

6. Gonorrheal orchitis may also occur due to local medication.
7. When complicated with tubercular diathesis gonorrhea is slow and difficult to eradicate.
8. Due to the tubercular diathesis, we cannot predict the complications that may occur or the intensity to which the tubercular element may be stirred.
9. For a complete cure the discharge must be re-established and cured scientifically.
10. The suppression will bring in the secondary and tertiary symptoms. It may not result immediately. It may take years. One can never tell how and what form the disease can break out.
11. About 94% of rheumatism has its origin in sycosis, prevalent in both the sexes.
12. If the sycosis at the primary stage is homoeopathically treated and cured properly there can be no secondary or tertiary state. These are the results of poor management of sycosis at the primary stage.
13. When the infection is passed on, in its first stage, the receiver also gets the primary state. If the disease is passed on in its second stage, there will be no primary stage seen in the receiver.
14. Anaemia occurs in the secondary and tertiary stages. Every cell and fibre is affected. This gradually progresses steadily and the entire organism is victimized profoundly.
15. The secondary state of sycosis has no period of commencement. Sometimes it is silent for even two years.
16. Almost all the secondary stages are inflammatory in some form or other.
17. An offensive odor itself is an indication of sycosis. The odor

is pungent musty or like that of a dead fish. Any amount of cleaning or washing will not eliminate the offensive odor.

18. His perspiration is extremely frank, more prominent in the axila, thighs and external genitals.
19. Sycosis scrubs and washes their body forever.
20. In males, cases of orchitis, epdymites, cystic troubles, sycotic arthritis, sub-acute rheumatism and gout can be seen. Females suffer more from the pelvic affections.
21. Warts are common in sycosis. Condylomata are a combination of syphilis and sycosis.
22. In the latent symptoms, a sycotic can very well remember the past events, but he cannot recall recent happenings. (In primary stage)
23. A sycotic is always very suspicious; most cunning and deceitful person; worst form of maniacs - A 'weather-cock'.
24. In the tertiary stage malignancy follows skin lesions. The internal organs like uterus, kidney, liver or heart get affected.
25. Similar to syphilis, the tertiary sycosis stage is very difficult to cure, as it binds itself with the life force. When complicated with psora also, it is very difficult to separate it.
26. Red mole, spider spot, etc. are sycotic tertiary stage result.
27. The sycotic malignancy develops at any age; in syphilis and psora it appears at about forty years of age.

Lecture - XXII

Disease and Drug Study in General

Our study should enable us to bring to our minds the picture of the diseases that torture the human race, as fully as possible. We cannot achieve this to any great extent from the Old School books. They do not treat psora, syphilis and sycosis in such a way as to bring the image of the diseases to our minds. The acute miasms are brought to our minds only in a limited way. The diagnostic or pathognomonic symptoms are brought out only with an aim of distinguishing one disease from the other. There is nothing to bring the image of the disease before the mind.

It is very important to go over the bulk of psoric symptoms given by Dr. Hahnemann. This will enable us to obtain an average as perfect as possible of psora. Take his "Chronic Diseases". Write opposite each symptom of psora all the remedies found from the proving to correspond to those symptoms. Now we have before our mind a list of the anti-psoric remedies. Now we know the disease symptoms and their corresponding remedies. This is what we should aim for and work. This exercise will provide a complete picture of the disease symptoms and also the corresponding remedies. Incidentally this is also a very sound way of preparing for the study of Materia Medica.

We should always see the disease in full and not from a few symptoms. This means we should see the disease from all the symptoms, pertaining to it, in the human race. Homoeopathy embraces the principle of totality. Hence in case of any disease it is improper to see it from a few symptoms and again improper to look upon a remedy from a few symptoms. We see the remedy image from all the symptoms including the peculiar symptoms. So psora must also be considered from its characteristics, the features that constitutes psora.

Remedies are adjusted as to appearance; the appearance of the remedy is expressed in Symptoms. This must be adjusted to the appearances of the diseases, which is also by way of symptoms. Once you have exhausted psora, go to sycosis and proceed in the same manner. Gather all the symptoms experienced by the sycotic - all their sufferings and all the ultimate. Group them as one and look upon them as one miasm. Take the Materia Medica and make an anamnesis. Take each symptom one by one. Write opposite each symptom the remedies that have produced that symptom. It will be obvious that the remedies, which run through most strongly, will be anti-sycotic remedies. In other words the remedies will be found to have the essentials of the disease or the sycotic nature in them.

We request the same process in the case of Syphilis. By going through the above exercise we will be able to bring before our minds the three chronic diseases torturing the human race. Armed with the complete details of the chronic miasms we can treat them.

While prescribing for a chronic patient, the symptoms constitute the whole basis of the prescription. We can theorize as much as we may like to, but writing out a prescription the symptoms alone guide us to the remedy. There are many angles from which we may look at the symptoms. We can easily get confused by the symptoms and also fall into error. This will be due to our taking the unimportant symptoms. Careful study of Materia Medica will

Lecture - XXII

teach us how to study the disease. This is so because the plan of studying the Materia Medica for the purpose of bringing the image of a remedy to the mind is the same we adopt in studying the disease.

A physician holding in his memory a disease or a remedy will be a failure. He has not learnt to think. He carries in his head only a mass of particulars, nothing to tie to. There is no order. It reminds us of a disorderly mob.

We shall now see a note of Dr. Hahnemann - 'Should it, however, be thought sometimes necessary to have names for diseases in order to render ourselves intelligible in a few words to the ordinary classes, when speaking of a patient, let none be made use of but such as are collective.' We ought to say, for instance, that a patient has a species of chorea, a species of dropsy, a species of nervous fever, a species of augue, etc."

We should be specific. Otherwise if we speak in terms of appearances and naming, the disease will not be correct. The homoeopath must not think in those lines. He must see the disease as an internal malady. It is all right to speak in terms of the name of a disease while conversing; fully realizing that speaking of this is only an appearance.

Now we come to paragraph 83 of the Organon. It deals with the study and examination of the patient and the qualifications necessary for comprehending the image of a disease.

Paragraph eighty-three of Organon reads as under: —

"This individualizing examinations of a case of disease, for which I shall only give in this place general directions, of which the practitioner will bear in mind what is applicable for each individual case, demands of the physician nothing but freedom from prejudice and sound senses, attention in observing and fidelity in tracing the picture of the disease".

So, we understand from the above that each case demands individualization with unbiased judgment and sound sense.

The old school prescribers and some persons calling themselves as Homoeopaths are absolutely incompetent to examine a patient. They are incompetent to examine Homoeopathy, to test it and say whether there is anything in it. Such persons are absolute failures.

One cannot test Homoeopathy, without first knowing how to get the disease image before their mind's eye and correct homoeopathic remedy to be selected. Some times we hear an allopath saying, "I am going to test Homeopathy on this patient who is vomiting." Ipecac produces vomiting. Hence homoeopathically it should also stop vomiting. But then even after this medication, the patient continues vomiting. Now the physician proceeds to proclaim Homoeopathy is a failure. Stop for a moment and think. Has Homoeopathy failed or the allopath failed? Homoeopathy is a solid science with very good and established doctrines. It is a God given science. Can God ever fail? In this test it is the miserable failure of the allopath. Whenever a failure occurs, it is the failure of the physician and not of the law. In this present day enlightened world, judgments are given out hastily. Though this is the way, commonly tests are made; this is not the right procedure. The persons like above do not know what to observe or how to select a remedy. There is a good list of remedies, which have vomiting. Here we should apply our thought and choose the proper remedy, which will be similar to this particular patient. That is the proper way.

"The examination of a particular case of disease, with the interest of presenting it in its formal state and individuality, only demands on the part of the physician an unprejudiced mind, sound understanding, attention and fidelity in observing and tracing the image of the disease, I will contend myself in the present instance with merely explaining the general principles of the course that is to be pursued, leaving it to the physician to select those which are applicable to each particular case."

Lecture - XXII

Let us analyze the above statement. The physician must be of unprejudiced mind. Unprejudiced mind is a forgotten issue today. There is almost no such thing. Seek out the doctors who profess to practice Homoeopathy and we will find them full of prejudices of various kinds. They will start rattling of what they believe in. One believes in one thing and the other believes in some other thing. A third one will swear on God and say that what he believes is the correct thing - you will find his belief is totally a different one far away from what the other one's professed. This again goes to prove that they all have different kinds of prejudices and beliefs. This is not the resultant of the facts, but it comes out from what each man has laid down as a fact. What each man wants to be so, in his view, is so. This establishes in him a prejudice. Since no two persons agree there are many different opinions, majority of which is false.

Take anything for that matter and speak to a man. You will find that man is full of prejudice. This state of prejudice exists in examining a patient as well. The physician approaches the patient with a prejudiced mind, as to his own theories. He has his own ideas as to how and what constitutes the correct method of examination. This results in his not examining the patient for the purpose of bringing out the truth and nothing but the whole truth. His prejudices make him snap the patient up, as soon as he tells his story. He will hammer him all over, from head to foot and then tell him what he suffers from. A prescription that has not any earthly relation to the constitutional state of the patient follows. Think out for a minute. Has this been a true and correct examination? The answer is a big **NO**.

It must be readily and truthfully recognized that a true man has no prejudices. Since he has no prejudices, he can listen attentively to his patient as well as others, he can examine the patient carefully and with skill and he can meditate. Can a judge go into a strong case with prejudice? You can well imagine what will happen. Do you know that a judge is prohibited to sit on judgment over his brother, over his wife, or over his other nearest relatives?

A Homoeopathic physician can attain an unprejudiced mind only by learning all the truth and all the doctrines of Homoeopathy. A physician is not in a rational state if he goes in with a prejudice for certain potency or a prejudice against certain principles, etc. He has lost his freedom with the patient, examines him in ignorance. If he cannot free himself from prejudice, how can he prescribe properly? When the physician understands soundly the doctrines of Homoeopathy concerning potentization, concerning Materia Medica, he goes into his case with full freedom. Now being in freedom he will be able to examine case in all its aspects and will listen patiently. He investigates the case collecting data about the patient and his ailments. He observes without prejudice, with wisdom and with judgment. He will and must go into the case full steam ahead and collect all the facts from everyone dear and near to the patient. He ignores no evidence. He collects all these without forming a judgment. Now, on this table lies the sheat of paper where his efforts to get a complete picture of the disease pertaining to this patient lies. It is all facts and only facts. No opinions. Armed with proper ammunition he now studies the case, the whole case. This is what is called approaching the case un-prejudicially. To proceed on these lines, the physician should have a deep and sound understanding, a clear knowledge of all the details relating to this subject and also to all his duties.

An allopath will wonder what earthly use is there in a homoeopath spending such a long time and taking down notes on his investigation. This is because the allopathic physician has no knowledge about the true Meteria Medica. Hence he does not see anything in it. See how a homoeopath works out his remedies? He first takes down all details, including things that may appear however insignificant putting them on the paper. He studies what he took down during the investigation and meditates on it and then choses the remedy most suitable under those conditions. An allopathic physician could not do this. He is not trained to imagine the disease picture on a canvass. This alone can help to fit the disease picture to that of the suitable drug in the Meteria Medica. He will also be ignorant of the homoeopathic medicine and would not know with which medicine he could compare the disease to. He goes by the name of the disease and the symptoms relating to it, which are visual externally. He does not go internally.

The unprejudiced mind can only exist on a foundation of sound understanding. A sound understanding can come only from proper education. Here reference is made to the homoeopathic education. The student should become well acquainted with all the doctrines, step by step, in the course of his education. Once taught what to give attention to, fidelity is absolutely essential. This faithfulness can only exist in the man who has no prejudice, by opening his mind to the homoeopathic principles and doctrines. In this connection all the homoeopaths work together following one pattern. When a student passes out of an institution he always carries the stamp of the institution, no matter where he is. That is a universal truth. He has passed through the sieves at different levels and thoroughly filtered off all prejudices and emerges out with great faithfulness and earnestness.

Now it is time to work out the plan in all its aspects for a faithful and careful examination of a case. The homoeopathic physician's top most and only mission is to cure - with minimum dosage of the remedy, rapidly and permanently. Keeping this in mind he should bring out the patient's symptoms in the very best possible way. This study is long and tedious with lot of difficulties en-route. Symptoms are the language of the nature to indicate the presence of disease internally. So disease is to be brought out systematically in terms of the symptoms. The intention is to match these or fit these with the drug picture in the Materia Medica. All the diseases known to man have their likeness in our Materia Medica. Hence it is very important for the physician to learn and know the art of perceiving this likeness. He must be able to distinguish the razor-sharp differences between subtle similarities. This is not an easy matter initially but with continual persistent application with patients will make one a master in this technique. All the senses must be alert to perceive the similarities as well as the most similar ones.

Summary

1. Our study of the disease must be able to bring to our minds the complete picture of the disease.
2. The Old School books present only the diagnostic or pathognomonic symptoms for the purposes of distinguishing one disease from another. They give nothing to bring out the image of the disease to the mind.
3. The homoeopathic books give out the symptoms in such a fashion as to bring the complete image of the disease.
4. A very sound way of preparing the study of Materia Medica is as follows:

   Take the "Chronic Diseases" of Dr. Hahnemann. Note down all symptoms given out by him, one after the other. Let us take up psora. Write down against each symptom the remedy/ remedies corresponding to it. Then proceed in the same manner in case of Syphilis and Sycosis. Presto! Now what do we have in our hands — a complete picture of each chronic miasm and a complete matching drug picture. This is what we want.
5. We should see a disease from all its symptoms. That is in totality.
6. Remedies must fit the appearances of the disease.
7. While a prescription is made for a chronic disease the symptoms are the basis.

8. He who has memorized the disease symptoms and the drugs will be a failure in homoeopathy.
9. We must be specific.
10. Each case demands individualization.
11. To test homoeopathy the person must be competent — the competency comes from his sound understanding of its laws and doctrines, disease image and drug image.
12. Allopathy does not follow these lines. They go by symptoms and by names of the diseases.
13. Where a homoeopathic physician is not able to cure a disease, it is the failure of the physician and not the failure of homoeopathy.
14. The physician must be unprejudiced.
15. Unfortunately, it is difficult to find an unprejudiced individual. But there are some like that and such people shine. It is because they work in freedom.
16. What each man wants to be so, in is his view, is so.
17. A homoeopathic physician should be above any prejudice - for, if he has any prejudice that may pollute his examination as well. Only with an unprejudiced mind, on examining the patient, he can bring out the truth and nothing but the truth.
18. A true man has no prejudices.
19. A true homoeopath will learn all the truth about homoeopathy doctrines. He has a sound understanding of the homoeopathy doctrines, potentization, chronic and acute disease and can attend the case with confidence and freedom.
20. An efficient homoeopath will collect all the data, even those appearing insignificant from all the possible sources. All these data are symptoms - these are put down on the paper in

black and white. He sits over these carefully considering each symptom and mediates on how it is connected to the disease. Armed with these he is perfectly in a comfortable position to choose the appropriate remedy. He knows the facts and has no prejudices.

21. Once a student is taught to what he must pay attention to, then comes fidelity. When the student passes out of a college of high integrity he will automatically inherit the college's stamp. He will become naturally faithful to his college principles throughout his life. So it is essential to be a student of highly principled institution.

22. The homoeopathic physician's uppermost and only mission is to afford a cure, with minimum dosage, rapidly, gently and permanently. He should always remember this in every case, new or old.

23. Symptom is the language of the internal disease. The homoeopath must understand them to be so and hence interpret them closely to the disease. This must fit to the drug symptoms given in the Materia Medica. Thus his choice of the medicine will be perfect to a "t". He must be able to distinguish the similarities, between two, very close to each other. There can be two similar but there can be only one similimum, which matches the disease picture perfectly.

24. The dedicated homoeopath can automatically be alert by constant, persistent practice and there will be no confusion. He must keep all his senses alert always which can be only possible for an unprejudiced mind.

Aphorisms & Precepts

1. A truth, on any plane, presented to different men is accepted or rejected by each according to the good or evil in his mind.

Lecture - XXII

2. The man who loves truth and humanity, lives in that idea, and it becomes a part of his nature, and can be seen in his looks and his life.
3. If you loose the attitude of mind, which, seeks the good of the patient you will loose your homoeopathy.
4. If homoeopathy does not cure sick people you are to despise it.
5. Those who say they have tested homoeopathy and it is a failure have only exposed their own ignorance.
6. So long as a man relies upon the senses to settle what is scientific and what is not, and does not use his understanding, so long will he be in confusion and sciences will oppose each other.
7. The Old School must know pathology before they can treat disease, and they must have a post mortem before they can know pathology.
8. Technicalities are condemned in homoeopathy. Only frame in your mind that you have seen a species of Scarlet Fever, a species of Measles, or a species of Tuberculosis, or Diabetes and speak of them as such; that the speech may be a true outward representation of internal thought.
9. You cannot depend on luck shots and guess work; everything depends on long study of each individual case.
10. Memorizers have no perception; they can only resemble what they see, and they see only the surface.
11. Memory is not knowledge until it is comprehended and used. Then grows the ability to perceive.
12. If you do not use your homoeopathy, you will loose it. This is a responsibility so great that where one has gone into the Truth and does not make use of his knowledge, he will become like Egypt of Old.

13. Leave out names when prescribing. They are only for the foolish and for the boards of health.
14. The disease is not to be named, but to be perceived, not to be classified but to be viewed that the very nature of it may be discovered.
15. Throw aside all theories, and matters of belief and opinion, and dwell in simple fact.
16. The human mind should not be burdened with technicalities. They destroy description and close the understanding.
17. Materia Medica never inspires perception. The physician must have the love of its use, and he becomes wise in proportion as he loves his use, and in proportion as he lives uprightly with his patients; that is, desires to heal them beautify their souls. Can the physician who does not love his neighbor as himself, get into this position?
18. Homoeopathy is an applied science not a theory.
19. If we could accept opinion we should go back to allopathy, because we find there only a record of man's experiments, a mass of heterogeneous opinions.
20. Man must be studied as he is, as he was, everything of man and of the human race in general, in order to understand disease.
21. The homoeopathic principles, when known, are plain, simple and easily comprehended. They are in harmony with all things known to be true.
22. Memory is the gateway to man. The outermost envelope of this Esse is formed to be a receptacle for the will, the understanding and the memory.
23. A prejudiced mind has his affections, his pet theory to subdue.

Lecture - XXII

24. A prejudiced mind decides without wisdom the way he wants to have it.

25. When the Materia Medica is fully learned, you see at a glance the image of the remedy. It looms up before you. You know it as a physician of experience knows measles or scarlet fever.

26. Only a few drugs will be similar enough to cure, and there will be only one similimum.

27. Perception comes with use.

28. The quiet, silent manner of perception is to be cultivated.

Lecture - XXIII

The Examination of the Patient

Let us see what paragraph 84 of Organan has got to say.
The paragraph reads as under: —

"The patient details the history of his sufferings; those about him, tell what they heard him complain, of how he has behaved and what they have noticed in him; the physician sees, hears, and remarks by his other senses what there is of an altered or unusual character about him. He writes down accurately all that the patient and his friends have told him in the very expressions used by them. Keeping silence himself he allows them to say all they have to say, and refrains from interrupting them unless they wander off to other matters. The physician advises them at the beginning of the examination to speak slowly, in order that he may take down in writing, the important parts of what the speaker says."

Let us now analyze the above point by point.

(1) The patient explains the history of his disease and sufferings to the physician.

(2) His close friends and relatives, who were with him during his sufferings, apprise the physician of the complaints he made to them. They also bring to the physician's notice as to how he behaved during his sufferings, and

(3) The physician also sees, hears and considers what his other senses remarked about the patient's altered or unusual character.

(4) Now he sits down and writes down accurately all that the patient (in his own way) and his friends told him in the same expressions used by them.

(5) The physician keeps silent and hears all, allowing them to say all they have to say. He does not interrupt them unless they wander off to other matters.

"Each interruption by him breaks the train of thought of the narrators and all they would have said at first does not again occur to them in precisely the same manner after that."

Dr. S. Hahnemann

(6) The physician instructs them at the beginning itself to speak slowly thus enabling him to take down the important parts of what the speakers say.

The above can be summarized as: The patient and the attendants narrate the history of the disease and describe sensation, symptoms and the behavior of the patient. The physician also observes with sight, hearing, touch and smell and allows the story to be finished without interrupting. The sufferings and the history are also heard from the patient himself.

Now, we go into the lecture, and see what Dr. Kent says in this connection.

To secure the correct image of the sickness is to preserve in simplicity the patient's statement in his own way. This does not mean that we should also make notes of every thing that he says. Wherever and whenever the patient digresses and is not to the point what he said is ignored and the patient is gently brought back to the subject. But when he talks about his sufferings in his

Lecture - XXIII

own way he is not to be interrupted. The notes are corrected for any grammatical mistakes alone. Where symptoms are used they should not be ambiguous. When a woman speaks her menstrual periods she may use various terms to represent it. Since we have recorded the same expression and vocabulary the patient has used, it is better to use the medical term "Menses" wherever the patient has used her own vocabulary. The terminology that we use should maintain the purpose of our work, i.e., to secure the image of the sickness only not causing ambiguity, in its absolute simplicity. We should be sure that our way of making the notes and the words we have used keeps the thought intact.

Once a proper record of a patient is made we should be able to refer to it during subsequent examination without being disturbed by the repeated statements of the patient. This is important. Equally important is the way that the points are noted down. They must be written down one after the other. When written down continuously it looks like a composition and will cause only confusion. That way of writing down will not help because there will be utter confusion in forming out the image of that sickness in the mind. When the mind is in full blast to hunt out something, there will not be any concentration in listening.

You have the habit of going through the newspaper. Have you stopped to think why the news is presented in columns? They are not provided in the form of essays. Why? The columns are in about 4 cms. width. With this presentation we are able to quickly read the short lines. Time is saved and at the same time the editor is able to bring out the impact more easily. There is lesser eyestrain and makes it easier reading.

Similarly we should also take a lesson from the newspapers. We must divide the page vertically in such a manner that when the patient talks to you, a single glance down the paper will give you everything the patient may talk. It is a good idea to divide a page into three columns. First column dates and prescriptions, second column the emphatic symptoms and the third column things predicated of the symptoms, as follows: —

I	II	III
Dates	Symptoms	Things predicated of the symptom < (Aggravation) > (Amelioration)
Remedy		

The patient has told all his sufferings in his own way. You have gone through all the things, which you can predicate of the patient's symptoms. Then you must make an enquiry of someone who has been with the patient. In most of the private patients there could have been a nurse, sometimes only a sister, or a mother or a wife. This person would have always been observing the patient, his behavior and all that he had to complain about. To say the least this person would have literally undergone what the patient felt, for all practical purposes — only that person was not the victim of the disease. This person will furnish a wealth of information about the patient's behavior and all that he complained of and also what that person noticed about the patient. The physician must respect this person and should listen to him with great alertness and concentration, and make notes on it. The physician, at the same time, should decide that the observer is not anxious and overplays his or her role.

If the observer were the patient's wife, the physician should use his discretion in accepting her words, for she in her anxiety and fear may intermingle her own notions and fears in her statements. In this instance it will be better to get the nurse if possible and counter-check the statement of the wife with that of the nurse. The exact words as told by the patient to her should be elicited. If this is achieved in acute sufferings it is always worth more than

Lecture - XXIII

what the nurse is able to convey, always remember that the more anxious and frightened the observer due to his/her personal interest in the patient it is less likely he or she will be able to present the truthful image. This is not because he/she wants to deceive. To that person the patient's sufferings appear greater when recollecting his words, thereby everything the observer reports may be exaggerated. This is what we said that the observer also for all practical purposes suffers with the patient. Emotions play a big role here. It will also work out better when a third person, disinterested in the patient gives out such details. The physician should collect data from two or three such disinterested persons for a better coverage wherever available or possible. From here the physician goes to his own observations and the notes made by him. He should describe the urine if there is anything in particular. Where the urine and stool are normal he may leave them at it.

Studies have been made for hundreds of years as to how to question a witness. They have settled upon certain rules for eliciting the best evidence. Homoeopathy has also set down certain rules for examining a case, which has to be followed with exactitude through private practice. Some students have memorized all this and some others fallen out. These students are defaulters because they have been violating everything they have been taught. Not knowing the principles they have gone to low potencies, making greater and greater failures. It is disgracing their teachers and also the God given science, they swear to follow. Such persons must realize their folly and follow the correct path.

Let us see what happens under such circumstances. The first sufferer will be the patient where a proper and careful examination is not made. But look out at it carefully. Finally the real victim of such a folly will be he himself. At the same time the science of Homoeopathy also gets a bad name. Dr. Hahnemann has provided us questions and way of examining the patient. But, then, it is only a guideline. Following this way will lead us in a certain direction.

The physician should question the patient, then the friends and must observe for himself the various factors; these must give sufficient clues to a proper prescription. If sufficient data could not be collected the physician should go back to the particulars. Constant and persistent practice on the part of the physician will gain experience and will be able to get at the truth. Store up Materia Medica so as to use it. Your knowledge will flow out as your language flows. While examining the patient, use the form of speech as your patient. This will help him give you the details properly.

The physician, during his course of examination, must not put any leading questions or put words into the patient's mouth, or biased his expression in any way. How do you do that? Simple, do not put any direct questions. If you do put any direct question do not record the answer. In all probabilities, for such a question, the patient will say "yes" or "no". If a patient answers yes or no you should immediately know that the question was badly formed. The patient may not answer a question - either he does not know or he has not noticed it. Never ask a question having choices. Such questions again are defective. When pain is involved ascertain the exact location and also the character of pain- e.g. tearing pain, pricking pain, etc., find out how long the attack was, if there is any discharge, its appearance.

How does one practice this art of questioning and become competent? Practice, practice and practice. Go over the questions framing collateral questions. Practice case taking. In boxing they do what is called shadow fighting. The boxer assumes that his competitor is in front of him and is fighting him. He uses all the techniques in fighting with the shadow. Similarly this shadow box fighting is used in sports in both out-door and indoor practice. By doing this you are virtually able to direct the game, almost in a predictable manner since every possible move of the opponent is worked out and fought against. Thus do shadow box fighting in case taking at every possible opportunity till you master the game. Use imaginary patients.

Lecture - XXIII

The patient must be relaxed and be completely free. There must not be any tension or stress in him. So basically make him take comfortable position as far as possible. Give him the physical comfort first and other things will take care of themselves. Do not hurry the patient. Give him all the time in this world. Be with him totally. Listen most attentively. Do not interrupt or divert the patient's attention in the least. Keep your clinic simple looking, but clean and orderly. Let there be nothing that could draw or divert the attention of the patient. Even a loud ticking clock could distract. Fall into a fixed habit of examination and let that be your second nature. Keep up your reputation and fulfill your highest use.

Say as little as you can. Let the patient do the talking and always assist him keep close to the line. By allowing this freedom to the patient both general and particular symptoms will be revealed. When a patient goes astray bring him back to the toe-line gently and quietly without disturbing him in the least. These techniques will take you a long way without trouble. Your batting average will be better.

All sleep symptoms are very important. Sleep is closely relating to the mind. The transfer from sleep to waking, from cerebrum to cerebellum is important. Old pathologists could not account for difficult breathing during sleep. Knowing the functions of the white and gray matter is important. The physician must possess a rational knowledge of anatomy. Homoeopathy does not discourage the study of anatomy and physiology. Essentially he must know the superficial and the real profound character. This permits the recognition of one symptom-image from another.

This subject matter is a very important one and several lectures had been dedicated to this subject. The student should well master this and follow the principles laid out here. Hence study this and the ensuing lectures on examination of the patient with great concentration. Follow the golden path and be a Homoeopath of reputation. If you do not do so at the earliest you may have to regret for this inaction later.

Summary

1. In this lecture the examination of the patient is dealt with. Paragraph eighty-four of Organon is explained.
2. In examination of the patient the following should be followed, step-by-step.
   (a) Note down all that the patient says in his exact words, which relate to his sufferings.
   (b) Collect as much data as possible as related by the attendant or friends or relatives close to the patient, who were present with the patient at the time of his sufferings. Data about the patient's behavior during that time, his complaints (as far as possible the words and exclamations as uttered by the patient) and any changes noted in the patient must be collected from them.
   (c) The physician sees, hears and observes the patient and notes down his own observations.
   (d) All the above should be carefully noted down and the case is studied.
   (e) All the time the physician collects the necessary data he is "all ears". He notes down without interrupting or diverting the person away from what he is saying. Whenever he goes astray the physician gently brings him back to the subject.
   (f) The physician requests the patient as well as the observers to speak slowly to enable the physician note down what all is important.

   A woman may use various terms for her periods — The

Lecture - XXIII

physician can make a note of these as menses. The physician's way of noting must be simple, plain and without any ambiguity.

4. Each point must be noted down one below the other. This will enable construction of the disease and drug image easily and without any confusion.

5. As far as possible keep the sentences small. Write them down in a newspaper column fashion. This type of noting down will help in seeing at a glance the various items noted, while the patient or the observer keeps talking.

6. Dr. Kent has suggested a three-column noting of the points:-

   First column: Date and prescriptions

   Second column: Symptoms

   Third column: Things predicated by the symptoms.

7. While taking down the notes from the observers who are close to the patient, certain precautions are to be taken. Due to anxiety and fear of the patient's sickness there is a chance for the near and dear to be emotional and they may not report truthfully. This has to be guarded against.

8. The physician should follow the rules given in Homoeopathy to examine the case. He must not take things for granted or take liberties with the rules. He has to follow them strictly and without prejudice.

9. Memorisers fail miserably. Those who take liberties with the law or rule makes the patient suffer and also spoil the name of Homoeopathy. They are the ultimate sufferers, in fact.

10. Following Dr.Hahnemann's directions by way of questioning will help us tread the path easily and help us go in a certain direction.

11. To write down a proper prescription we need as much data as possible. To reach this goal the physician must question the patient, diligently. There should be no leading questions, then the patient's near and dears, without interruption from his side. At the same time he must keep his senses alert.

12. The above comes with constant persistent efforts.

13. The physician is to use the same form of speech as the patient and keep him relaxed throughout the examination. Thus we will be able to collect much information about the disease.

14. Rules to be followed in case taking: —

   (a) Do not ask a direct question.

   (b) Do not put a leading question.

   (c) Never ask a question with choice answers.

   (d) If the patient gives a one-word answer like "yes" or "no", the question is badly formed.

   (e) The patient may not answer a question - then it means he does not know or he has not noticed it. Do not press for an answer. Frame this question in other words and present it a little later.

   (f) Where pain or discharge of any nature is present seek the exact locality and also their nature, character and its appearance.

   (g) Find the length of the attack.

   (h) The patient must be comfortable and relaxed throughout the examination.

   (i) Never interrupt the patient, bias his ideas or break the continuity of thought.

   (j) Whenever a patient goes astray, take care to bring him back to the line of thought, in a gentle, easy manner.

- (k) Do not ask any uncomfortable or embarrassing questions at the beginning of the examination itself. If at all you have to ask such a question ask these questions casually and in such a manner that the patient will co-operate. Let such questions be asked once you know the patient is very comfortable with you.

- (l) Never hurry a patient.

- (m) Be with the patient totally and be very attentive for any golden nugget the patient may drop most casually.

- (n) Keep your clinic in a clean and orderly way. Keep your consultation table clean and void of anything that may distract the patient.

- (o) Let the patient do the most talking.

- (p) Always retain in your mind that your top-most and only mission in life is to cure, with minimum medicine, rapidly, gently and permanently. Nothing else matters.

15. All sleep symptoms are very important.

16. The physician must have knowledge of anatomy and physiology. Knowledge of the superficial and the real character permits the easy recognition of one symptom image from the other.

17. The student of Homoeopathy must do a lot of homework. He has to do shadow box fighting whenever possible and improve his technique of case taking minute by minute. Only constant, persistent and sincere practice of this will give him more and more confidence. This love of humanity and a single pointed mission to cure will carry the physician a long way in his profession. His work will be above average.

Aphorisms & Precepts

1. "It is no proof of man's undertaking to be able to confirm what he pleases; but to be able to discern that what is true is true, and what is false is false, this is the mark and character of intelligence."

   Emanuel Swedenborg

2. The external man is but an outward expression of the internal sickness.

3. A physician's attitude is performing his duty to the sick, is different from that of any other person. He has a different sphere from that of the ordinary man. This is a thousand times amplified in homoeopathy. One who has entertained that peculiar "circumcision of the heart", always looking to the good of his patient, never thinking of the criticism of man, acquires an ability to say what is right to do. He establishes a garment of righteousness.

4. This opens a field of tedious labor, and many failures, but if once in a while you succeed in curing one of these lost ones it is well.

5. The physician, who violates his conscience, destroys his ability to perceive.

6. What appears to be intuition comes from using that which is in the understanding.

7. Eternal Principles, themselves, are authority. The law of similar is a Divine Law. So soon as you have accepted the law of Similar, so soon you have accepted Providence, which is law and order.

8. Man's unbelief and opinion do not effect truth. The experience, which the homoeopath has, is experience under law and confirms the law and by this order is maintained.

Lecture - XXIII

9. It becomes your solemn duty to heal the good, bad and indifferent.

10. Homoeopaths have a consciousness of what life is, what the life force is, what nature of disease is, and can apply to all theories of the world our measure and test them. They can realize the philosophies. The whole aim of homoeopathy is to cure.

11. The value of the service is nothing; your use is first and so long as you have this in mind you will grow.

12. The physician, who ceases to study a case before he sees what the patient needs, is neglecting that case. He falls into a habit and it becomes second nature to prescribe without reflection.

13. The physician must be sober, candid and able to receive.

Lecture - XXIV

The Examination of the Patient (Contd.)

The examination of the patient is a very important limb in Homoeopathy. Dr. Kent has treated this subject in four lectures. Just imagine the great importance of this topic. Homoeopathy does not use microscope or any of the so-called state of the art, expensive investigative apparatus. The only ammunition that the Homoeopath has is his investigative procedure according to the law and doctrines of the science. He relies only on facts. He does not treat the disease. He treats the man. The proper examination of the patient is the foundation of the case. No wonder Dr. Kent has dealt with this in an extensive manner. We learnt some point in this connection in the previous lecture. Now let us proceed.

We have the sickness and the Materia Medica. The sick man exhibits several symptoms and Materia Medica several remedies. The examination must proceed with due respect to the nature of the sickness and with due respect to the nature of the Materia Medica.

Some symptoms have reference to pathology and diagnosis. Others have reference only to the Materia Medica. Now what do we do with these? We should consider the symptoms carefully, constantly and weigh them in the mind. We can thus establish their grades as to common or peculiar symptoms. When all the symptoms are common symptoms, the Materia Medica is left out. Either the examination has not been conducted in respect of the Materia Medica or the symptoms taken down did not exist at all. Let us see it in this way; the key to the prescription is the symptoms. Where the symptoms do not exist or if it had not been found by the doctor that makes no difference as far as the cure is concerned. No prescription can be made.

Let us consider the opposite case. The symptoms have reference to pathology, diagnosis, prognosis and the Materia Medica. It will only be proper later to talk about incurable disease, pathognomonic symptoms, obscure case and the Materia Medica symptoms, etc.

The physician has to proceed thus - he takes all the symptoms and arranges and classifies them. Now he will be able to categorize as peculiar, most general and that are common. All these categories appear in every complete case. These also appear in every proving of every remedy. Homoeopathic knowledge and homeopathic sense including keen observation will help to pick these grades easily and at a glance. Every case can be seen to have common symptoms. Where there are no peculiar symptoms or are absent, one cannot expect any cure. Every curable case can be successfully treated by homoeopathy. But the catch is to know how to apply it. It is the purpose of the physician to judge the symptoms as peculiar or common. Where the patient has presented an incoherent statement the physician must ascertain whether the patient is intoxicated or delirious or there has been a brain breakdown and insanity. The physician must be alert to such an extent that even a flashing of the eye must be noted. He can get loads of information from that eye flash. The nurse cannot convey these details.

Expressions count a lot. See an actor. He displays his emotions through his expressions - the eyes to be more exact. Similarly agony, dismay, etc., is displayed by the eyes - the facial muscles complement the eyes and the expression is all over the face.

A patient has a staring glassy eyes we should think why this is so. Has there been a head injury, does he suffer from the shock, intoxicated or affected by typhoid fever or is he got a disease due to which the mind is stunned? See what a single expression leads the physician to? The natural immediate question will be " how long has the patient been in bed? " If the patient is above reproach his being intoxicated is out of question. On the other hand if the patient has been down with fever for many days, tongue quoted, abdomen sensitive, etc., he has typhoid fever. If the physician is well acquainted with the nature of disease, he will immediately know about the state of the patient. He will immediately recognize whether the patient resembles apoplexy, coma, opium poisoning, etc.

Earlier we have said that the physician must be alert. He must be like an electric bulb. It should light up the moment the switch is on. Similarly, the physician should apply his mind to the task of ascertaining the patient's condition and what relation the symptoms maintain to the Materia Medica. If there was Opium poisoning it should immediately strike the physician to administer an antidote for it. If the patient is suffering from apoplexy, the physician should take down the symptoms, carefully in relation to the cerebral clot to prevent further inflammatory symptoms relative to that state and the remedy. The patient may be intoxicated and have apoplexy at the same time. Every symptom has its own value, especially in acute and serious cases.

Children sometimes sleep so soundly that they cannot be aroused. The mother gives *Cina*, saying that worms are present. Cina's symptoms have symptoms of stupor, difficulty in arousing and falling back to sleep. This *Cina* does not work and the child slips into coma, nose flapping, the chest heaving, brows wrinkling, rattling in the chest clearly indicating the child is going into a cerebral congestion state. The physician under these circumstances must examine the case from every possible angle and find out the nature of the disease to know what to expect. If the physician neglects this course of action, he is not a true homoeopath. Homoeopathy deals with the internal man, so superficial approach to the disease will simply not do. Homoeopathy is much more deeper. The Homoeopath must proceed systematically to fulfill his only mission, to cure. He has a lot of homework to do. After noting all the symptoms, the physician must study attentively the character of the fever- whether the fever is intermittent - or was it a sudden attack, etc. The physician must know sufficient of the case to make a judgment.

In Homoeopathy, we learn much about the significance and the aspect of each motion of the human being. Hence the reliance on the diagnostic symptoms as diagnostic symptoms will decline. We learn to place more value on the symptoms and treat symptoms as symptoms. The regular and careful study of the symptoms will boost the ability in diagnosis and prognosis. Every case we handle will teach us something more.

We see a waxy face. Scores of cases immediately spring into the mind. But by fast elimination process we are able to conclude that is not a case of cholera, hemorrhage, etc. and finally we pinpoint the cause of this waxy face. We can predict the time for a cardiac compensation to break-out in Bright's disease; a peculiar tremulous wave that belongs to the facial muscles and neck muscles, a tremulous jerk of the tongue, putting it out half the way, the pale, cold, semi-transparent skin with cold sweat. The most important thing is to know instantly the cause, for the treatment will be different. Remember the name is not important.

Symptoms have respect to remedy and diagnostic conditions. When there is a morbid anatomy, symptoms will also be present.

Lecture - XXIV

But that cannot indicate a proper remedy. Where there are no other symptoms present, no remedy can be found.

There are many things, which interfere with the examination of the patient. Taking some irrelevant medicine or tampering with the symptoms is by far the most important which changes the symptoms and causes confusion to the physician. It is common to see a patient in the clinic come and rattle off a great number of symptoms. He will also say that he took a dose of such and such remedy, which gave him no relief. This is a very serious situation. Why? What has happened? The rule in Homoeopathy says that there are many similar remedies but only one similimum. In this case the patient has taken a remedy that was not a remedy for his problem at all. The unsuitable remedy has interfered with the symptoms and caused havoc. This also has interfered with the process of finding out the homoeopathic remedy. In acute diseases this is very bad. In acute disease both the drug and disease symptoms must be prescribed for, collectively. In chronic diseases the method is different.

The taking of a powerful medicine causes confusion. The complete true disease picture is changed by it. Now what are the options the physician has in his hand to deal, in a situation like this? He has two options - one is to wait for the inappropriate drug to finish its course of action; two, if the name of the drug is given by the patient at best the physician can administer an antidote to the drug. Sometimes the wait will be long one when the original disease symptoms emerge or reveal themselves, and the nature of the disease discovered. In some cases the patient might have come in with the original disease symptoms. The physician himself might have bungled the issue by giving a wrong or unsuitable remedy. Be it the patient drugging himself or a bad prescription, the confusion created are just the same.

A little amount of patience and the nature to wait on the part of the physician is a trait. Some physician's mix up their cases and prescribe for their own drug symptoms. Such people have no idea what-so-ever of waiting for the true image of the disease to develop itself and present the relative symptoms, which leads the physician to the nature of the disease.

By drugging, the symptoms change and disease is masked. The taking of drugs, drinking too much of wine, drinking toddy or great exposure and anything that will change the symptoms in any way will obscure the real disease. An intelligent physician could effect a cure only when this cloud passes away. Symptoms are the language of the disease present. So the physician must get at the bottom of the language of nature when it is hidden behind a mask because of medicines that cannot be identified.

Any meddling will definitely affect the originality of the case. Unfortunately there are persons who call themselves homoeopaths - they have no cure to offer but only confuse and create problems. The patient is also dissatisfied. Sometimes the patient, of robust constitution, in spite of the meddling can recover. Here the physician is ignorant as to which remedy cured since he has administered several remedies. Only a very robust constitution can take such a beating of this homoeopathic villainy and get well in spite of their indulging in wine, in eating, etc. Coming to think of it. We have to wonder as to how their recuperative powers succeed in throwing out the disease.

We do not meet with this situation in ordinary cases. One aspect about waiting is what to do in that waiting period. Most of the patients are in no mood to wait. Psychologically they cannot entertain this proposition. So, what is the course for the physician? He is in a platform where he has got to wait for the remedy to run its course. But the patient is in no mood to wait. He wants the physician to give him something to keep his mind at peace - that the physician is continuously treating him, and taking care of him. At the same time the physician is bidding time to see the outcome of his remedy. What can the physician do, under such

Lecture - XXIV

circumstances? Placebo - call it by other names like sacrum, etc. - placebo is a great savior for the homoeopath.

The twentieth century chamber's dictionary defines placebo as a medicine given to humor or gratify a patient rather than to exercise any curative effect. (Latin — "I shall please"- placere, to please)

Placebo is given to please the patient and set him up in peace. He feels the physician cares for him. The physician is also happy that he has given time for the remedy to run its course and he can see the results of the remedy. So, keep placebo in your medicinal arsenal always.

So, after the wait the true image of the disease emerges making things easier for the physician. In some cases, someone known to the patient or the patient himself who might have vague knowledge about some homoeopathic remedies might have thought of a drug as suitable to his condition. He might have taken this drug. To the amazement of the patient he might have felt cured. He comes to the physician and narrates this occurrence. Think for a moment. Has the patient been cured by the drug he took? If not, how did his suffering vanish? The fact is this - that drug that the patient took has really got scattered. Now another image is going to emerge, of which the physician can collect nothing! The new symptoms that crop up may run into a long long list - but what is the use? What remedy does the physician see or think of? Absolutely nothing - the case is now jumbled up. It looks as if several drugs proving had got mixed up, all together. Symptoms are intermingled here and there. There is no distinct pattern or image.

Homoeopathy, right from the beginning is a matter of individualization. Each case is a new case. When there is a jumble of symptoms, all mingled up and no distinctiveness, how can the physician analyze these? What then is or will be the way to tackle this problem?

When the patient came to the physician and narrated his case up to a particular date things worked out as planned. The physician was able, up to that date, to ascertain things that occurred. Only after that date the things went haywire. So a definite image up to that date is concrete and without any confusion. In homoeopathy we relate that nature of the disease to the nature of the drug or remedy. So up to that date we have the symptoms that presented the image of the remedy that was administered. Only after that confusion had set in. Now the physician can again administer the same drug and that may yet act. Initially, due to the confusion set up in the system, this drug may not act. Patience and waiting are the attributes of a good homoeopath. So after the administration of the remedy just wait. The remedy will act. It may not be out of place here for me to remember a saying "If the diagnosis is proper the cure can be had".

A remedy may go on acting after its administration, which was prescribed upon the symptoms in the past. A remedy may also fail entirely. In such conditions it is wise to wait a while and order will be restored. The remedy which was indicated, previous to the drugging will act. To explain the above a little more by an example, consider the following case. A physician says, "I was able to contain a patient's symptoms with *Thuja*. Then the symptoms changed and I administered such and such a medicine. Oh God! What a marvelous results I got. I never saw such good results as I did up to that period". Here we should continue with Thuja.

Examine the above case. Carefully study the image of the case where the chaos set in, and the order was lost. We have to seek the image at that point and find it out. "On the contrary, the symptoms that were present prior to the use of such and such medicine/s or several days after the discontinuance present us the true fundamental notion of the original malady."

Lecture - XXIV

Our main idea or the purpose is to obtain the original form of the malady. Sometimes we may have to trace it through a lot of troubles. Whatever the trouble, we cannot afford to skip it since we have to reach the bottom and have to see the beginning of this malady, in accordance with all laws of Divine Providence, must have conformed to some remedy which will cure it. Just prior to the changes in the symptoms up to such and such date was clearly pointing out to a remedy. Since the new confusion set in everything got jumbled up only confusion persisted. The result was that nothing could and be examined enabling any distinction. Often it is possible to take up the thread and get at the indicated remedy even where it is twenty years before. If the remedy was not administered then, that alone will be the most appropriate remedy to cure that condition. There will be no other.

From that period the patient would have been suffering due to the action of the drugs. A time lapse of twenty years is no reason why that remedy be thought of now. Look at it this way. The patient has not been cured. That has been only changed and modified - the patient is the same person, the sickness is the same. So that disease requires the same medicine now. What reasons do you have to hunt for another remedy? Let us assume that drugs have complicated the disease. The chosen remedy may not prove useful. In this case, however, the other drugs have to be antidoted. Then give the same medicine and the patient will be cured.

The physician must observe throughout the progress, to know the disease at its beginnings, the manifestations during the early period, its symptoms and its endings. Let us take an example. You get a case with most violent pains along the course of the nerves in an adult patient. You try administering remedies - but the relief is only temporary. From the investigation of the early childhood of the patient that he had eczema with symptoms similar to *Mezereum*. Also you note the patient's present violent neuralgic pains also conform to the *Mezereum* neuralgic pains. *Mezereum* is the remedy for this patient. On its administration the eczema of his babyhood re-appears and the patient is in his path to recovery. *Mezereum* came to the mind because of the old scald head and now its nature coincided with the neuralgic pains also.

Let us take another example. Instead of *Mezereum* we will think of *Sepia*, which has a likeness of that scald head. His present symptoms also bear a strong similarity to *Sepia*. You put the patient on *Sepia*. According to the law, the last appearing symptoms vanish, with *Sepia*. The eruptions on the head and the eruptions behind the ears now re-appear. Now the patient is cured.

In our day-to-day practice, we do come across many similar instances. All these go to prove what has been said earlier. If this sort of practice is followed incessantly and also carefully studied, collecting everything that was in the beginning your cures would be very very striking. Do not place much importance on the masking of the symptoms by improper repetitions and careless closing of the remedies.

Now we proceed to paragraph ninety-four of Organon. It reads as under:

"While inquiring into the state of the chronic disease, the particular circumstances of the patient with regard to his ordinary occupations, his usual mode of living and diet, his domestic situation, and so forth, must be well considered and scrutinized, to ascertain what there is in them that may tend to produce or to maintain disease, in order that by their removal the recovery may be promoted."

A footnote is given here. It is - in chronic disease of females it is especially necessary to pay attention to pregnancy, sterility, sexual desire, accouchements, miscarriages, suckling and the state of the menstrual discharge. With respect to the last named more particular, we should not neglect to ascertain if it recurs as to short intervals or is delayed beyond the proper time, how many days it lasts,

Lecture - XXIV

whether its flow is continuous or interrupted, what is its general quantity, how dark is its color; whether there is leucorrhoea (whites), before its appearance or after its termination but especially by what bodily or mental ailments, what sensations and pains it is preceded, accompanied or followed; if there is leucorrhoea, what is its nature, what sensations attend its flow, in what quantity it is, and what are the conditions and occasions under which it occurs?

Let us now analyze the above paragraph:

(1) While examining a chronic case we must consider the particular circumstances under which the patient is.

(2) The physician should also learn what the patient's occupation is, how he lives and his domestic situation.

(3) The physician must check up the patient's domestic relationship, any wrong way of living or life style, hygienic condition, etc. If these are the causes for his disease or maintaining it, these should be rectified or removed.

Now let us proceed to the lecture.

Look at life. What does it consist of? Nothing but circumstances! All our activities are circumstantial. All business is governed by circumstance. The circumstances have a control over the actions and reactions, symptoms and their symptoms. The body is entwined with the circumstances. Every function has a relationship with the circumstances. All our natural functions of life are connected to the circumstances. Without these we would have nothing to prescribe upon, we have nothing to ascertain the images by; there would be nothing to form the symptoms. From the above what do we surmise? The circumstances of life and man's habits cannot be separated from one another. They should be studied in conjunction with one another. The purpose of the study must be to going into even the slightest particulars.

Here on a practical basis when examining a female patient the physician must also consider points relating to her eating habits, stool, her menstruation, her bathing, her dress, her other habits, etc., since all these things are all natural to her. These are the circumstances under which her symptoms may or may not come. The footnote of this paragraph of Organon is explanatory by itself. So, please go through it again.

The woman has got to be properly educated to enable her understand. It may look absurd to her. But when the physician wants to know more about her stomach or headache he asks her under what circumstance does these appear or how her dress or how the whether affects these, how these have been affected before, during, after her periods, etc. This may look absurd or useless exercise to the patient unless she is educated, what role these things play in her ailments.

There is also another set of circumstances - a group of circumstances that is different relating to ordinary occupation. Every person will be governed by some circumstances more particular than those in general. As an example a patient might have been standing in a store all day. This might have resulted in a prolapse. May be she may lead a sedentary life, or her occupation may have hazards which might promote dermatitis, etc. When we talk of modes of life, they may mean so many different things. They are beyond the natural conditions and circumstances of life. Modes of life are important because it is an exciting cause for the disease. These things do drive things in a certain peculiar direction, disturbing the economy.

Domestic circumstances play a big role in the life and health of any person and are more so in the case of females. In her case the circumstances may vary from A to Z. Any circumstances can upset her or her health. She may feel that her husband is intemperate with her sexually. There may be a domestic situation that cannot be cured and hence endured. Any such thing must be

Lecture - XXIV

carefully examined and the chances of removing it. Things that cannot be eradicated will develop psora, in a peculiar direction. So, from all the above we do learn that all the circumstances ought to be very carefully examined and anything which could give birth to and keep up or maintain the disease is to be eradicated permanently. Once these circumstances, which are controllable, and having a chance to be eradicated must be eradicated and this facilitates a cure.

Summary

1. The proper examination of the patient is a very important limb of Homoeopathy.
2. Homoeopathy does not make use of expensive technical investigative apparatus. Microscopes are not used.
3. The sick man exhibits symptoms - the Materia Medica has several remedies.
4. Symptoms are common and peculiar - two types.
5. In an examination if only common symptoms are present the Materia Medica is left out. In this case the examination has not been conducted in respect of the Materia Medica or the symptoms noted down did not exist at all.
6. Symptoms are the key to a prescription.
7. The physician notes down all the symptoms - arranges and classified them. He categorizes the symptoms as peculiar, most general and common.
8. Where there is no peculiar symptom, cure may not be possible.
9. At the time of examination, the physician has to ascertain that the patient is not intoxicated or delirious.

10. The physician must be alert - even the flashing of the eye will give loads of information.
11. Expressions count a lot.
12. The physician's mind must be always alert to the situations and quickly discern the nature of the disease.
13. The physician must be able to determine his course of action at lightning speed on judging the condition of the patient. He must relate the disease symptoms also to the drug symptoms in Materia Medica at an equally fast speed.
14. Each symptom is extremely valuable - so do not ignore or overlook even those that may appear insignificant.
15. In Homoeopathy the symptoms are treated as symptoms.
16. We do not go at a disease by its name - the name is used only for conversational simplicity. When it comes to the actual case it is only symptoms.
17. The patient meddling or tampering with his symptoms may end up in difficulties. Drugging loses the originality of the disease. It causes confusion. The cause for drugging could be due to the patient's action on inadvertency of the physician.
18. The physician's mind must be always alert to the situations and quickly discern the nature of the disease.
19. The physician must be able to determine his course of action at lightning speed on judging the condition of the patient. He must relate the disease symptoms also to the drug symptoms in Materia Medica at an equally fast speed.
20. Each symptom is extremely valuable — so do not ignore or overlook even those that may appear insignificant.
21. The physician should have patience.
22. Placebo is one of the ways to buy time.

Lecture - XXIV

23. The physician should wait and gather the beginning of the disease.
24. Homoeopathy is individualization, from step one.
25. Where there is confusion due to drugging, the physician must go back and study the condition prior to the confusion. Prior to the confusion the patient should have been stable by the administration of a suitable remedy. When confusion has set in even if it is several years after, the physician must go back to the remedy prior to the confusion. It may take some time to rope in results - but that remedy will cause the reappearance of the beginning of the disease, and we are on our path to success.
26. The environment, habits of life, occupational circumstances (occupational hazards), etc. play a vital role in the health of a person.
27. Wherever a circumstance is there as an exciting cause or a reason for maintaining cause for a disease we should see whether that can be permanently eradicated to bring back the patient into harmony. Such external removable cause must be attended to immediately.
28. In examining a female patient the physician must go into the peculiarities particular to the females. In this connection female patients may have to be educated, sometimes.
29. Occupational circumstances also play a big role in health and disease.
30. Domestic circumstances play an important role. This also has to be taken into consideration.
31. Circumstances, which are exciting causes or those that maintains unhealthiness, wherever possible must be eradicated, for a cure.

Aphorisms & Precepts

1. The Homoeopathic physician must continue to study the science and the art before he can become an expert. This will grow in him until he becomes increasingly astute and he will grow stronger and wiser in his remedy selection for sick people.

2. The physician cultivates his eyes for everything that it is possible to pass judgment upon and must write down everything that is unnatural, everything that is expressive of illness.

3. The expressions by which we know that he has been sick for a long time we know by our study of pathology and anatomy. These are the results of the disease, but the primitive disease is evidenced by the symptoms, the morbid sensations.

4. The healthier the patient becomes, the more likelihood there is for an eruption upon the skin. The vital energies must be sufficient for this. A cure progresses from within outward.

5. In cases without symptoms, the patient must be kept on Saclac until you can discern some general, such as aggravation of symptoms in the morning, or at midnight. If the patient is only 'tired', without guiding symptoms, you may know that it is liable to terminate in some grave disorders - consumption. Bright's disease, cancer or the like.

6. All things that change the aspect of a case should be avoided.

7. Unless the inner nature of the remedy corresponds with the inner nature of the disease the remedy will not cure the disease but simply remove the symptoms, which it covers; that is, suppress them.

8. The physician must be possessed of a knowledge of the

human desires, must be a reader of human nature, not only as it relates to the sick room but in health.

9. Never prescribe for a chronic case when you are in a hurry; take time. Never give a dose of medicine until you have duly considered the whole case.

10. The most villainous doctors are always hunting for something strange and peculiar. Those out of the way symptoms and strange pains are not what we prescribe or and will seldom serve you. The generals are the ruling symptoms and are what the *patient says*, the individual himself.

11. The more you cultivate Homoeopathic methods, and the finer you discriminate, the better you see, and the more you can understand.

12. When a remedy has benefited a patient satisfactorily, never in your life, change your remedy, but repeat that remedy so long as you can benefit the patient. Do not regard the symptoms that have come up.

13. There are general, common and peculiar symptoms. The general is used in the sense of the general of an army, and the generals command all other symptoms and really control the patient.

Lecture - XXV

The Examination of the Patient (contd.)

The ninety-second paragraph of the Organon throws some more light on the examination of the patient. Let us see what this paragraph tells us. It reads as follows: —

"But if it be a disease of rapid course, and if its serious character admit of no delay, the physician must content himself with observing the morbid condition altered though it may be by medicines, if he cannot ascertain what symptoms were present before the employment of the medicines, — in order that he may at least form a just apprehension of the complete picture of the disease in its actual condition, that is to say, of the conjoint malady formed by the medicinal and original diseases, which from the use of inappropriate drugs is generally more serious and dangerous than was the original disease, and hence demands prompt and efficient aid; and by thus tracing out the complete picture of the disease he will be enabled to combat it with a suitable homoeopathic remedy, so that the patient shall not fall a sacrifice to the injurious drugs he has swallowed."

Let us analyze the above paragraph and then draw the gist of it. We go point by point.

Where

(a) The disease is rapid in its course

(b) And due to its serious character which brooks no delay

(c) The physician has no other go but content himself with the observing the morbid condition

(d) The conditions might have been altered by medicines taken by the patient

(e) Where the physician is unable to ascertain the symptoms, which existed before the medicines were administered

(f) In order that the physician may be able to form and apprehend a complete picture of the disease in its present condition - (here the original malady is complicated by the drugs taken)

(g) Due to the inappropriate drugging

(h) Is generally more serious and dangerous than the original disease and hence demands immediate and efficient support from the physician;

(i) This will help the physician to trace out the complete disease picture, this in turn will help him combat the situation with suitable homoeopathic remedy and get the situation well under control

(j) Thus saving the patient from disease.

The Organon paragraph is stripped down completely by the ten points. Go through them once again, point by point. What is the main point or gist of the above, which Dr. Hahnemann is attempting to hammer into our thick skulls? Think for a moment.

The point Dr. Hahnemann trying to make is, "Malady complicated by drug symptoms is more difficult to either prescribe for or cure than the original malady which is not complicated by drug symptoms."

Now let us go into the lecture and see how Dr. Kent deals with it.

Generally when the patients are with the physician, they always draw the physician's attention to the commonest things. We have seen earlier that there are certain symptoms, which point out a remedy. Can you think what they are? I will tell you - they are the strange and peculiar symptoms of the patient. We have said earlier that the physician must be a good observer. In any particular case, due to the physician's observatory ability, he would have got some points to guide him to the appropriate remedy. Somewhere in the whole process this slips. But the persistent physician brings it back and to the patient this symptom might have been so unimportant. The patient when hears of it tells the physician "well doctor, I always had this and I never thought it would have any significance to my disease." The furious (?) physician asks the patient why he did not tell him this earlier. The cool patient replies "well doctor it is so trivial that I supposed that it did not matter."

When the patients are so confusing, how can the poor physician prescribe properly? All remedies have many ordinary and common symptoms. In such a confusing platform, the physician does not have the guiding remedy and takes chance with several remedies. Now what happens? Think of it. The inappropriate remedies play havoc. The patient comes back uncured, month after month, and year after year. Due to the inappropriate drugs many symptoms are withheld, and seem to be so obscure and so difficult to obtain. Dear friends, these are the very symptoms that the patient thinks are insignificant and trivial which lead the physician to the remedy. What seems to be insignificant and trivial is the very characteristic of the disease. These are the ones essential and necessary for the choice of the appropriate remedy.

Let us look at an illustration. A patient with the following symptoms comes into the clinic:

(1) Pallid face

(2) A rather sickly countenance.

(3) Tired and weary.

(4) Subject to headaches.

(5) Disorders of the bladder and disturbed digestion.

With all the physician's ability of questioning we get nothing that is peculiar. Many symptoms are written down. The patient is not cured and visits the physician month after month; *Sulphur*, *Lycopodium* and many other medicines are administered. By a little more prodding or by observation we find the patient chilly or hot-blooded. We are able to get a little closer, but not have yet hit the target. One day, the patient drops a golden nugget. He says "doctor the urine smells like horse urine." Oh God what a bolt from the blue! Now we know it is *Nitric acid*. We are aghast. We wonder at God's ways of guiding us. The physician asks the patient "well how long have you been experiencing this?" the patient replies " I have had it always; I did not think this amounts to anything relating to my disease." We examine the symptoms of *Nitric acid* and we find all the common things belonging to *Nitric acid* and all the features of the case matched to a 'T'.

The guiding symptom here was "urine smelling like that of a horse". The keynote of *Nitric acid* is also this. Now look at this from other angles.

(1) The urine smells like that of a horse.

(2) Many more symptoms are there in addition to the above.

A remedy is given for horse urine like smell. This symptom will be corrected, but then what about the many other symptoms the patient is suffering with and many other drug symptoms? With a remedy for the first symptom above when cured, the patient will return with the other. The symptoms in our illustrative example

Lecture - XXV

also match with the drug picture. So, along with the first symptom given above, the rest also matching the drug is able to provide a cure. So the physician should see that the selected drug covers the patient's symptom for a complete cure. Use the keynote and see whether that remedy has all the other symptoms the patient has.

In the above case the physician could have as well given Sac-lac, till the right remedy was found. Many a times when we ask the patient specifically what the urine smells like, the invariable reply is, "Frankly I do not know or I have not observed it". But the same patient comes one day or the other and say it was like the urine of a horse. This is because the patient is accustomed to his long-sufferings. Hence they pay little or no attention to the lesser symptoms, which are often the characteristic of the disease. These are decisive in choosing the appropriate remedy.

No doubt ascertaining the symptoms from patients could be a laborious and lengthy process. There is a common belief that educated patients are able to tell their symptoms in the best manner. The ignorant class does a much better job. They do not disguise their symptoms and give out even little details in an excellent manner. Their expressions coincide with the language of our remedies. Our remedies are recorded in simple language to a great extent. This simple language is often observed better in simple-minded people, or uncultivated people. It is not so in the case of an educated or aristocratic persons. These people are not accustomed to think like simple-minded people. This can be observed in our clinics almost every day.

People who are conveniently placed in their lives and those who have more education are more excitable. They have a lot of fear in their minds and consult many doctors. A typical example of this was Mr. X. He had a chronic disease. He was never satisfied with any doctor. He switched on from one doctor to the other. In the process he gained a lot of knowledge about his disease.

Whenever he went into a fresh clinic, he used to rattle out a long list of famous doctors whom he had been to. He would explain his case with as much technicalities as possible to the doctor. What has happened now? Just think. The doctor spent his valuable time and could not ultimately collect any useful material to help him choose a proper remedy. *This is a typical sycotic personality.*

It is with great difficulty that the doctor can bring him around and that too gradually. He has to be opened out very gently to make him roll out his sufferings to the doctor. Plus this he has been drugged recklessly. Such people have spent lots of money for their treatment at various clinics - extremely frightened about their disease - suspicious of each treatment whether it will do him good or not. Because of this, such people go from doctor to doctor. So an intelligent, dedicated homoeopath will handle him like gunpowder. He has to be extremely gentle and unobtrusively collect the symptoms and build a great confidence in such a patient's mind. The physician cannot rush in such cases. At the slightest provocation or the shade of doubt in the patient's mind, the patient will run off to another doctor. Here let me remind that the only mission of the homoeopath physician is to cure the patient - not to drive him away.

Let us look at Organon, paragraph ninety-six. It reads as under:

"Besides this, patient's themselves differ so much in their dispositions, that some, especially the so called hypochondriacs and other persons of great sensitiveness and impatient of suffering, portray their symptoms in too vivid colors and in order to induce the physician to give them relief, describe their ailments in exaggerated expressions."

In this paragraph, Dr. Hahnemann has given us a footnote. It is as follows:

"A pure fabrication of symptoms and sufferings will never be met with in hypochondriacs, even in the most impatient of them -

Lecture - XXV

a comparison of the sufferings they complain of at various times when the physician gives them nothing at all, or something quite un-medicinal, proves this plainly; but we must deduct something from this exaggeration, at all events ascribe the strong character of their expressions to their excessive sensibility, in which case this very exaggeration of their expressions when talking of their ailments become of itself an important symptom in the list of features of which the portrait of the disease is composed. The case is different with insane persons and rascally feigners of disease."

Analysis of the ninety-sixth paragraph of the Organon:

(a) Patients differ much in their disposition

(b) There are some who are hypochondriacs; and some persons of great sensitiveness;

(c) They are impatient and sufferers;

(d) They portray their symptoms in very vivid colors

(e) They have a tendency to greatly dramatize their symptoms in a big way

(f) This they do to gain the sympathy of the physician and to induce the physician to give them relief.

Dr. Hahnemann suggests here that the physician should not be taken for a ride by the exaggerations and over dramatizing of their symptoms of this type of patients.

Now let us slip into Dr. Kent's lectures. Dr. Kent says about this paragraph that there is another kind of patient mentioned here. These types depict their sufferings in lively colors and make use of exaggerated terms to induce the physician to relieve them promptly. This is especially characteristic of the native Irish as a class. They will exaggerate their symptoms, really and sincerely believing that the doctor will give them stronger medicine if they are very sick and will pay greater attention to them. These types of people have a feeling that if they did not exaggerate violently and dramatize more, perhaps the doctor may turn them off by administering some simple remedy.

The next is the group of sensitive persons who exaggerate the symptoms. This is an insane habit and belongs to hysteria. When such exaggerators come to the clinic, the physician is virtually helpless. Homoeopathy seeks the truth, the complete truth only - it is detrimental to get too much or too little. The entire coloring, either by the patient or by the doctor will end in failure. This exaggeration in itself should be considered as a symptom, by itself. Now how will the physician note this symptom in his case taking?

Whenever a patient is found to exaggerate a few symptoms into a large number, just note down in the case sheet as "tendency to exaggerate the symptoms". If you go through our Materia Medica we do find a few medicines for this tendency.

This is misleading and confusing because the physician is not able to determine the symptoms that the patient has and what symptoms the patient does not have. We must know that no person consults a doctor unless he has a symptom. Generally no person constructs a case out of imaginative symptoms and that too to exaggerate the symptoms and the sufferings. No healthy person or sound in mind will do such an act. With this idea well planted in our minds, when a person comes into the clinic, with such a "tendency to exaggerate the symptoms" the physician must take this itself as a symptom. The possibility is that this will be the first and only element that can be considered of that which the patient may utter. Now the physician has a great responsibility. Can you imagine what it could be? Well, the physician is to measure the exaggeration carefully and weigh it with great discretion and wisdom.

"Even the most impatient hypochordriac never finds or invents sufferings and symptoms that do not have a sound foundation. The truth of this statement can be very easily ascertained or

Lecture - XXV

confirmed by comparing the other complaints that the patient conveys at various intervals. The physician must only give him that which is non-medicinal during this period. The physician must not be sentimental, loose his balance or hasty in administering any medicine. The physician will be able to appreciate the wisdom in this advise in the course of his practice."

Dr. Hahnemann's plan was not to give any medicine. He also received and compared the various symptoms that the patient gave from time to time. The practicality of this can be understood by persistently following Dr. Hahnemann's sound advice.

These patients cannot memorize the various symptoms. He collects the various symptoms from other sources but by watching and comparing from time to time, allowing the examination is far apart for him to forget. By comparing the earlier said symptoms and those now the patient tells, the physician can accept those things that he repeats. See the logic behind this. When the patient repeats the same symptoms again and again there must be some truth.

So, the advice for the physician of any age and experience who are misguided by patients of above type is:

"Know something about the nature of symptoms that ought to appear."

We have got one more hidden lesson in the above. Can you guess it? Read the paragraph starting "by comparing the ....there must be some truth. Contemplate - are you able to infer what it is? Well, it is the importance of maintaining records. Do not short list this or under-estimate the value of this.

In the examination of a case, there are several difficulties. One such difficulty or obstacle is laziness. You will wonder how laziness could affect this process.

(a) The patient is too lazy to note down the symptoms as they appear.

(b) The patient not understanding the importance of symptoms in getting his disease cured is too indolent. He forgets to remember it when with the physician. His indolence has taken its toll. His indolence does not permit him to write down the symptoms at home as they appeared.

Something very important is lost here. The patient must be firmly instructed to write down the symptoms as and when they appear. It is wise not to put any reliance on the patient's memory aspect. Human memory fails at the right moment. So the physician must insist the patient to write down his symptoms as and when they appeared - if the patient does not do it, the physician should refuse further treatment. The physician must educate the patient to enter the symptom on its appearance - he must not wait till the night to record the symptom that comes in during the day. The symptoms must be recorded or entered the moment they appeared. They must be written in simple easily understandable English with no technicalities involved. The patient must record his sensations at that time, the location, the time of the day of its appearance and disappearance and also the modalities. The following diagram will also help to a certain extent.

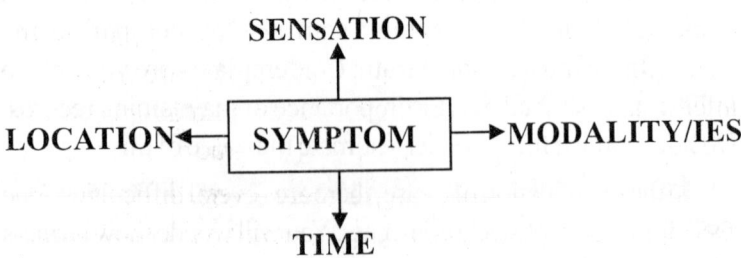

This four-pronged approach of the symptom will go a very long way in finding a remedy for cure.

Lecture - XXV

So, now you see how laziness, indolence and forgetfulness on the part of the patient proves a great obstacle in the process of examination. So, the homoeopath must not allow this default, at any time of his career.

In other aspect, which proves a big hurdle in the process of examination, in fact the greatest hurdle, preventing the patient to speak out his true disposition. Can you guess what it could be? I have given you a big clue; guess what it could be.

The biggest hurdle is the patient's self-modesty and a sense of shame and guilt. A patient came into my clinic one day. He was well dressed and appeared to be a person of the society. He came into the clinic alone. He gave several symptoms. The way the patient spoke appeared suspicious. There was look of guilt in his face and a sense of shame in his mind. All the time he acted like a school-kid who had committed some grave mischief and faced trial. Though you could not place the finger on the pie, one thing was sure - the patient's mind did not permit him to tell the truth and unload his burden.

Sometimes an advertisement is flashed on the television screen for condoms. The customer tells the list of all the items he needs in a loud voice - but when he comes to the item 'condom' he just whispers it to the shopkeeper. This is due to just self-consciousness and false modesty.

So, some patients have a lot of self-modesty and guilt when they acquire a sex transmitted disease. They feel they have committed a big crime not suited to their status. To tell this out is very shameful to them. Hence they do not tell the truth.

Patients deny having been affected by gonorrhoea or having been exposed to similar circumstances. In this society even asking for a condom in a shop, appears to be below the dignity of the customer, as if he has committed a heinous crime. With such false-modesty and shame how will a patient come out openly?

In the early stages the human race was innocent. But now the various guilt and shame have increased from generation to generation. The viles have increased. The result is the self-modesty; sense of guilt and shame has knit itself into the human race. Humility and simple thinking have vanished; ego has become a part of every person. Lust, greed and jealousy have gained control of the human race today to a very great extent.

If these viles had not knit themselves into the human race as a part of life the situation would mean truth and frankness. Under that condition women would frankly discuss their menstrual and sexual problems with the physician without any reservation, with perfect freedom. Even things concerning will and intelligence would have been discussed freely and an easy solution got for all the troubles.

Wait for a moment and think - are the matters so simple today? As a matter of fact it is not so. The physician can draw out these symptoms through mistaken modesty and with great difficulty only.

When the patient visits the doctor, modesty must not be allowed to interfere. It must be laid aside. The most innocent in mind very easily cast aside this modesty. Homoeopathy is based on truth and only on truth. Such innocent people tell the truth and stick to frankness.

The wife must tell everything to the physician about herself and her husband whichever appears to be abnormal. Under such a circumstance the physician has little or nothing to ask beyond listening to the truth. When looking back, many physicians could remember several patients - especially women, who appeared so embarrassed, on their first visit to the physician, having to talk about their symptoms. They forget almost everything. It would have taken several visits to the physician, for them to open up and frankly convey their symptoms.

Sometimes it is very difficult for the physician to make the patient comfortable. Such a case must be patiently handled and

Lecture - XXV

considered carefully. The physician has to ease the patient and gain his/her confidence and slowly bring around the bashful patient. Looking back at your several years of practice, you will realize a great accomplishment of yours.

We have known about many good traits that an efficient and true homeopth must possess. Here we have some more. A physician must have:

(a) A good share of circumspection and tact. A well-known standard dictionary defines circumspection as the ability to look around on all sides, watchfully, cautious, prudent, to examine. Tact, in the same dictionary is defined as adroitness in managing the feelings of persons dealt with nice perception in seeing and doing exactly what is the best in the circumstances.

(b) Knowledge of the human heart, prudence and patience.

(c) Must be able to form a true and complete image of the disease in all its details.

The dictionary defines prudence as wisdom applied to practice attention to self-interest, caution.

Patience is defined as quality of being able to calmly endure.

(d) He must live the life of his neighbor.

(e) He must be known as a man of honor.

(f) He must be believed totally and respected as a candid man.

(g) He must not be careless, lazy, trivial or jocular. The qualities will prevent the physician from going into such a state of homeopathy that will enable him to understand and grasp his Materia Medica or to be conversant and familiar with his science. This will prevent the physician to command the respect of the people or community. Further such a person cannot take a case properly as it ought to be.

Dr. Hahnemann had a wonderful knowledge of the human heart. This is a very important thing - knowledge of the human heart and knowledge of other things in a man.

It would appear there are many men who do not have the slightest knowledge of the human heart. Such people have not traveled into their own interiors, felt their own heart impulses, ever they have just lived their lives wildly. What do we do to know the human heart well? We should constantly examine into oneself and always ascertain what one's impulses are; what one is compelled to do under differing circumstances; what impulses one should control in oneself in order to become a man. Where and when a man has lived according to his heart's desires, without any restraint, he is unworthy of any respect. On the other hand when and where the man had controlled such impulses he is worthy of a great respect. Where a physician practices this constantly, will become well familiar with the human heart. Such a physician will have sympathy knowing fully well what constitutes the language of the affections.

Summary

1. Examination of the patient is one of the most important pillars in finding the cure. This art must be well learnt for being an efficient and successful homoeopath. Our benefactor Dr. Kent has allotted four lectures for this subject. So you see its importance.

2. Paragraph ninety-two of Organon leads us. It says that a disease in its original condition is much easier to prescribe for and cure than when it is complicated by severe drugging.

Lecture - XXV

When the original malady is complicated with the drug-induced disease it becomes extremely difficult for the physician to prescribe for and cure. It may be so serious that it demands immediate medical attention and is very serious.

3. Dr. Kent then goes into the types of patients that one will meet almost every day in the clinic.

   (a) The patients who tell the doctor the commonest symptoms - but out of their utterances it is impossible to get any strange or peculiar symptoms. These are the symptoms that lead the physician to the correct remedy. After several visits this type of patient tells a symptom. They might not have given out that symptom earlier in spite of the physician's asking. But now it comes through. The physician notes it down having a sigh of relief, as he is able to see the light after all. These patients when asked why they did not tell earlier, they say - well doctor, I had it for a very long time and I thought it was not significant to my case.

   (b) There is another tribe. They come to the doctor with an 'I know all' attitude. These are the educated and cultivated people who use high sounding and bombastic words. These can be broken down only in fragments and installments to note down the case. Compared to these, simple folk are very frank and they use simple words making the physician's work much more easily.

   (c) There is another class by itself. Such people jump from doctor to doctor. They know so much about their own disease. Every time they visit a doctor they unroll a long list of prominent doctors they went to. Our current physician spends fairly long time with them and on summarizing finds he does not have any constructive material on his hand that guides to the remedy. Such people are to be handled extremely carefully - they say steel hands covered with velvet gloves - without raising any doubt in the patient's mind. At the very slightest provocation he will run away to another doctor.

(d) There is another group - we can call them a chatterbox type, perhaps. They come to the physician and tell their symptoms in each step, they gain momentum. The entire case is zoomed up to such an extent that the physician gets boggle-eyed and literally reels totally confused. Irish people are considered to be excellent exaggerators!

Now, these types feel that only by giving an exaggerated version of their symptoms a strong dose of medicine to relieve them immediately will be given. Otherwise the physician could turn them out with some simple remedy.

Out of these people, the physician gets only one main symptom - tendency to exaggerate the symptoms.

(e) The other class of hypochondriacs is there they build up their own symptoms and in their own way. They can be handled only in one way. Maintain a proper record from the first day of visit and go on entering what all he says. The physician will find almost everything new and unconnected in each visit - but he will find a few symptoms repeated again and again. Well such symptoms do really exist and the physician has to take cognizance of such symptoms only.

In all the above cases it is wise to give Saclac till the physician gets something that leads to a remedy. In any case of emergency the physician could act most suitable to the circumstance.

This also leads us to a teaching. "Know something about the nature of symptoms that ought to appear."

4. Obstacles that prevent proper case taking are as follows:

   (a) Laziness on the part of the patient. These lazy people do not pay heed to the physician's suggestion that they note down the symptoms as and when they occur. It should contain the location, sensation, time and modalities. The lazy people do not understand the great importance of this. So, laziness is a hurdle to be jumped over.

   (b) Indolence does not permit him to write down the symptoms.

   (c) Forgetfulness — another big fence to jump over. If a symptom is not noted then and there as it appears, due to forgetfulness it gets lost. This is also the case when with the physician. They forget the symptom and hence it is not conveyed.

   (d) False self-modesty — this prevents the patient from conveying his symptoms - more so in case of a sexually transmitted disease.

   (e) Shame and guilt feeling. The patient thinks that it is under his dignity to have contracted a problem, which is always discussed in a hush-hush manner.

   (f) If the physician does not make the patient calm and comfortable and if the patient is not at ease he will not convey the truth.

There is only one way to win over these obstacles. The physician must help the patient to ease out and be fully comfortable and have a lot of confidence in the physician. On many occasion each physician has accomplished this knowingly or unknowingly-just go through your own history and you would be surprised how many times you have done this in the past.

5. Qualities a good and efficient homoeopath must possess:
   (a) A good share of circumspection and tact.
   (b) Humane, prudent and patient.
   (c) Capable of forming a true and complete image of the disease in all its details.
   (d) Must lead a simple life - a life of high thinking and simple living.
   (e) Be a man of honor.
   (f) Be totally believable, and candid.
   (g) He must not be lazy, careless, trivial or jocular.
   (h) Must be quite conversant and quite familiar with his science, Materia Medica.
   (i) He must command the respect of the community by his behavior and demeanor.
   (g) He must be a man of sympathy and have a feeling for the welfare of the community and follow his heart than his brain.

Aphorisms & Precepts

1. It is no proof of man's undertaking to be able to confirm what he pleases; but to be able to discern that what is true is true, and what is false is false, this is the mark and character of intelligence.

   —**Emanuel Swedenborg**

2. Truth, on every plane, is a sword, that wounds deeply and blood flows freely.

Lecture - XXV

3. A truth, on any plane, presented to different men, is accepted or rejected by each according to the good or evil of his mind.

4. Hahnemann's was an unusual life. He was as circumspect as a woman, and that is saying a great deal. He had a duty to perform, and could do it. He was clean, honorable, noble a man of integrity to himself and his family.

5. A physician's attitude in performing his duty to the sick is different from that of any other person. He has a different sphere from that of the ordinary man. This is thousand times amplified in homoeopathy. One who has entertained that peculiar 'circumcision of the heart' always looking to the good of his patient, never thinking of criticism of man, acquires an ability to say what is right to do. He establishes a garment of righteousness.

6. Principle teaches you to avoid suppressions. A homoeopath cannot temporize. Those sufferings are necessary sometimes to show forth sickness in order that a remedy may be found.

7. If you do not make use of your homoeopathy you will lose it. This is a responsibility so great that when one has gone into the truth and does not make use of his knowledge, he will become like Egypt of old.

8. A profane man can have no more idea of sentiments of a gentle, highly religious woman, than can a lobster.

9. Man's unbelief and opinion do not effect truth. The experience, which the homoeopath has, is experience under law and confirms the law and by this order is maintained.

10. A man whose services are worth having can starve in the gutter, in order that he may be good, for the love of his neighbor; and he will acquire this power, this perception. Such a physician may realize what it is to have a duty to perform.

11. The human mind should not be burdened with technicalities. They destroy description, and close the understanding.

12. A physician above all men if not innocent should be anything else but a doctor. A bad man has only one course, vicious ideas of the human heart.

13. Homoeopaths have a conscience of what life is, what the life force is, what the nature of disease is, and can apply to all theories of the world our measure and test them. They can realize the philosophies.

14. In proportion as man thinks against everything, his country, his God, his neighbor, he wills in favor of himself. Therefore this forms man into the nature of his affections.

15. Man today, is destroyed as to his interiors, so that truth looks as black as smoke, and false philosophy as bright as the sun.

16. Never amuse the patient with things that will injure him.

17. Man must keep on plodding as long as he lives. He must be patient and toil on, candid, kind and gentle as a lamb, ready and willing.

18. The more ignorant the physician the more he will do.

19. Don't change the slightest symptom, observe everything. Receive the message undisturbed and get it on paper, there is no other way for a physician to perform his function and do his duty.

20. An inappropriate prescription may be the stepping-stone to breaking down.

21. A man who prescribes from a keynote for everything mixes the case up, and has to wait a longtime to see the sickness as it really is.

22. Hahnemann was always in a state of humility; he never

attributed anything to himself.

23. How is it that bread and meat nourish the human body? We cannot say. How the homoeopathic remedy cures the disease will never be known, but the direction in which life flows into the body and the direction of cure can be known.

24. Belief has no place in the study of homoeopathy. The inductive method of Hahnemann is the only way.

25. Ten years of practice will be a revelation to you, so that you will understand people and their minds. You will almost know what they are thinking and will often take in a patient's constitution at first glace.

26. The body becomes corrupt because man's interior will was corrupt.

27. Positive principles should govern every physician when he goes to the bedside of the sick. The sick have a right to this if it can be had.

Lecture - XXVI

The Examination of the Patient (Contd.)

Two disease images may exist in a body at the same time. This should not confuse one. A chronic patient may also be suffering from an acute disease. The physician may think of considering the totality the symptoms to select an appropriate remedy. If he mixes the symptoms of both acute and chronic disease together, he will be confused. He will not reach the right remedy. What is the way out to the physician? The physician must separate the two. He must prescribe for the group of symptoms that constitute the image of the acute miasm. The chronic symptoms will not of course be present when the acute miasm is active. The reason for this is, the acute disease symptoms will either suppress or suspend the chronic symptoms. Not recognizing the fact, the physician in his enthusiasm, could gather all the symptoms that the patient might have had in his lifetime. On the other hand while collecting the chronic symptoms together it will suffice to just note down the patient had typhoid or measles or other acute miasms. These diseases are not a part of the chronic miasm. The symptoms of the acute are totally separate and by themselves.

Never attempt to prescribe for two distinct miasms. It will end up as an error.

An illustration: a patient suffers from intermittent fever. He has been treated with quinine, arsenic, and low potencies of various other drugs. Can you guess what has happened as a result of this? You are right; the case has become complicated. Naturally the present symptoms would have changed from what existed previously at the beginning stages. The total disease picture is changed now. The physician now looks at the current symptoms - taking it to be a species of malaria. He also antidotes all the drugs that the patient had. Can you now imagine what must have happened? There is a big surprise — the case opens up in the most surprising and wonderful manner. The patient reports after about a week and says, "Doctor, the symptoms at the beginning of the disease have returned. This was how I was".

On investigation, the present symptoms are as follows:

(1) Chill at about 5.00 p.m. with accompanying symptoms.

(2) This chillness lasts over a good portion of night.

(3) His day is well and eventless.

(4) Next day 11.00 a.m. chillness starts.

(5) Next day is a well day and eventless.

Now examine carefully this case. The observation is:

(a) The two chills begin at different places,

(b) The heat of each begin at different places,

(c) The symptoms of the two attacks are totally different.

Two malarial miasms exist in the body at the same time and hence two different sets of symptoms. Each differs from the other. You now see that these two can co-exist. Each one has its own timings and expressions. They do not interfere with each. The big

Lecture - XXVI

doses of quinine can complicate the case and shatter the scene and nobody can tell anything about it.

Now the physician is at a quandary! How is he to handle the situation? Attempting to prescribe the same remedy for both the groups would not help. The physician in such a case, be wise to follow this pattern of action, viz., 1) choose the worst disease first, 2) ignore the other one totally for the time being.

It is not right to give one remedy for a disease and another for the other disease when both co-exist. On treating as suggested above i.e., singling out one and covering it carefully with an appropriate homoeopathic remedy, you can observe the first one disappear. The other one will come on as if the patient had not been given any remedy at all.

It is suggested to go patiently in the case of curing or combating the second one. The patient generally improves after one disease has been cured or removed. The second, which was left alone, will become more and more apparent day by day. After that prescribe for it also and the patient will be cured. Remember - wait for the medicine to take hold and act. Time heals!

The line of action suggested above - when an acute and chronic disease co-exists in the same body is the soundest one and is according to the doctrines, perfectly. NEVER prescribe for any two conditions unless they are complicated with each other. Remember that acute is never complicated with the chronic. Always the acute suppresses the chronic, so they never become complicated, or complex.

The allopaths may talk about the sequelae of measles, scarlet fever, etc.; they know nothing about it and their pathology teaches them nothing, what is true concerning it. We as homoeopaths know that, what comes after all self-limiting diseases have already run their courses is not due to the disease itself. The sequelae of measles or the scarlet fever is not due to either measles or scarlet fever. It is due to a prior state of the patient. A psoric disorder may appear after scarlet fever or measles. This psoric disorder must be treated as psora.

These sequelae, regardless of the disease, which stir them up are psoric. This crop up at the convalescent time and that is the time when the human body is weakest - without much resistance to fight back. We spoke above of treating the acute disease. The better it is treated, the remoter are the chances of any sequelae. When measles and scarlet fever do strike and are treated properly by and large we have very little problems to face afterwards. So, sequelae is only due to the way of the physician handing the diseases. He must be careful and cautious. Sometimes we do come across cases where the constitution happens to be extremely psoric; the decay could have advanced. In case of a malignant scarlet fever in such a patient it is extremely difficult to find a proper remedy - the finest of the physician in the world could make an error. All said and done when a good treatment is meted out properly sequelae need not be anticipated. The sequelae in an improper treatment could be sore eyes, running ears, etc.

From all the above what do we understand? We understand one thing. In such a case or such cases, it is very very important to be able to separate and distinguish one thing from another clearly. As a physician you should know what you are prescribing for. As a rule you cannot and must not prescribe any antipsoric remedy to prevent any sequelae following scarlet fever when the scarlet fever is running its course. Follow what was mentioned earlier. Always in such cases, prescribe initially for the acute attack, and its symptoms. We have also said earlier that it s a wise thing on the part of the physician to know all the symptoms which the chronic patient has. This is so because the physician must know what he is to be expected and wait for the close of the acute disease - wait for the old psoric manifestations to blossom out. Often a new group of symptoms may rear its head.

Lecture - XXVI

At the close of the scarlet fever certain troubles may be seen. The physician must not take it to be part of the scarlet fever itself; he should understand that this is because of the low state of economy. The dropsical condition in Bright's disease must have to be connected with the psoric state. When looked at this in this manner this will lead you to a constitutional remedy. If the physician views it as the Bright's disease, he will be making a grave error.

We have talked earlier about ultimate. Ultimate are the results of the disease - they are not the disease themselves. Ultimate indicate what has happened due to the disease in internal man. We have also spoken of the un-importance of naming a disease. This is done so for only reference or a convenience. If the physician makes a wrong turn and picks up the habit of prescribing for the ultimate, he is deviating from the laws and doctrines of homoeopathy. The physician is hereby warned! So please do not sink in the slush of prescribing for ultimate. You have heard about Bright's disease. You have also known about remedy *Apis*. The book says about the *Apis* that it is a wonderful remedy for Bright's disease, which follows scarlet fever. Do not make a mistake here administering *Apis* for Bright's disease, which follows scarlet fever. The disease is an ultimate of the scarlet fever. Understand this well.

With a little amount of observation and contemplation and persistence any physician can properly see the disease and the ultimate as two different identities. One cannot mistake one for the other. Now you have been once again told what not to do in homoeopathy. Work diligently with confidence following the laws and doctrines. Homoeopathy is a trusted and reliable science when properly followed. No two opinions about it.

I once knew a person who was doing some so-called homoeopathy. Similar persons like him are the ones who make homoeopathy be named a fake science and homoeopaths are quacks. May their tribe vanish from the crust of this world! We will see how these people function.

Such persons commit the grave error by attempting to fit the remedies to the complaints or states of the patient. Look what he does and how he does it. He goes to the bedside of the patient. He already knows what is wrong with the patient. How? Simple - he has dealt with similar cases. He knows what to do and how to handle this case. He knows what remedy must be given because in his last similar case also he gave the same remedy.

Our prayers to God — 'Oh Lord! Forgive these children of Yours for they know not what they are doing.'

We have been repeatedly saying that

(1) Homoeopathy is individualizing all the way.

(2) No two people are alike.

(3) Each one in disease is affected in a peculiar way - no two cases are alike.

(4) Do not treat by the name of the disease - the names for homoeopaths mean nothing.

(5) Treat the man, not the sickness.

Well, my dear brethren, what happened to your basic senses? Have you forgotten the foundations? Go back to your study and refresh yourself. Come back to the world after that; give yourself to the world. Remember this - the world has given you so much, how have you reciprocated? Try and make the place a better place for your brethren because of your presence. This is the principle a good homoeopath has to follow among many others. So knowingly do not commit mistakes. When you do, take responsibility and correct and never, NEVER repeat the same mistake again. Even in the previous lecture we have spoken about the many good qualities that a homoeopath must possess.

Lecture - XXVI

So far we have covered ninety-nine paragraphs of Organon. Now we shall proceed with the other paragraphs and see what we could learn from these paragraphs as well.

Paragraph one hundred of Organon reads as under:

"In investigating the totality of the symptoms of epidemic and sporadic diseases it is quite immaterial whether or not something similar has ever appeared in the world before under the same or any other name. The novelty or peculiarity of a disease of that kind makes no difference either in the mode of examining or of treating it, as the physician must in any way regard the pure picture of every prevailing disease as if it were something new and unknown and investigate it thoroughly for itself, if he desire to practice medicine in a real and radical manner; never substituting conjecture for actual observation, never taking for granted that the case of disease before him is already wholly or partially known, but always carefully examining it in all its phase; and this mode of procedure is all the more requisite in such cases, as a careful examination will show that every prevailing disease is in many respects a phenomena of a unique character, differing vastly from all previous epidemics, to which certain names have been falsely applied - with the exception of those epidemics resulting from a contagious principle that always remains the same, such as small-pox, measles, etc."

Now let us analyze the above paragraph as under:

(a) Epidemic and sporadic diseases called by the same name frequently re-appear in this world.

(b) In investigating these diseases and the totality of the symptoms, it does not matter whether or not something similar had appeared in this world earlier or before.

(c) Always the mode of examining or treating it does not matter either.

(d) The physician must always treat the pure picture of the prevailing disease as if it were un-known and new.

(e) The physician has to do this if he desires to practice medicine in a real and radical manner.

(f) He must not substitute conjecture for actual observation.

(g) He must never take things for granted that the case of the disease before him as already wholly or partially known.

(h) He must examine the disease in all its phases.

(i) When the physician conducts such a careful manner he will find that the present prevailing case is a case of unique order.

(j) They differ vastly from all the earlier and previous epidemics.

(k) Again the paragraph says the disease might have been falsely applied.

(l) Of course there are always exceptions. The paragraph exempts the disease from the above diseases such as small pox, measles, etc. The diseases exempted are those that result from contagious principles, which are the same and permanent at any given time.

Now let us see the gist of this paragraph. The names of the disease do not matter. In case-taking it means much more than that. The physician has to investigate each case as a new one. If he assumes that he had dealt a similar case and he uses the same medicines, he is gravely mistaken. This considering each case as a new one includes the individual case as well as epidemics. Diseases that result from contagious principles are the same and permanent

Lecture - XXVI

at any given time are exempted from the above rule.

Now we shall see how Dr. Kent has handled this in his lecture. He begins his comments as follows:

"With regard to a search after the totality of the symptoms in epidemic and sporadic cases, it is wholly indifferent whether anything similar ever existed before in the world or not, under any name whatsoever."

Dr. Kent wants the physician to hammer this point in their minds. He goes some more steps ahead. He wants the above to be underscored half dozen times with red ink, painting in the wall with big bold letters with an index finger high-lighting it. When the great genius puts so much importance to the above point is it not the duty of the present day physicians to mark it down and make this point their own? Let us learn from the experience of great people. Let us pay heed to their valuable advice.

Dr. Kent has treated paragraphs of the Organon in an exemplary manner. He has highlighted certain points in the course of his lectures. Well, this paragraph is one such. We shall proceed to what more he has got for us!

A physician is to keep out of his mind during the course of the examination of the case, one important thing. He should sheet out any other earlier case that was similar or appeared too similar to the present case. We have seen that one of the qualities to be possessed by any homoeopath is he must be unprejudiced at any stage. If in the present case he muddles up an earlier so-called similar case this will prejudice his mind. The physician's progress across the proper route will immediately be blocked or diverted. The best and the most sincere effort to wipe out the prejudice will be a negative attempt. So, treat each case as a fresh new case. Deal with it on its merits and de-merits. Under this circumstance when dealing with a fresh case deal with it as a new case and work in water-tight compartment as the saying goes.

The physician must examine the patient with an unprejudiced mind. He will have only this case and deal with it with full attention to all details as if that is his only case in life. He will not be distracted. Never, NEVER work with a remedy in your mind. The drug picture will haunt you so much that the mind will be prejudiced and confused. This may even prove fatal. It is always a good principle to take down the case in black and white. Once this is done examine it carefully in relation to the remedies. Where the selection is between three or four remedies get back to the patient and now see which one of these three or four remedies match the patient very closely; choose it.

We spoke earlier that fitting the remedy to the patient is against homoeopathy laws and doctrines. But under the above circumstances only the physician is permitted to fit the remedy to the patient.

It is most important to get all the symptoms down on the paper. Once this is done analyze the symptoms and search for an appropriate remedy. Why must be the sickness analyzed thus? What is its importance? Once all the details about the disease are collected the analysis is made. This process will reveal peculiar symptoms that will relate to remedies. Let us elaborate this a bit further. Sickness in each individual has something peculiar according to the person. These are strange and rare. We will be wondering at these things - these are the very things that must be compared with the remedy and which are peculiar to remedy. This knowledge is very valuable than an extensive knowledge of a morbid anatomy. Knowledge of the symptoms and understanding the nature's language is a great asset. Learn the following principle well: 'we ought to regard the pure image of each prevailing disease as a thing that is new and unknown, and study the same from its foundation, if we would really exercise the art of healing'.

Lecture - XXVI

The physician as we have repeated several times in our earlier lectures must have a great ability to perceive what constitutes the miasm. What happens if the physician is not alert and perceives - if he is dull of perception and careless? The physician would not be clear in his judgment and intermingle symptoms that are not belonging together.

Dr. Hahnemann was a person of wonderful perception. He was able to perceive things at a glance. Every physician should constantly sharpen his perception diligently and constantly practice perception. Dr. Hahnemann has developed his skills. This was possible because he was a hard student of Materia Medica. The homoeopathic adage goes as follows:

"Read and learn a remedy daily from the Materia Medica - on Sundays learn two remedies".

Dr. Hahnemann examined the remedies carefully - he virtually saw them, he felt them and he realized them. How many physicians are so conscentitious and so dedicated to homoeopathy, today? No wonder Dr. Hahnemann was so successful.

Learn well the following: "Never substitute hypothesis in the room of observation, never regard any case as already known."

Now we understand why it does not make any difference whether a physician has seen a similar disease before or not. The homoeopathic physician is very well acquainted with the signs and symptoms of the man and a different disease is only a change in the combination of them - only a change in their manner, form and representation.

Every sickness has an order within itself. It is the responsibility of every homoeopathic physician to find that order. The homoeopathic physician is always alert and hence need never be taken unawares.

Summary

1. Two diseases can co-exist in a body, at the same time.
2. A chronic patient may also suffer from an acute disease at the same time.
3. The symptoms of both should not be mixed together.
4. The acute disease will suppress or suspend the chronic one.
5. Keep the acute case symptoms totally separate.
6. Never try to prescribe for two distinct symptoms.
7. Consider the expressions and timings as two distinct features in two diseases.
8. Never administer two different remedies for two different diseases at the same time. Single out the one first and treat it. After it disappears wait for some time and treat the other one.
9. The above principle is same to all cases where two diseases co-exist.
10. Under proper care and attention there cannot be any sequelae.
11. Sequelae are psoric in nature regardless of the disease that stirred it up. Sequelae crop up at the time when the human body is weak and at the time of convalescence.
12. Acute diseases are never complicated. Chronic diseases can be complicated with each other.
13. In case of sequelae what comes after the self-limiting disease is not due to the disease since such a disease would have already run its course and exhausted itself.
14. Where the constitution is already psoric and decay has advanced, finding a remedy under that condition is extremely difficult.

Lecture - XXVI

15. The physician should know and be aware of what he is prescribing for.
16. Do not prescribe any anti-psoric, to prevent a sequelae when the disease is running its course.
17. The physician should always know the chronic case symptoms well and have the disease picture clear in his mind. Only then he will know what he is to expect.
18. Bright's disease must be connected with psora. This will be the proper way.
19. Ultimate are the results of the disease - they are not the disease themselves. Learn to see the disease as disease. Ultimate are not to be confused as diseases.
20. Do not fit the remedies to the diseases, or the complaints.
21. Treat each case as a new case. Let not your experience or any previous dealing with a so-called similar disease interfere here. Keep it at bay.
22. Certain homoeopathic principles are given in this lecture. The names of the disease does not matter; case taking is beyond that. Each case should be treated as a new case. The physician must not allow his previous experience interfere in the case taking and of the selecting of the appropriate remedy in the present case. Each epidemic is also taken up as a new case. Diseases, which originate from the contagious principles, are treated as the same and not as new cases.
23. Regarding the search of the totality of symptoms in epidemics and sporadic cases, it is wholly indifferent whether anything similar existed before in the world or not under any name whatsoever.
24. Earlier experience of handling a so-called similar disease must not contaminate or confuse or dilute the present case-

taking. This may prejudice his mind. He cannot come at the right remedy with a prejudiced mind.

25. Never approach a case with a remedy already in your mind. This also will prejudice the decision.

26. Fitting of a remedy to the case can be done only in one condition. If after proper case taking we arrive at two or three or four remedies, then we can see whether any of the chosen remedies can fit the case. The remedy, which fits most closely will be the selected remedy.

27. Capacity to understand the nature's language and a perfect knowledge of the symptoms of any disease is a great knowledge. It is better than knowing more about the morbid anatomy.

28. Learn the remedies well enough till you are very well versed with them. They must be literally able to speak with you - not appear as lifeless print in a book or sheet of paper. Feel them in all their properties. You must be able to touch them. **Realize they are your friends and treat them with love and respect. That is how Dr. Hahnemann was familiar with the remedies. So, be dedicated to them.**

29. Learn well the following: "Never substitute hypothesis in the room of observation, never regard any case as already known."

30. What a sound advice. Constant practice will teach you the importance of these suggestions; your case taking would just become much more easier.

31. The homoeopath knows that a change in the combination of the man, yes only a change in them or in their manner form and reputation is disease.

32. Nature has clamped orderliness in every sphere. This is true in the case of sickness also. Every homoeopath must find

that order. A physician is always alert and he need never be taken unawares.

Aphorisms & Precepts

1. The more idols a man has the less able is he to receive the truth.
2. So long as man is capable of believing that diabetes is disease, and that Bright's disease is a disease, so long will man be insane in medicine. His mind is only directed towards the results of disease.
3. You must see and feel the internal nature of your patient as the artist sees and feels the picture he is painting. He feels it. Study to feel the economy, the life and the soul.
4. Every ignorant man thinks that what he knows is the end of knowledge.
5. It is the imperfect machine that causes death. The Vital Force is the Soul, and cannot be destroyed or weakened. It can be disordered, but it is all there.
6. Throw aside all theories, and matters of belief and opinion, and dwell in the simple fact.
7. You must be able to recognize every ambassador of the internal man.
8. The physician must see and feel, as the artist does his picture. He must perceive, by his knowledge of the human heart, that good woman's state whose religious melancholy he could not otherwise understand.
9. The personal stamp is upon every disease and upon every proving, and the individual must be permitted to stamp himself upon the disease as well as upon the proving.

10. There are no two things alike in the universe. This is so of diseases and of sick people, of thousands of crystals of the same salt. No two stars are alike. When this thought presents itself to the mind of the physician, he can see that no remedy can be a substitute for another.
11. A disease may be suppressed by a medicine as well as by a stronger dissimilar disease.
12. Homoeopathicity is the relation between the symptoms of the patient and the remedy, which will cure.
13. One sick man is to be cured, not the disease.
14. Man must be studied as he is, as he was, everything of man and of the human race in general, in order to understand disease.
15. One, who is not acute in observation, goes through life, seeing only indifferent similarity. Most men only know only the toxic power of a drug.
16. Individualization is blocked by this inability to distinguish between the finer features of sickness and of medicines.
17. The whole aim of homoeopathy is to cure.
18. It is inconsistent and irrational to think that there are several active diseases in the body at the same time.
19. Perception comes with use.
20. The quiet, silent manner of perception is to be cultivated.
21. The physician must be sober, candid to receive.
22. It is all-important to see the remedy in its nature as a sick being.
23. If you think names you will think remedies, you cannot help it.

Lecture - XXVI

24. Any physician with pathological notions in his head, if he finds no organic disease, is apt to think his patient is sick only in the imagination.

25. The prejudiced mind is not content to write down simple facts and symptoms but says, "I will examine the organs and parts, and see if congested or inflamed, and then I shall know what to do."

26. We must think what makes the patient sick; not what causes changes in his liver, kidneys and his other organs.

27. The physician is not called upon to cure the results of disease, but the disease itself. All pathological changes must be regarded as the results of disease since all disease is dynamic.

28. We cannot see all symptoms in disease. We can see the expression of the face but cannot know what that represents. There is nothing in the outer man that does not have its beginning in the inner man.

29. Don't change the slightest symptom, observe everything. Receive the message undisturbed and get it on paper; there is no other way for a physician to perform his function and do his duty.

30. How dare you meddle with that image? How dare you meddle with those symptoms? There is intelligence at the end of the wire.

31. It is the same if the physician prescribes for this and that group of symptoms. Avoid this, for it is not healing the sick.

32. Sickness exists on varying planes. Acute diseases occupy an outer plane and do not take so great a hold upon the life. The chronic diseases reach what we may call the innermost potency of man.

33. Two sick people are more unlike than two well ones.

34. The physician cultivates his eyes for everything that it is possible to pass judgment upon and must write down everything that is unnatural, everything that is expressive of illness.

Lecture - XXVII

Record Keeping

A physician should always endeavor and cultivate the habit of knowing thoroughly acute as well as chronic miasms. First of all the picture of psora must be mastered from all the symptoms that we can gather about it. Where can we gather all the symptoms covering psora? Dr. Samuel Hahnemann has already done the spadework for us and recorded his collections in his book, "Chronic Diseases". Similarly we proceed with syphilis. We collect as much symptoms from the books, from clinics, from observations and all other possible sources that could be thought of. Then an anamnesis is conducted for sycosis. Once these are collected and learnt well, the images of the three basic miasms will be vivid in our mind. We will be able to recall these images whenever we need or feel like reviewing them. Now, herein we have a grand picture of the miasms tormenting the human race from time immemorial.

We have spoken a lot about psora in eighteenth and nineteenth lectures under the heading chronic diseases. If we recall those lectures or refer to those lectures we can clearly see that psora is the very foundation of human sickness. It would even appear as if the human race is an enormous leper. Add to this syphilis and the picture is grim and the entire scenario has changed from bad to worse. Now to this muddle add sycosis. See what you have got on your hand, now? We have a picture indicating the extent of human disease or sickness.

The next step is to proceed to the acute miasms. Again what is the procedure to be adopted? Yes, the same process as above. We get the information from books, from observation making use of every channel and source that could provide us with more and more information. All the information, thus gathered must be very carefully noted down in a paper in such a way that recalling would be easy. Moreover just the thinking of the list must be able to bring the image of the miasms vividly on the mental screen without missing a point. What we mean here is, so much love and labor should have gone into this process that it becomes a part of you.

Smallpox features are few and can be easily brought to the mind. Similarly with acute miasms, infectious diseases, cholera, yellow fever, etc. The disease that has up to now appeared either in an epidemic or endemic form must be covered like this. At a snap of the fingers the images must flash boldly and vividly in the mental screen. It may be said of them that they all are true diseases seen by examination based on the totality of the symptoms.

We can find the old books deal exhaustively and clearly through symptomatology, the images of the disease. This is the best way of collecting information. Most of the patients either do not convey their symptoms in nature's language or on occasions some physicians do not allow them to do so. Many times the patient goes on telling his symptoms and this interferes with the physician's prescription writing. Whatever the reason the mission of case taking has proved futile.

There are many clinics nowadays who are able to say what remedy was administered, when and for what symptom. This they do very methodically. Come to think of it. At the outset it may appear a wasteful exercise. A clerk noting such details in one place — call it by any name you like as ledger, case sheet or even in the computer now a days.

Lecture - XXVII

There are several reasons - all-important ones - for keeping records — and also referring to them frequently. A homoeopath is a compassionate and considerate person. Let us see how this record keeping and the above qualities of the physician play a very important role.

A patient has stuck to a particular homoeopath for three or four years continuously. The doctor has maintained a complete record of this patient from day one of his visit to the clinic. Entries are made at every visit details of his symptoms then, remedies given or Saclac, details about any fever the patient might have had etc., etc. Now the patient has been brought out of the woods - but still he is not cured. In that condition assume the patient for some reason visits another homoeopath. This compassionate and considerate physician to whom the patient went for the past four years is worried - not worried because of loss of revenue from the patient. He is genuinely concerned about the welfare of this patient. He is worried how the other homoeopath can proceed further with the treatment without knowing the background of the case till then. This is on the part of the physician who has hitherto attended upon the patient. Now think of the other side of the river. The homoeopath, if a conceited person will jump at such an opportunity and grab the patient for what he is worth, and will proceed to add to his bank balance.

There is also another possibility — when the patient parts company from the earlier doctor and goes to another homoeopath. The new doctor is a very conscentitious person. What will he do? The moment he understands the patient wants to come to him, he will 1) feel concerned for the patient 2) feel the responsibility towards the patient and also the ex-physician thus - the ex-physician has done proper work and maintained perfect record of every step of the case. This goes to prove that he has done so much good to the patient. So there is no reason for the patient to desert his previous doctor and consult him or come for treatment to him. Such a conscentitious physician will very gently and unobtrusively and in the least offensive manner suggest the patient to be with the previous physician.

In a chronic disease the physician must always feel his duty to serve the patient on the basis of treatment.

We all know about ships and aeroplanes. Have you ever stopped to think for a moment how a ship or aeroplane reaches one place from another? Yes, navigators navigate them. But how do the navigators do their jobs? They have compass to direct them. Will the compass alone be sufficient to reach the destination? They need a chart and then the most important thing called rudder.

For a homoeopath and his patient a record of the progress or degress is shown by the chart or record sheet. At any given time it will give out the medicines or remedies administered. So without a proper record, you are in a sea of confusion, without a compass or rudder.

Dr. Hahnemann says, "he can then study it in all its parts, and draw from it the characteristic marks." So, this helps for the physician to have the nature of the disease continuously in mind. Once the image of the disease has passed from the mind, its very nature is gone. Pay heed to the advice of the master. Maintain proper record. This also helps the physician to review any case at any particular time.

There is one other angle to this. In a particular case the physician has made a prescription and administered a remedy on a particular date. There is an aggravation. Unless it is recorded how will you know about this at a later date - how severe it was and how long it lasted — what happened after this, etc. Perhaps there might have been no change at all. There might have been some change, if so what changes came in, how it came about, when it came about, what happened after this, etc. must be recorded. Now we know how the disease has proceeded. This will also indicate to the physician how to proceed further. If there are some changes, which come and go no medicines can be administered. This is because such symptoms cannot guide anyone as what to do.

Supposing a commotion has occurred. When the commotion has occurred and is running its course, no medication can be done, because the symptoms are changing place - they come and go, may be one to three weeks after the administration of that medicine. Remember and follow the rule 'wait' and watch. The next dose of medicine need be given only when the symptoms do no reappear or set in order. Such conditions come to play after an administration of a pretty high remedy, that is high enough to take hold and when the case falls into order. That is the time the patient needs another dose of remedy.

A patient had several symptoms running for a period of say three to four years' visits the town. He comes from outstation and he has become worse. The homoeopathic physician is called in. Under these circumstances what is the physician supposed to do? The physician gives a dose of remedy and the patient becomes better. After some time the patient wants to know the remedy and writes to the physician. The doctor remembers that he attended on him but forgets the case and does not remember what it was. What a shameful and confusing situation? Now you see the importance of maintaining proper records?

Dr. Kent was in contact with another staunch homoeopath in a far away place. Whenever there was need for any patient to go out of town to that place where the physician was, Dr.Kent used to send a report of all the treatment afforded to that person to be carried to the other physician. Similarly the other physician also reciprocated this action with his patients. Now, both the physician's were staunch homoeopaths following practice in the footsteps of the master and interested in the welfare of their patients. Just contemplate - what a marvelous condition and co-operation! All these things are nothing but in the pure interest of the patient's welfare and towards some contribution to the science. It is the duty of any physician to furnish such details when the patient leaves the city to go under the care of another physician. It is the duty of the physician to direct the patient to an efficient physician wherever and whenever possible.

The maintenance of proper records is a preliminary step in practical homeopathy.

Summary

1. A physician must always be fully familiar with acute and chronic miasms.
2. Details are to be gathered from all available sources - be it books, clinics observations, etc. This must be done for all the general miasms, psora, syphilis and sycosis.
3. The physician must have a vivid, detailed image of all the miasms and it must be stored in the mind in such a manner that it could be brought to the mental screen at a flash.
4. Psora is the fundamental miasm and if psora were not there the other two miasms would not have been ushered.
5. The same procedure is to be adopted for acute miasms as well. This holds good for epidemic or endemic diseases.
6. Record keeping is a very important feature of homoeopathy. This helps to review any disease at any given time clearly giving us the progress of the disease, remedy administered, the after effects, progress and decline of the disease, etc. It also helps the physician to plan his course of action at every step. Records are like compass and rudder for ships.
7. Always wait and watch the action of the remedy. When a commotion is underway do not administer any remedy. Once

Lecture - XXVII

having given a remedy go for the next dose only when the earlier symptoms are set to order.

8. It is the duty of any proper physician to provide the record sheet whenever the patient is going out of town or so. It will help the other physician to proceed further for the benefit of the patient.

9. Maintenance of proper records is the preliminary step in homoeopathy practice.

Aphorisms & Precepts

Aphorisms and precepts relating to record keeping could not be found. Hence some selected at random are given below.

1. When derangement localizes itself upon one particular place it is for the purpose of tearing that organ all to pieces. If it sets up a discharge, that is a sort of safety valve and the other organs are protected.

2. In vaccination when a new disease comes on, the former is suspended during the time, and comes on again even though the crust had not formed. This is related as most wonderful, but this the homoeopath understands. Syphilis makes symptoms of scrofula to disappear the same way and after mercury subdues the syphilis, then the scrofula comes back. One occupies some hidden precinct in the economy while the other is active.

3. Structural changes are not the basis for a prescription, but the symptoms, which existed before the structural changes appeared.

4. We see the difference between short and long acting remedies from this. Short acting remedies are only capable of corresponding to the outermost degree of man.

5. When a case comes back in a few days with all symptoms changed, unless they are old symptoms, the prescription was inaccurate and unfortunate.
6. In old incurable cases, when we give a remedy that fits the whole condition the result is one of three things - first aggravation of the symptoms with the advance of disease, second no action and third Euthanasia.
7. When we recognize the fact of the long years of existence of chronic cases also that they are often inherited for several generations, if a cure is made in the course of two or three years, it is a speedy cure. It takes from two to five years to cure chronic diseases. (See the importance of record keeping?)
8. There are general common and particular symptoms. The general is used in the sense of the general in the army and the generals command all the symptoms and really control the patient.
9. The most natural thing to do is to remove external obstruction, but anything that comes from within must be treated from within.
10. Confusion comes from losing one's head, prescribing on few indications and giving medicines when no medicine should be given.
11. The increase of conditions show increase of sickness, the increase of symptoms often shows diminution of disease.
12. There is a plane of nutritional and a plane of dynamics. The normal individual who receives it on the plane of nutrition appropriates common salt, but the sick one who needs it eats it constantly and it does not make him well because he needs it on a higher plane.
13. When Hahnemann speaks of disease it would seem to be limited to disease activities.

Lecture - XXVIII

The Study of Provings

The first portion of the Organon contains the doctrines in general. From this lecture onwards that knowledge can be put to practical use in Homoeopathy. This covers the oldest established rules and principles. At this stage, it is better to refresh us, with these doctrines. The first is the theoretical aspect of Homoeopathy. The next step is practical application. In this stage we make use of the earlier knowledge and study the sickness in the homoeopathic way. This method is totally different from the study of sickness in our old school. But until this time, the doctrines have not revealed their main objective. It becomes obvious only when we reach the third step. The third step deals with the use of Materia Medica.

How is this study of sickness conducted? We take you back to our previous lecture. The symptoms are gathered from our sick patients. We have also seen in our earlier lectures that the symptom is the language of nature, which indicates the existence of the sickness. The totality of symptoms constitutes the nature, quality and all there is to know the disease completely.

Now how are we to apply these principles and arm ourselves with sufficient ammunition to combat human sickness? In the old school, we are aware that there is no plan fixed for acquiring the knowledge of medicines except by experimenting upon the sick. Dr. Hahnemann condemns this practice. He says it is dangerous. It subjects the human sufferers to many hardships due to its uncertainty. This system has been in vogue for more than a hundred years. There has been no principle or method to help in curing the sick. The proving was made without a study of the disease. As a contrast see how Dr. Hahnemann worked. He worked out and built the Materia Medica, then examined the patient and checked up the drug picture with that of the sickness. But now a days, Homoeopathy has been established. So is the Materia Medica, and the examination of the patient precedes the examination of Materia Medica. Yet they go hand in hand for study purposes. Dr. Hahnemann would really be turning in his grave because of the present day practice!

Think of the conditions that existed at the time of Dr. Hahnemann. There was no Materia Medica. Dr. Hahnemann had to build one. At that time, there was no proving, none to examine, etc. Are we not blessed doubly and lucky? We have the instruments before us to examine; we have the proved remedies.

Dr. Hahnemann was disgusted with the old school method. Children were sick. He was terribly affected and sad about this. He placed his faith on the Providence and prayed for these little children. He was of the conviction that the Good Lord had not brought them into this world to suffer and then to be made worse by the violent medicines. Dr. Hahnemann tuned his mind towards God and sought for the solution. Dr. Hahnemann reached a state of acknowledgement of his ignorance and that man's own opinion did not matter and must be cast away. This realization made him humble and he also acknowledged the Divine Providence. It may not be out of place here to state that Dr. Hahnemann was always in a state of humility; he never attributed anything to himself.

When a person is in a state of humility his mind is thrown open. When a man is in a position to trust him, he makes himself a God; he makes him the infallible; he looks to himself. When the state of humility is not there, his mind is closed. He cannot see beyond himself. When a man realizes within himself that he is nothing and just a failure, he blossoms out like a flower. Numerous examples can be given. So, always remain in a state of humility and be receptive. The very opposite of this state closes your mind; you are turned away from knowledge.

You can see drop-outs in schools, in career, etc. Dr. Kent in his years of teaching experience has seen many people who dropped out of Homoeopathy study and practice. They were all in some degree or other capable of practicing the science. Yet they did not do so. He made a small research on this. He always noticed that such a dropout had no humility. This was so in all such cases.

When one turns his attention into self and relies upon self, closing his mind, his mind is deprived and closed to the avenues of knowledge. He also looses the power of clear perception. We have been repeatedly impressing that a homoeopathic physician must perceive. He must develop this faculty by diligent and constant practice. If his mind is closed to this avenue how can he do it?

Man has the capacity to think. This is his greatest asset. If not used properly or unused, this very same great asset proves to become the greatest liability as well. We will see how, presently. Sailing in the path of least resistance is the natural way of living. Our navigator in this boat is none other than the Providence Himself. When a man pulls himself from this stream he becomes discontented and unhappy with him. His ego and pride shoots up. He forgets his humility. He becomes headstrong. A man must be governed by the mind not by his brain. We had a professor in our college, a very well read person. Often he used to advice the students to be with the Providence and be governed by their minds. He used to say, "A man who is governed by his brain will always be a successful scoundrel."

So once the man looses his natural balance, in our context, feels he is the master of everything and knows everything. He feels there is no need for him to study further or refresh what he has studied. Today almost everything is progressing by leaps and bounds. What we read in our younger days about fifty years back in stories has become a reality today. Remember those childhood stories where the witches used to see what is happening in the world in a magic mirror. Remember the picture of a witch traveling to the moon on a broomstick. They were stories for our fathers and us. But now a reality for us! We have them in the form of Televisions, Rockets, electricity, etc. They used to say that whatever we have studied is just a fistful of sand but what is to be learnt is as big as the world itself. Remember whatever materializes in this world is what existed already. There is nothing new. Only man could not see it. Providence helps or plans this materialization as and when he thinks is the right time. Man by himself is absolutely helpless and cannot lift the smallest thing unless Providence wants it to be so.

We were talking about things progressing by leaps and bounds. Whatever was 'something' today morning is already obsolete by the evening. The new entry is also pushed back and something new emerges. When things are like that, so fast, a man has to be constantly on his toes and keep track of all progress only by widening his knowledge constantly. He cannot feel he knows everything. He has got to be an eternal and constant student. This opening up can occur only when one realizes the absolute power of the Providence and totally surrender himself to that power. Come on now, adopt total surrender and see how you glow in His care.

We have now seen what self-conceit can very generously offer us. Do you not feel it is a wrong attitude and you are blinded? You are unable to use the means of cure and that means we cannot get properly acquainted with the Materia Medica.

Lecture - XXVIII

We have been talking so much philosophy above. What has prompted us to do it here? Close your eyes and think for a moment. This lecture hitherto looks like a theological lecture, not a homoeopathic philosophy lecture. Are we trying to convert the homoeopath physicians into clergymen? In our earlier lecture XXV, we have outlined some of the qualities a good homoeopathic physician must possess. In addition to this list we have also mentioned about this subject at various lectures. Refer to all these and contemplate. In addition meditate on this aphorism: "You cannot divorce Medicine and Theology. Man exists all the way down, from his innermost spiritual to his outermost Nature."

Now you are able to see what we are driving at? A homoeopath and a clergyman have to be pure, always in a state of humility and a state of innocence. They do not do anything that will label them "conceits". The persons who have dedicated to the cause of science are those who are in the greatest degree of simplicity. They are the most wise and the most worthy. These people had to struggle tremendously to keep self under control and thus they have reached this state of great simplicity.

What does knowledge do to a man? Sit quietly for a few minutes and think. Extensive knowledge makes a man simple. A fully filled pot will not splash or spill. This knowledge makes him simple and gentle too. Extensive knowledge makes a man realize how little he knows and he is only a speck in the ocean. On the contrary look at a man who is not well read but read all the same. His little knowledge makes him gibber around like a monkey. He shows off and tries to impress people around. The lesser he knows the more he tries to show himself off as a bigger scholar. We have seen such personalities in many places. Have people not looked at such persons disdainfully. They need our sympathy.

The person who feels he is only a speck in the ocean, so small and practically invisible is the one who knows more. You can be certain about this. To achieve this he must be a constant student, learn from all possible avenues, keep himself always in a state of gravity, in a state of thirst for knowledge and in a state of innocence. Such a person will never say, "Oh that thing? I know it fully well and I am the authority in that line."

An incident in my college days comes to my mind. In those days my mind was interested in electronics - Transistors were yet to make their appearance - and mechanical/electrical gadgetry. I had plans for a multi-filament bulbs, clock controlled electric switches for gadgets and a light coupled typewriter keyboard. I had made several experiments - but could not perfect any of them! I went to a National Science Research Institute to see how far I could go with these. The co-ordinator I met was a motherly looking old lady. I spoke to her and she saw all my drawings and put me on to another person. He also spent some time with me and made his own notes. He retained my drawings etc., and sent me away. I was in a room with another employee of the same research institute. I told him of the day's happenings. He told me to collect my drawings etc., the next day and not to speak of items with anyone - he said people there were so capricious that they will grab the ideas but use it as their own. They were jealous and greedy.

Why I brought it down here is because, in this scientific world jealousy and hatred are very prevalent. But then are they real and good scientists working for the benefit of the society. They cannot be. A real scientist, or people who will control this upsurges of the mind alone are fit to be real scientists and enter the field of Homoeopathy. He must be innocent. He must be willing to learn from all sources and in all opportunities wherever truth flows. Once a person reaches this frame of mind a physician could go ahead into the study and examination of the Materia Medica.

Remember here, each scientific man today is trying to find something he can claim as his own. Such a man cannot understand

Lecture - XXVIII

Homoeopathy. He worships himself. Has dwelt on the externals so long that it is impossible for him to think rationally.

Dr. Hahnemann did not have a Materia Medica to start with. He had to build one up all by himself. He could not go to books, read and meditate upon them to find the remedies and compare with the images of the human sickness. There was no study material available to Dr. Hahnemann. He had to build up the Materia Medica from nothing. What a frustrating experience it ought to have been to know that this knowledge was not available on the face of the earth. He earnestly felt that a true and pure Materia Medica must be formed. It had to be formed by observing the action of the remedies upon the healthy human race. He started the trials on himself. The first proving was his taking the Peruvian Bark and noting down the effects upon himself. The Peruvian Bark or Cinchona or China was thus the first homoeopathic remedy to be born.

Dr. Hahnemann searched as many literatures as possible to know more about the effects of China that had been discovered accidentally. He compared notes with these points and the effects of China on himself. He accepted those points, which were in harmony. China closely resembled the intermittent fevers. China had most abundant relation of similitude to intermittent fevers.

From the above, a question arose into the mind of the master. Can it be possible that the law of cure is also the law of similar? If that were so, can similar cure sickness symptoms when they correspond to drug symptoms? This law got more and more reinforced and appeared more and more definite by each drug that was proved thereafter. Thus each remedy was proved and one by one our Materia Medica was built up. This was known as Hahnemann's Materia Medica Pura and Materia Medica of the chronic diseases. Just imagine the voluminous work and the labor involved in compiling it. This work was very thorough. Many additions have been made to it since then by many other stalwarts of Homoeopathy.

The best way to study a remedy is to make a proving of it. How are we to do it? We select a group of healthy members. Each member would take a dose of remedy. For a week each one would note down all the symptoms he or she experience, very carefully and methodically. The present condition and the condition many months back is noticed, examined and listed properly. Then the entire group once again combines the list and referring to each other's symptoms experienced they make a comprehensive list of the symptoms they experienced which are in harmony. From the group symptom we treat it as a single person's symptoms and now we have the complete and through picture of the drug or remedy.

In proving, a master prover is decided upon by the group. He will prepare the substance for proving. The other provers will not be informed of what the substance is. He puts into a vial the first or earliest form of the drug. This could be the tincture or 30th potency. Each prover is given a vial of this. They do not know what the substance is. They make their own notes of the symptoms each one experience. They are requested not to compare their notes with others. Nor do they discuss their experiences with the others. Each one notes down the reaction to this substance on their own chronic symptoms - they note down whether that symptom is cured; or exaggerated; or whether interfered or not; without being increased or diminished, it may be looked upon as one of the natural things of that particular prover. But when it occurs on the natural way all natural things of the prover are eliminated.

Let us assume this substance takes a marked hold of a prover. Generally all his chronic symptoms will subside. When the hold is only partial it may create a few symptoms. These few symptoms are added along with those the other of provers experienced, will be considered to draw the chronic effects of the drug. So, now we have the effect of the remedy upon the human race.

Lecture - XXVIII

We will presently see the method followed. Each prover gets his vial of the substance, from the master prover. One single dose is then taken and waits to see its effect. Where the prover is sensitive, to that particular drug, a single dose will produce symptoms. Such symptoms must not be interfered with and allowed to progress or decline in their own way. The instructor knows about the medicine. So in an acute remedy like *Aconite* he may inform the group that if any effects do appear because of this drug it will happen in the next three or four days. It is not necessary to wait for a longer time in the case of *Aconite*. Consider certain other remedies - like *Nux vomica* and *Ignatia* might require a longer time. Anti-psorics like *Sulphur* will need a much longer time. When proving *Silicate of Alumina*, the class will have to be informed to wait at least for a period of thirty days. This is because its prodrome period runs to about thirty days.

Homeopathic laws are natural. The human race has either forgotten or has batted an eye about these natural laws. But the animals and children have not done so. Watch a cat - it patiently waits and watches before catching its prey. Watch a crane - this also waits very patiently for the fish. This waiting and watching is an important aspect. One cannot overlook this. In Homoeopathy this is a very important trait to be adopted and followed - after all it is but natural. We have spoken about this in our earlier lectures. Go back and refresh what is said there. Refer back to lecture XXVI. We have mentioned about this in some other lectures also.

In our very early lectures we have mentioned about each disease having a prodromal period, period of progress and period of decline in acute diseases and only prodormal period, period of progress in chronic diseases.

The homoeopathic remedies also have a picture. This drug picture corresponds to the disease picture if the disease is to be cured by that remedy. From this what is it that you are able to draw here under the present contest? The remedy also has its own disease picture and this picture is proved in the provers or proving of each remedy. That means the drug-induced disease should also possess a prodromal period before it gives out symptoms. Keep this in your mind.

From the above two paragraphs, we are able to surmise that in the proving of a remedy it should be allowed its prodromal period of taking hold and acting. It is very important and also basic to wait until the possible prodrome of any given remedy definitely elapses. In short acting remedies the action will come in faster.

Here the stress is made on the following: When studying the Materia Medica and the miasms, one must always bear in mind the prodromal period, period of progress and the period of decline. You may as well go back to lecture V and refresh yourselves on this.

In the proving classes, the master will usually be able to indicate the waiting time - whether short or long. This is better available for it will tell the prover when to take the next dose. This instruction will help the class also to know whether the drug taken up by them for proving is acute or chronic.

Let us assume that the first dose has been taken. It has not produced any effects or symptoms in spite of having been given the time to act. Now what does this situation mean to you? The possibility that can be drawn out of situation is that the prover is not sensitive to the remedy taken up. What do you do then? Do you remove the prover from the group? If done so, you loose a prover - getting another prover might not mean much - but you will have lost a lot of ground, which is not worth it. Then what do you do with this insensitive prover? Simple - Create the suitable conditions and make him sensitive to that remedy.

Let us have a look at the effects of poisons. Assume a person is poisoned by Rhus. After this poisoning, such a person becomes many more times sensitive to Rhus poisoning, than before. Similarly

Lecture - XXVIII

consider a person poisoned by Arsenic. They become extremely sensitive to Arsenic after that first effects wane away. However, if they continue to keep on with the initial effects, then sensitivity to it reduces. Under such a circumstance the dosage has to become progressively larger and larger to take effect. This is a common rule with the poisonous substances, which affect the human system markedly.

Now, we get back to the class of provers. This particular person knows he was not sensitive to the remedy, since he has not reacted to the medicine by means of a simple dose. Here, we should also make a note of one point - In a proving group of about forty provers there will be only one or two persons who can make the proving from a dose of thirtieth potency. What are we to do now? We can do two things to make the proving and to intensify the effect. Dissolve the medicine in water and have the insensitive person take a dose of this every two hours for the next twenty four to forty eight hours. Stop this administration the moment symptoms arises. How does this solve the solution? The prodromal period is hereby shortened. The frequent administration of the remedy appears to intensify the effect. Now as soon as the symptoms start coming out, further administration of the medicine becomes unnecessary.

You may feel whether this is proper and no danger will come out of administering a remedy this way. It is perfectly o.k. Then where and when does danger lurk around? It is dangerous to take the remedy for a few days and then stopping the remedy; then again start taking it after a few days.

We shall take the case of *Arsenicum*. We find the prover not sensitive to it. You wait for thirty days nothing has happened. He is given *Arsenicum* in water for three or four days. The symptoms emerge. Now wait. Nothing will happen so long as it is discontinued. The symptoms have started to emerge and now you wait. Wait till the *Arsenicum's* effect wears off. Allow it to come and wear off by itself. Never interfere with it. If at all there is any interference it must be only to truly antidote the *Arsenicum*. At this point do not interfere with the process by giving another dose. This will be a most dangerous thing.

The *Arsenicum* symptoms show, say in about a week or few days. You prefer to do this better and more thoroughly. So you give more *Arsenicum*. See what happens now. The *Arsenicum* diathesis is engrafted upon the prover's constitution. This diathesis can never be cured. You have broken right into the cycles of that remedy. It is a very dangerous thing to do. Do you realize this? On rare occasions this error has crept in and those provers who were unfortunate victims had to carry the ill effects of proving throughout their life. What a sorry state of affairs! So, now do not give another dose of the medicine during proving without waiting.

If left alone, this Arsenicum effect would have passed off leaving the prover better after it. Earlier it was mentioned that when a medicine takes hold the symptoms would be removed. This shows that when a proving is conducted properly it will improve the health of anybody. The disharmony is set right and things are set to order. Hahnemann suggests that one should make several proving.

There is another set of people in the class. Such people will not get any symptoms, no matter however bad the remedy is abused. If it were *Arsenicum* only a crude dose can bring in some effect. When you see the symptoms they are only the toxic effects. But then this cannot help the proving. The toxic results of poisons are proving of the grossest order. Here, we do not get finer details. An example for this could be had from *Opium*. *Opium* is administered in large doses it immediately poisons. Only the grosser symptoms like the stertorous breathing, the unconsciousness, and the contracted pupils, the mottled face and the irregular heart. Now look at the above a bit closely. These symptoms do not provide any finer details. All that is given out is only common things. This does not serve our purpose.

Then comes reproving of the remedies. This is of a very great value. In those days the Vienna Society did not endorse Dr. Hahnemann's proving fully. The Society refused to accept that it was possible that such wonderful sensations of the people could be revealed. Dr. Hahnemann had selected the 30th potency for his proving. The society was not in agreement with this potency. So, this society decided to test the 30th potency. The society was an honest one. Remedies like *Natrium mur.*, *Thuya* and others were proved. It was found that symptoms gathering from 30th potency were very strong. The Vinenna Society tested and reproved the polycherts of Hahnamann and fully proved them. The *Natrium mur.* 30th potency proving was a great revelation. But one person Mr. "S" was prejudiced right from the beginning. He was gracious to acknowledge that he was wrong. But he continued to use potencies lower than the 15th potency. Mr. "S" prejudice was so strong that he could not accept 30th potency. Dunham says that though they were able to obtain better results they could not accept the 30th potency. Dunham humorously commented about this non-yielding tendency as - "they are ossified in their cerebral convolutions as well in their bony structure". In other words he meant that their minds were so set and inelastic they could not accept to expand. The mind is closed and hence the understanding.

Paragraphs 107 to 112 of Organon are now explained. We quote below each paragraph:

Paragraph 107: "If, in order to ascertain this, medicines be given to sick persons only, even though administered singly and alone, then little or nothing precise seen of their true effects, as those peculiar alterations of the health to be expected from the medicine are mixed up with the symptoms of the disease and can seldom be distinctly observed."

The gist of the above paragraph is as follows: —

In proving we must select only healthy persons. The reason is this. If a sick person is chosen and the medicine to be proven is taken by him, true results cannot be had. The reason is that along with the symptoms of the remedy to be proven, the existing sickness symptoms may also mingle and hence the true proving cannot be done.

Paragraph 108: "There is, therefore, no other possible way in which the peculiar effects of medicines on the health of individuals can be accurately ascertained - there is no sure, no more natural way of accomplishing this object, than to administer the several medicines experimentally, in moderate doses to healthy persons, in order to ascertain what changes, symptoms and signs of their influence each individually produces on the health of the body and of the mind; that is to say, what disease elements they are able and tend to produce, since, as has been demonstrated in paragraphs 24 to 27 all the curative power of medicines lie in this power they possess of changing the state of man's health, and is revealed by observation of the latter.

Dr. Hahnemann gives a footnote to this paragraph. He laments that other than Albrecht von Haller no one else had thought of this natural, absolutely necessary and the only genuine mode of testing medicines for their pure and peculiar effects in deranging the health of man to learn what morbid state each medicine is capable of curing.

The gist of this paragraph and read along with the footnote tells us one important thing. Dr. Hahnemann says that the only sure way to ascertain or prove the real power of medicines is to administer them in moderate doses to healthy persons. Observe the bodily and also mental symptoms they produce in the humans to ascertain their curative powers. In Homoeopathy the curative power of the remedy is its power to bring about a morbid change in the prover's health when the medicines are given in minute doses.

This paragraph also refers to the drug proving. Please review the above paragraph once again and understand it.

(1) Administer the medicines in moderate doses.

(2) Administer them only to healthy persons.

(3) Wait and observe the actions of the remedy.

(4) Though he says as moderate doses initially he comes down to minute doses at the end. (Here remember the Homoeopathic law of curing - gentle permanent cure with minimal dose; so this minimum dose must be a minute dose.)

Paragraph 109: "I was the first that opened up this path, which I have pursued with a perseverance that could only arise and be kept up by a perfect conviction of the great truth, fraught with such blessings to humanity, that it is only by the homoeopathic employment of medicines that certain cure of human maladies is possible."

The above paragraph has two footnotes; one says that there can be no better way than homoeopathy to cure all diseases. It is as simple or as impossible to draw more than one straight-line between two given points. True homoeopaths and followers of Dr. Hahnemann should educate the people on this. The second footnote refers the papers wherein his observations were documented and recorded.

The gist of this paragraph is that Dr. Hahnemann is conveying the idea and the fact that he was the originator of homoeopathic drug proving. The discovery was made with a lot of perseverance. He also says that maladies can only be cured by homoeopathic way.

Paragraph 110: "I am, more-over, that morbid lesions, which previous authors had observed to result from medicinal substances when taken into the stomach of healthy persons, either in large doses by mistake or in order to produce death in themselves or others, or under other circumstances, accorded very much with my own observations when experimenting with the same substance on myself and other healthy individuals. These authors give details of what occurred as histories of poisoning and as proofs of the pernicious effects of these powerful substances, chiefly in order to warn others from their use; partly also for the sake of exalting their own skill, when under the use of remedies they employed to combat these dangerous accidents, health gradually returned; but partly also, when the persons so affected died under their treatment, in order to seek their own justification in the dangerous character of these substances, which they then termed poisons. None of these observers dreamed that the symptoms they recorded merely as proofs of the noxious and poisonous character of these substances were sure revelations of the power of these drugs to extinguish curatively similar symptoms occurring in natural diseases, that these pathogenic phenomenon were imitations of their homoeopathic curative action and that the only possible way to ascertain their medicinal powers is to observe those changes of heath medicines are capable of producing in the healthy organism; for the pure, peculiar powers of medicines available for the cure of disease are to be learned neither by any ingenious, a prior speculations, nor by smell, task or appearance of the drugs, nor by their chemical analysis, nor yet by the employment of several of them at one time in a mixture in diseases; it was never suspected that these histories are first rudiments of the true, pure Materia Medica. Which from the earliest times until now has consisted solely of false conjectures and fictions of imagination - that is to say, did not exist at all."

The gist of this paragraph is: —

Dr. Hahnemann speaks here about the poisons. The physicians have recorded the pernicious effects on healthy individuals. These could have been taken by them either accidentally or to commit suicide. Dr. Hahnemann found that results of his own experiences or these poisons on himself coincided with the previous records already recorded by these physicians. The experience of Dr. Hahnemann also included himself and various other healthy individuals.

Those physicians did seldom realize at the time of their recording the facts that they had unknowingly recorded the curative properties of the poison when given in small or minute doses.

The curative power of medicine of any remedy cannot be ascertained by speculation, smell, taste, appearance or chemical analysis.

Paragraph 111 reads as under: —

"The agreement of my observations or the pure effects of medicines with these older ones - although they were recorded without reference to any therapeutic object —and the very concordance of these accounts with others of the same kind by different authors must easily convince us that medical substances act in the morbid changes they produce in healthy human body according to fixed, external laws of nature, and by virtue of these are enabled to produce certain, reliable disease symptoms each according to its own peculiar character."

The gist of this paragraph is: —

"It was said earlier that the obnoxious effects recorded by the physicians also agreed with those recorded by Dr. Hahnemann. From this we can surmise that the medicinal substances produce some morbid symptoms according to their peculiar character, in healthy persons."

Paragraph 112 reads: —

"In these older prescription of the often dangerous effects of medicines ingested in excessively large doses we notice certain states that were produced not at the commencement, but towards the termination of these sad events and which were of an exactly opposite nature to those first appeared. These symptoms, the very reverse of the primary action - see paragraph 63 of Organon - or proper action of the medicines on the vital force, are the reaction of the vital force of the organism its secondary action - (see paragraphs 62 - 67), of which, however there is seldom or hardly ever the least trace from experiments with moderate doses on healthy bodies, and from small doses none whatever. In the homoeopathic curative operation the living organism reacts from these only so much as is requisite to raise the health again to the normal healthy state - refer paragraph 67."

The gist of this paragraph: —

In paragraph 112, Dr. Hahnemann gives us the differential actions of massive and moderate doses.

What or how will a massive dose affect the humans? Dr. Hahnemann tells us that in administering a massive dose it was always adverse to the vital force. This is also called the counter-effect or after-effect of massive doses. Now when medicines are administered in moderate doses the medicines will produce the primary action on the vital force, just sufficient to restore the body back to its normal health. In this case, there is no secondary action. Please refer to paragraph 62 - 67 for refreshing yourself on the primary and secondary actions.

Now, we will see what Dr. Kent says about these paragraphs of the Organon.

The poisonous influence of a drug does not appear to flow in the direction of his life action. But when the reaction comes in, the poisonous influence, which have been lingering flows into the vital action stream. The symptoms arising there from are the best ones. So it is necessary and important to take such a portion of the drug that will just disturb and at the same time will not suspend since it will flow into the stream of vital order, in the order of the economy. It must be capable of establishing a symptom, without suspending

Lecture - XXVIII

any action; similar to a larger dose of Opium we talked about earlier.

Whenever a suspension of the dynamic economy occurs the activities of the economy gets be-clouded. Taking this point in our mind administering a large dose of any remedy to palliate pains and sufferings is not advisable and is dangerous. When do we have a suspension? A suspension of the vital order occurs when a medicine is administered which does not flow into the stream of vital influx.

Homoeopathic medicines administration is done for only one purpose — for healing or curing - in higher purposes. In lower potencies they disturb. Crude drugs are never restored to proving. They are to be used only for momentary or temporary experimental purposes. Crude drugs should not be followed up. We cannot attach any importance that is made out of crude drugs proving. This can give us only a vague or fragmentary idea. The proving that where those from strong doses get added with the smaller doses is to be taken into account.

Certain prescription suggests using a particular potency for the primary effect of a drug and another potency for the secondary effect of the same drug. This is not needed. In many apoplectic cases homoeopathic drugs have saved the patient from death. In some cases there have been patients with flickering pulse, eyes glazed, countenance besotted, stertorous breathing coming on, frothing at the mouth. In such cases *Opium* CM. has been administered - the patient has gone into a sound sleep, remained quiet and rests. Woke up to consciousness and were well on the road to recovery. *Alumina* also has a similar state of stupor resembling apoplexy. Hence *Alumina* and *Opium* becomes antidote to each other.

There was an apoplexy case, which was puzzling many physicians. The patient was found in a profound stupor. The previous physician had administered *Opium*. It stopped the stertorous breathing, but the patient could not regain consciousness. A close investigation revealed that one half of the body was paralyzed and not moved for several days. That side also had fever. The other half was well and there was no fever in it. The natural condition of any paralyzed part is coldness. Here in this case the paralyzed portion was having a fever - not the usual coldness, and the other half was normal. Here this fever was unusual or peculiar. Going through Materia Medica carefully *Alumina* was found suitable to the case. *Alumina* in high potency was administered - the fever subsided on the paralyzed side and the patient became conscious.

Summary

1. The first part of Organon is dedicated to the Homoeopathic laws and doctrines. The other portion gives out the practical application of the laws and doctrines.
2. The language of nature is the symptoms. The totality of the symptoms gives us the true picture of the sickness.
3. The examination according to Dr. Hahnemann is to precede the Materia Medica.
4. Dr. Hahnemann had no Materia Medica. He built one slowly and surely.
5. Dr. Hahnemann was aggrieved to see young ones suffering. He prayed to Providence for their well being and knowledge to combat their sufferings.
6. This taught him to be always in a state of humility and attributing everything to the blessings of Providence.
7. By the constant state of humility Dr. Hahnemann opened his mind to knowledge.
8. When one turns his mind into self and relies upon self, closing

his mind to the external impressions, his mind is deprived and all the avenues for knowledge is closed.

9. Man must always be in league with Providence - more so when he is a homoeopath.

10. The first proving done by Dr. Hahnemann was on himself with Peruvian Bark — (or *Cinchona off.* as we call it).

11. One by one he proved himself and also with a band of his sincere followers. Materia Medica pura and Materia Medica of the Chronic Diseases were born. These form the instruments we have, to examine.

12. Proving is done on healthy humans. Proving done with crude medicines is not to be taken into account. For each proving the prover has to wait for its prodromal period. There must be a group of people to prove - both males and females. Each one makes a note of the various symptoms they experience. Then the entire group of provers meets together and where the notes coincide with, all are compiled. These group symptoms are taken as an individuals' symptoms, and that is the Drug Picture. It is recorded properly. All use the same potency.

13. Some of the provers may be insensitive to the drug and will not show any symptoms. Then the remedy to be proved is mixed in water, administered every two hours or so for 24 or 48 hours. This is stopped as soon as the symptoms emerge. They are noted down in their true form.

14. In a group of forty provers there might be only two people who may start the symptoms as per the gestation period. Others may not show out any symptoms. The frequent administration of the remedy shortens the prodromal period. The intensity of the medicine is increased.

15. In certain cases people may interfere with the symptoms once it emerges. It is not right. To make the drug induced symptoms better further doses might be introduced or administered. This may engraft a Drug diathesis in the system and there may be no cure for it. The prover may have to suffer throughout his life.

16. There is still another group of provers wherein no symptoms could be seen from potency. Then the administration of the crude drug alone may bring about some symptoms. They will only be toxic effects. These are of the grossest order and are useless for proving.

17. It is good to re-prove the remedies. We get confirmation of earlier records.

18. A short acting remedy is acute, longer acting is chronic.

19. In proving each prover must be true and record the symptoms as they are. The group must not compare notes in the absence of the leader. It should be compared together.

20. The conditions for proving a remedy are:

    (a) Administer medicine in moderate doses

    (b) Only healthy people are taken as provers

    (c) Wait and observe the actions of the remedy — do not rush in to administer further doses

    (d) The moderate dose could also be the minimal dose capable of bringing out symptoms.

21. Dr. Hahnemann was the first one to assure that the homoeopathic remedies could cure human maladies. People have to be educated on this.

22. Many physicians recorded the effects of poison. In certain doses they did not kill, but brought back the health.

Knowingly or inadvertently these people had made notes. These have proved useful. Dr. Hahnemann's notes have also coincided with these.

23. When homoeopathic remedies are administered in such qualities to react with the human organism they restore the health.

24. Massive doses are adverse to the vital force, always. This effect is known as the counter-effect or after-effect of massive dose.

25. Where the medicines are administered in moderate doses, they are able to produce the primary action on the vital force in just sufficient quantities and is able to restore the health back. Here we need not think of the secondary effects of the remedy.

26. Whenever a suspension of the dynamic economy occurs, the activities of the economy are affected. A suspension occurs when a medicine, when administered, does not flow into the stream of vital influx.

27. There is no need to give one type of potency for primary effect and another for the secondary effect.

28. While administering a medicine and in case-taking do conduct a careful investigation and seek for unusual peculiar symptoms.

Aphorisms & Precepts

1. All susceptible provers will bring out the image of the remedy. The prover catches the drug disease from one or two doses just as people do Scarlet Fever or the Grippe.

2. Never leave a remedy until you have tested it in a higher potency if it has benefited the patient.

3. There are degrees of fineness of the Vital Force. We may think of the internal man as possessing infinite degrees and of external man as possessing finite degrees.
4. You cannot count twenty-five decent proving since Hahnemann. They leave out what they call imagination and put in morbid anatomy.
5. The finest degrees of sensation are to be perceived for these changes constitute the nature of the disease. If drugs could not produce these changes they could not cure. This is the foundation. If you would discover whether the law of similar is the law of cure you would need to draw upon this store of finer symptoms.
6. It is only after a careful and complete study of the finer proving of drugs and the same of the finer features of the diseases that a law can be demonstrated.
7. There is much more to be learned about disease from the medicines, because disease is more obscured by the culmination.
8. The word disease really means the signs or symptoms before organic disease has taken place.
9. The lower potency corresponds to a series of outer degrees, less fine and less interior than the higher.
10. In acute miasms the whole disease is found in one individual, in chronic miasms this is not so.
11. We potentiate to render the remedy simple enough to be drawn in by the influx of Vital Forces.
12. Lower potencies can cure acute diseases because acute diseases act upon the outermost degree of simple substances and the body. In chronic disease the trouble is deeper seated, and the degrees are finer, hence the remedy must be reduced

to finer or higher degrees so as to be similar to the degrees of chronic disease.

13. Hahnemann was always in a state of humility; he never attributed anything to himself.

14. Here we have on the one hand, the action of disease upon the healthy and on the other hand the action of drugs upon the healthy. We find one a duplicate of the other. Is this not peculiar?

15. Every action in homoeopathy must be based on a positive principle.

16. The one who understands the nature of these remedies will remember most about their peculiarities.

17. The remedy pervades the economy silently and completely with its prodromal period; then comes the evolution of the disease, which runs its course.

18. It is worse than useless to give a second dose until the effect of the first dose has ceased.

19. If you can feel in your old age that the well proved remedies are all your friends, you should feel a state of humility that you are an instrument of such service.

Lecture - XXIX

Idiosyncrasies

Idiosyncrasy is defined in our dictionaries as below:

Chamber's Twentieth Century Dictionary: Peculiarity of temperament or constitution; crotchet or peculiar view, any characteristic of a person.

Practical Glossary of Medical Terms: Peculiarity of temperament of an individual e.g., a susceptibility to a special drug.

Gould's Pocket Medical Dictionary: Individual peculiarity.

The usual explanation for idiosyncrasy is an oversensitiveness to one or few things. Dr. Hahnemann speaks of idiosyncrasy in paragraph 117 in his book of Organon. We shall see what he has got to say about it. The paragraph is reproduced below - then our usual analysis and the gist of the paragraph follows.

Paragraph No. 117 reads as: —

"To the later category belong the so-called idiosyncrasies, by which are meant peculiar corporeal constitutions, which, although otherwise healthy, possess a disposition to be brought into a more or less morbid state by certain things, which seem to produce no change in many other individuals. But this inability to make an impression on everyone is only apparent. For as two things are required for the production of these as well as all other morbid alterations in the health of man - to wit, the inherent power of the influencing substance, and the capability of the vital force that animates the organism to be influenced by it - the obvious derangements of health in so-called idiosyncrasies cannot be laid to the account of theses peculiar constitutions alone, but they must also be ascribed to these things that produce them, in which must lie the power of making the same impressions on all human bodies, yet in such a manner that small number of healthy constitutions have a tendency to allow themselves to be brought into such an obvious morbid condition by them. This shows that these agents do actually make this impression on every healthy body, that when employed as remedies they render effectual homoeopathic service to all sick persons for morbid symptoms similar to those they seem to be only capable of producing in so-called idiosyncratic individuals."

Now let us analyze this paragraph:

(a) Idiosyncrasies — the persons who are in this state have peculiar constitutions. By and large they are healthy to a certain extent. They slip into more or less morbid state, which appears to create no impression, or any change in many other individuals.

(b) The inability or failure to make any impression on everyone is just only apparent.

(c) To create a morbid condition two things are necessary — the power of the influencing substance and the capability of the vital force to suffer the influence's pressure.

(d) The peculiar constitutions alone are not responsible; the things that create them as well are responsible, as these possess the power to create this morbid condition on all human bodies.

Lecture - XXIX

(e) Yet only a small number of people are affected though they have a healthy constitution.

(f) Such agents do affect all healthy people; it is revealed to us by one fact — when employed as remedies in homoeopathical method they are very effective to cure the all-sick persons.

(g) This curing occurs because they possess the same symptoms of the sick, though they are capable of affecting only the idiosyncratic persons.

In the beginning of the paragraph a reference is made to 'latter category'. What are this latter category people? It is those persons who belong to the explanation given under 'a' in the analysis of the paragraph.

The overall idea is to convey what idiosyncrasy is and how that affects the different constitutions with different susceptibilities.

To elaborate the above a little more: some people otherwise healthy are peculiar in certain ways in their constitutions. Such persons get affected easily whereas these things do not affect other healthy people. These people are susceptible to some morbific agents.

Two things are needed to create disease symptoms in every person — the medicine must be having the capacity to influence and it must be able to influence the vital force. The morbid symptoms are obvious in a small percentage of people and not seen outward in the rest. It does not mean the substance does not have the power to affect all and does so only in a small group. The inherent power is evident from the fact that when a homoeopathic dose of that remedy is administered to all sick people it works, when the symptoms and the drug picture agree.

An example provided by the master is, some are morbidly affected by the smell of a rose. Different things similarly affect some others. Some do not exhibit any morbid symptom at all. This is idiosyncrasy. Some are susceptible and some immune.

Before going into the lecture let us gather some more knowledge about idiosyncrasy. Dr. Kent in his Lesser Writings says: "this term is used by allopaths to define a special hypersensitive state present in a particular patient. Some people are more irritable for certain drugs. For want of a better term or explanation idiosyncrasy is used for susceptibility. Disease does not exist in the absence of idiosyncrasy.

Now let us turn our attention to the lecture.

Homoeopathy and idiosyncrasy are clearly related. Idiosyncrasy is an over-sensitiveness to one or a few things. It is not the same as general susceptibility in feeble constitutions. Therein the patients are susceptible to all things and also over susceptible and over impressed even by simple annoyances. The old school related the idiosyncrasies to certain patients known to the physician as over-sensitive. Such oversensitive cannot be given Opium for his pains, due to the congestions it produces, because of dangerous symptoms. Due to the patients oversentiveness to the drug and even a small dose complicates, the physician is compelled not to administer it. Some other patients cannot tolerate quinine for his chills and fevers. The primary action of quinine makes the patient terribly sick. The same quinine can be given even in 15 grains to some other patient without any problem. One who is idiosyncratic to quinine cannot take even a quarter grain of quinine without any over-action of it. This is known as quinism.

A homoeopathic physician has knowledge and can recognize a wide range of susceptibilities. There may be a chronic idiosyncrasy due to a chronic miasm and an acute idiosyncrasy from acute miasm. In every community there are many people who are susceptible to the hay fever at the slightest provocation, many cannot bear the smell of flowers and fall sick, some become sick

Lecture - XXIX

smelling a rose. This affection due to rose is known as rose cold or rose fever. Dry lavender flowers and a few other things in her room affected a patient. She used to go about searching for these items in her room. Another patient used to have diarrhea because of peaches in her room. The reason for stating all these here is to know the importance of susceptibility of only a small number of people. Others are not affected similarly. We can also infer their susceptibility to the remedy that will cure. Where an idiosyncrasy is absent, then the patient will not be susceptible enough to be cured. The patient's sensitivity to the drug to cure him is very analogous to the idiosyncrasies mentioned above. Think about susceptibility man has to the remedy that cures him in high attenuations.

Idiosyncrasies are congenital as well as acquired. Idiosyncrasies of congenital variety and those resulting from poisoning are very difficult to cure. Take Rhus tox poisoning for example. Those who handled Rhus tox and as a result got poisoned are very sensitive to it. If they go within a quarter of a mile from the vine, in a few days they will come down with Rhus poisoning.

A very high potency of Rhus tox, in this case may sometimes remove that susceptibility. They may need a dose of *Rhus tox.* CM or MM and this may check the acute poisoning. But in the case of a congenital idiosyncrasy to Rhus tox, Rhus tox doses may palliate the person a few times; finally even that will cease to act. Such congenital idiosyncrasies are very tenacious and will persist in spite of our very best endeavors. They will persist to the end of the victim's life. If at all it could be eradicated, this could be achieved by only the use of an anti-psoric.

Hay fever comes around and is supposed to be caused due to the over-sensitiveness of the patient. This is due to the irritants that develop at that time. It is attributed to the hay, which lies in the fields after cutting, and sometimes to the weeds that grow during that season. They may be able to drive out the things that they are susceptible to. What is at the bottom of all this? It is psora - yes, psora is at the bottom of these idiosyncrasies.

Often idiosyncrasies develop in patients who have just come out of typhoid fever. The chronic miasms are responsible for these. In scarlet fever psora is prior to the sore eyes. We have already talked about sequelae in our earlier lectures. Kindly go back to lecture XXVI and refresh yourselves. These are all miasmatic and also the out-cropping of chronic miasms.

There are persons who are sensitive to all things - over-sensitive to high potencies, over-sensitive to smell, oversensitive to taste, over-sensitive to light and several others. This is a constitutional state and the patient is born with it. In some cases we cannot observe this sensitiveness. It is not in the nutritional plane.

Some people crave for common salt at the dining table. They need or desire a lot of salt, yet eating so much salt does not appear to satisfy them. They consume a lot of salt, remain sick. They grow thinner and thinner all the time. We mentioned in above paragraph about nutritive plane and the dynamic plane. Here in this case what we see is the nutritive plane wherein the patient takes crude form of common salt along with his food. To such a patient, what happens when a dose of CM potency salt is administered? The patient will become sick and there will be a violent aggravation.

In the above, we see food sustaining a curative relationship upon a higher dynamic plane. We have seen that the human race, when diseased, is affected in the dynamic plane. The cure also lies in the same plane. So when potentized common salt is given as a medicine in this patient, salt now enters from the nutrition plane to a dynamic plane. Human diseases can be combated only at a dynamic plane since they are also dynamic force.

Remember that 'the dynamic plane is more interior or above

Lecture - XXIX

the nutritive plane; it presides over it and commands it. This is the plane of proving.'

We will see another instance i.e. Calcarea. We have seen many infants withering and emaciating for want of calcium. An allopathic physician may provide calcium to these infants in various ways - an example is lime-water in milk. The more lime water they are given the less bones they make. These are the children who are slow to form the bones, and teeth, fontanalles taking a very long time to close. The allopath has administered calcium in an improper form. Here bone salt inanition and non-assimilation of lime is the problem. The allopath is attempting to combat in a nutritive plane, all the time feeding lime in crude form.

Now a single dose of very high *Calcarea* will promptly help the child assimilate all the lime it needs from the food it takes. The remedy has been given in a dynamic plane.

This causes the proper digestion of the food and assimilation of the lime from the babies' food possible. See, from nutritive plane to dynamic plane.

We see in such non-assimilating patients *Calcarea* or *Natrium mur.* could be indicated. An intelligent physician can always locate which one is needed. Now, we are well aware that a CM potency medicine of lime can build bones in a body. But then why was this administered which culminated in what we wanted? The answer is this. There is no mystery or miracle behind this. What has happened is that the internal disorder has been corrected. This is resulted in causing outward forms of body to get into order. Look what is the principle to be learnt in this. The correction of the internal disorder established or establishes that the nutritive principle from internal to external.

By all these, we can see the wider ranges that idiosyncrasy and susceptibility has in the field of homeopathy. This is the same what we meant in an earlier paragraph that a homeopathic physician has knowledge and can recognize a wide range of susceptibilities.

A new word is coined - it is 'homoeopathicity'. Let us see what this word means and elaborate on it. Homoeopathicity means the relationship between the homoeopathic remedy and the patient who has been cured. We have administered a homoeopathic remedy to a sick person. He is cured by that medicine. See what has happened. The appropriate homoeopathic remedy has acted properly; it has cured the patient; this has proved that the remedy was related to this case. This relationship when sustained is called the homoeopathicity; i.e., its homoeopathicity has been demonstrated amply.

We have normal homoeopathicity, a normal state and an exaggerated state, where the patient is oversensitive to the curative remedy. Then it only establishes a curative relationship but before this state the patient's symptoms are exaggerated. This condition is called an exaggerated state. The similitutde of any remedy is its capability to cure. It is known as simillimum, a remedy appears to be similar before it cures. The same remedy is known as the simillimum once it has cured.

Now we shall consider the difference of a crude poison taken in the nutritive plane and the same poison taken in the dynamic plane. The poison upon the nutritive plane is not very deep, is more superficial, and relates more to external things, to the body tissues. The poison taken on the dynamic plane lasts a lifetime. The miasms also possess the same nature. Poison taken upon the nutritive plane may have a life-long effect upon an individual. This is because of the person's susceptibility. Let us take up the case of Arsenicum. Small does of Arsenicum will establish in the individual arsenicum poisoning. It will last his lifetime.

The same Arsenicum is administered in the dynamic plane. The drug is given in a higher potency. This sinks much more deeper

Lecture - XXIX

than the nutritive plane. Only when the patient is susceptible can the higher potency affect thus, in dynamic plane. In the nutritive plane susceptibility is not required. Any individual can be brought under the influence of poison when it is given on the nutritive plane.

There is another difference. Inert substances and the substances we can use as food on the nutritive plane may very well be poisonous on the dynamic plane to such individuals who are susceptible. In such individuals no substance can be exempted as non-poisonous, in higher and highest potencies. For them in those potencies all substances are poisonous. So, these are the distinctions between crude and dynamic poisons. Remember these distinctions well when you think or work on poisons, and idiosyncratic persons.

We have talked so much about idiosyncrasy and susceptibility. Stop for a moment and assume that no idiosyncrasy or susceptibility existed in this universe. Can you see the condition of the universe or the human race? Simple, there could be no sickness. When there is no sickness can there be homoeopathy?

The foundation of all contagion and all cures is susceptibility. Susceptibility has been dealt earlier under our lecture XIV. It is strongly suggested that you go back to that lecture and refresh yourselves. Then proceed further with this lecture.

We can see that the cause and the cure, the cause of sickness and the cure of sickness have the same target. It is the humans. They flow in the same direction due to the simple and immaterial substance. When disease is in a primitive substance or first substance the cure of the disease must also be in the simple substance. That is homoeopathy. In olden days it was thought that all substances capable of extinguishing the vital force or whichever overpowered the vital force were all poisons. That itself was a very crude idea of poison. Poison is one which can impress itself upon an individual's economy to cause death or capable of creating a disorder to the human economy. This definition of the poison applies to both dynamic and crude poisons.

Poisons present an external as well as internal problem. Quantity affects the external and the quality affects the internal. In the dynamic plane it is not the quantity but the quality that affects. Crude substances are considered by weights and measures.

Set your thinking on these lines. This subject leads one to the study of protection as well. Man is protected from sickness by homoeopathy and its use. There are many physicians and nurses who have sacrificed many things in their life and dedicated themselves to serve the patients of yellow fever, typhoid, diphtheria, small pox, etc. They are extremely busy in their work. They have taken or chosen to be in this environment because of their love to serve dedicatedly. Such persons who take delight in this work will be protected by their love of service itself. They have no fear. Fear by itself is an overwhelming factor to make one diseased. Sometimes they do fall sick - very occasionally - it is because they may slip into fear. But they emerge out of it soon.

The second protection that we talked about is homoeopathy - the homoeopathic remedies, when we work in an epidemic, we observe certain remedies are used more often than the rest. What does this mean to you? It means that this one remedy suits more to the nature of sickness. At the same time one can also observe that for prevention of disease a remedy of lesser similitude will do its work. But for curing it should suit well. We notice that this lesser similitude remedies are used daily for prevention - to prevent the people from getting sick. This teaches us one more lesson. We must look forward to homoeopathy to protect us as well as to cure.

Summary

1. This lecture deals with idiosyncrasies of the patients.
2. Idiosyncrasy means individual peculiarity.

Lecture - XXIX

3. Dr. Hahnemann has enlightened us on this subject in paragraph 117 of Organon.
4. Some persons otherwise healthy are peculiar in their constitutions. Certain things affect these people easily whereas the same things do not affect other healthy people.
5. Some are susceptible and some are immune.
6. Idiosyncrasy is not the susceptibility that is seen in feeble constitutions.
7. A homoeopath can recognize a wide range of susceptibilities.
8. Idiosyncrasy is over-sensitiveness to certain things.
9. An acute idiosyncrasy springs from acute miasm and a chronic idiosyncrasy from chronic miasm.
10. Idiosyncrasy can also lead the physician to the remedy.
11. Idiosyncrasy can be congenital or acquired.
12. We can infer the patient's susceptibility to the remedy that will cure.
13. The patient's sensitivity to the drug to cure him is analogous to the idiosyncrasy he has.
14. Congenital idiosyncrasies and idiosyncrasies to poison are very difficult to cure.
15. In congenital idiosyncrasy from the symptoms we can infer a remedy that can suit the problems. The medicine has to be given in a high potency. This medicine will not actually cure the patient - at the most it could act as a palliative for a few times. After that the body becomes immune to this remedy and it will not act.
16. Sequelae are psoric. They are the out-cropping of chronic miasms.
17. In congenital idiosyncrasies the sensitiveness can only exist in the dynamic plane

18. Some people crave salt and eat a lot of salt. Here it is in the nutritive plane. This eating of more and more salt indicates they are sick and in need of salt - but salt consumed in the nutritive plane fails to save them. But the same salt in a high potency will reach his inner self and cure him. That means the remedy works on the dynamic plane.
19. Where the disease is in a dynamic plane the cure must also be in the dynamic plane.
20. Homoeopathicity is the relationship between the homoeopathic remedy and the patient who has been cured.
21. A remedy appears to be similar before it cured. It is called the simillimum once it has cured.
22. Crude poison, in a nutritive plane is not very deep, more superficial, relates to more external things and to the body tissues.
23. The same poison potentised and taken in the dynamic plane runs much more deeper, and lasts a lifetime. But then this can occur only when the individual is susceptible.
24. Some individuals are susceptible to all things and in their case nothing can be exempted as non-poisonous.
25. The susceptibility is the basic for the contagion and the cure.
26. Cause and the cure, the cause of sickness and the cure of disease are in the dynamic plane. When disease is in a primitive substance the cure must also be in the same.
27. Poison creates a disorder to the human economy or causes death. This applies both to the nutritive and dynamic planes.
28. Man is protected from disease by homoeopathy and its use.
29. For the prevention of sickness in an epidemic a remedy of less similitude is enough for protection from getting sick.
30. Homoeopathy protects us and also cures.

Aphorisms & Precepts

1. There are degrees in susceptibility. The old school calls a certain kind of susceptibility 'idiosyncrasy' though they have failed to find out what this is.
2. Think how susceptible man is to sickness, when the Rhus vine will poison him when he is on the windward side, half a mile away.
3. An individual may be susceptible to nothing else; gross, coarse vigorous in constitution; yet there is one thing he is susceptible to, and that is what he needs.
4. Primary and secondary effects of remedy have confused some. You need not worry over this. You only need to know that certain symptoms follow each other. Primary and secondary actions reverse themselves in different individuals.
5. Homoeopathic remedy only becomes homoeopathic when it has established its curative relation; the relation between two dynamic influences.
6. Homoeopathicity is the relation between the symptoms of the patient and the remedy, which will cure.
7. Man is susceptible to all things capable of producing similar symptoms to those, which he already has.
8. A crude drug may poison a patient, when the substance potentised would have cured him. The individual comes in contact with too much of something he is sensitive to and gets sick.
9. The same susceptibility is necessary to prove a drug, as to take a disease. That is the homoeopathic relation. Hence we see what contagion is.
10. Only a few drugs will be similar enough to cure, and there will be only one simillimum.

11. Susceptibility is prior to all contagion. If an individual is not susceptible to smallpox, he cannot take it, and will not receive it though he goes near the worse cases, or eats a smallpox crust.

12. When an individual is made sick by the crude substance, and even by the lower forms of simple substance as in Rhus poisoning it shows that he needs that substance on some plane. The dose has been yet too large to cure.

13. The old definition used to say that anything capable of extinguishing the vital force was a poison. This cannot be denied today, but we may say now, that anything capable of engrafting itself upon the economy so as to produce incurable injury is a poison.

14. When two remedies antidote each other, it cannot be said that one is more powerful than the other. It is like an alkali neutralizing an acid, the one added last seems more powerful, but this is only in appearance.

15. Increasing the dose cannot increase the homoeopathicity. If it is right at all, you can increase its homoeopathicity by elevating its quality towards its interior nature so that it corresponds more perfectly to the vital force.

16. It is all-important to see the remedy in its nature as a sick being.

17. Disease is a proving of the morbific substance. It is not true that there is one law for disease and another for drug effects, but the degree of susceptibility governs.

18. Now when a person susceptible to Rhus gets a whiff of air from a vine, he at once has the disease fastened upon him, and is not subject to further poisoning though he lie under the tree from which he was poisoned until he recovers.

19. The dynamic plane is more interior or above the nutritive

plane. It presides over it and commands it.

20. There is a plane of nutrition and a plane of dynamism. The normal individual who receives it on the plane of nutrition appropriates common salt, but the sick one who needs it eats it constantly and it does not make him well because he needs it on a higher plane.

Lecture - XXX

Individualization

In our earlier lectures we have told that homoeopathy is an art and science. It is also a matter of individualization through and through. We are refreshing a few things here.

(1) No two humans are alike.

(2) Each individual is susceptible to certain things; is susceptible to sickness and equally susceptible to cure.

(3) There are no two things alike in the universe. This is so of diseases and of sick people, of thousands of crystals of the same salt.

(4) No two stars are alike.

(5) No remedy can be substituted for another.

(6) Individualization is blocked by the inability to distinguish between the finer features of sickness and of medicines.

(7) No two remedies are absolutely equal in their similitude.

(8) Every person and animal has an atmosphere.

(9) Two sick people are more unlike than two well ones.

All the above leads us to one thing - no two people are alike, so also their disease. We also see that no two remedies are equal in their similitude — only one remedy can match a disease.

How do you comprehend this - taken as one unit? Homoeopathy is based on sound principles that have been repeatedly proven themselves again and again. It is very clear and simple. Compare, individualize, observe the razor-sharp differences in the nature, which are most similar. We have mentioned no remedy can be substituted for another remedy. Two remedies may appear very similar - but one cannot do for the other.

We have said that a homoeopathic physician discriminates - and also individualizes, how? He must be capable of individualizing things, which are widely dissimilar in one way, yet similar in many other ways.

Let us consider here the drugs *Secale* and *Arsenicum*. They both are chilly in nature yet different. Let us see how? The *Secale* patient does not want to be covered and wants all the covers off. He also desires the cold air. But in the case of *Arsenicum*, the patient desires all things to be hot. Though both these are chilly the remedies are wide apart. To put it more perfectly the two remedies are completely dissimilar to the general state, while wholly similar as to particulars.

We shall take up certain other symptoms and see how *Secale* and *Arsenicum* are similar but dissimilar.

In homoeopathy we do not call the sufferings by any name except for convenience. We shall take up a case of peritonitis. The symptoms are:

    (a)   Distended abdomen.

    (b)   Restlessness.

    (c)   Often vomits and passes blood from anus.

    (d)   Horrible burning with distended abdomen.

Lecture - XXX

(e) Thirst unquenchable.

(f) Tongue red and dry.

(g) Pulse lightning like.

If this patient wants to be fully covered and wrapped up, wants his food and drinks to be hot *Arsenicum* will fit like a T.

Consider the above patient. He kicks off all his covers and does not want them. Prefers to be in cold conditions, wants only cold applications, desires the windows to be open, is unable to tolerate the warm room here is a clear indication of *Secale*.

What does all these indications reveal to us? When there are two similar remedies we should be able to see the subtle differences and match the remedy and the disease. This also goes to show us in two cases of peritonitis two individuals are not identical in their symptoms. Again we repeat homoeopathy is an applied science where individualization plays a very important role.

We can see that Materia Medica is full of such sensitive and subtle sensations — all based upon individualization. For this great contribution to homoeopathy should we all not be ever grateful to the master and all the volunteers who suffered for us as provers? Gratitude and thanks giving nature should be a part of the homoeopathic physician.

Generals are very important. Without this we cannot practice homoeopathy. Generals help us to individualize and also to observe the distinctions. Between two remedies gather all the particulars - compare the generals and we see that one strong general rules out the other and helps us to pick up another.

Homoeopathic physician should perfect their questioning skills with the sound idea of individualization.

We see two remedies — pick out a common symptom. How can we separate them? Materia Medica helps individualize once we master the art of individualization. The generals of one remedy are so different from the other. It will easily become distinguishable by constant practice. Once we practice this art to select the remedy can we ever think of substitution? We practice to discern like this and we are able to select the remedy best adapted to the patient's constitution. Here there is an advice. The suggestion is to try one by one in the list alphabetically till you hit the bull's eye. The explanation is though the remedy has never been known to produce that symptom may be able to cure the case since it is more similar to the generals of that case than any other. This is the art of applying and using the Materia Medica. Many patients have rare or strange things that it has never been found in any remedy. It is necessary to examine the entire case fully and completely to find out which remedy of all the remedies is most similar to the patient.

Remember here — one sick man is to be treated - not the disease. So study the patient. The symptoms are not apart from the patient. When we study the patient and treat the man we are bound to be successful.

We now go to paragraph 118 of Organon. It reads as:—

"Every medicine exhibits peculiar actions on the human frame, which are not produced in exactly the same manner by any other medical substance of a different kind."

There is no need to analyze the above paragraph as we usually do with the other paragraphs. We shall go to the gist straight away.

"Each medicine produces particular actions on the human body. No other medicinal substance can create the identical similar effect on the human body."

It is very clear from the above that only one medicine is capable of a particular symptom in human body. Then where is the question of substitution? It is individualized. See how natural the homeopathic doctrines happen to be and also how easily comprehensible.

We meet cases, which are so mixed up, and confusing, we are not able to see any distinctions. With all these confusions we

Lecture - XXX

should know that there is one remedy most suitable to that case. We may know which one it could be or not. But one thing for sure is, there is no substitute for this particular remedy - which particular remedy differs from all the other remedies just as the patient differs from the rest of the individuals. This is what we meant by 'no two men are like'.

This single remedy may look it is not needed; it may not appear to be indicated even, but all the same this is the remedy that is needed in this case. The physician might have overlooked some point and missed this remedy by a mile. So we go back to something we already spoke about. Wait and watch. Once again this is a proof that one cannot substitute another remedy.

We now take up paragraph 122 of Organon. It reads: —

"In these experiments — on which depends the exactitude of the whole medical art, and the weal of all future generations of mankind - no other medicines should be employed except such as are perfectly well known, and of whose purity, genuineness and energy we are thoroughly assured."

On analysis of the above paragraph, we have:—

(a) Weal means state of well being in this context. We see that on the medical experiments the whole medical art and the well being of the future generation of mankind depend.

(b) Only perfectly well known medicines must be used.

(c) These medicines must be pure, genuine and be capable of producing results.

What are the medical experiments we are talking about? We can take them as proving. In homoeopathy alone healthy individuals prove the remedies. We are able to get the drug picture as well as the symptoms it can combat. In allopathy the remedies are administered to rats, dogs and monkeys first. Can these poor animals convey any feeling or sensation to the experimenter? The experimenter has to see the ultimate and draw his own conclusions. According to his conclusions he decides to take it to the humans, for trials and consumption. Such sad is the state of affairs.

Homoeopathy is an applied science. It is based on solid laws and doctrines. There is no assumption or opinions. Only facts count here.

With the above foundation we continue with the lecture. So interpret the above once again:—

"In circumstances of this nature on which depend the cirtitude of the medical art, and the welfare of the future generations, it is necessary to employ only medicines that are well known."

Purity is of great importance. Remedies, which are proved, must be kept unmodified. They must be preserved with full care as they are proved and maintained properly to enable them possess their full energy.

Whenever and wherever we use a fully proved remedy we should see to it that the substance we have taken up must be as close as possible to the substance that was taken up for proving. Only then we can expect the same results as in the proving. This must impress the fact why we must not deviate from the original substance even by a hairbreadth.

Several years back we had an opportunity to go and stay for few days with one of my relatives. In their backyard they had a few papaya fruit trees. Each tree bore a lot of large papaya fruits. Everyday we had these very sweet fruits. The time for us to leave for our native town came. We thanked the host profusely and started. The host gave us a pocket of papaya seeds with clear instructions as to how to grow them as he had done. The first thing we did on reaching our house was to prepare the ground as per instructions and planted the seeds. The plants came up according to our expectations. The trees started bearing fruits. The fruits were not that big. The color was not as deep. The taste

Lecture - XXX

also was not the same. All of us were very disappointed and felt that love's labor was lost. We consoled ourselves that this was the first crop and the next crop would measure up to our expectation. Not only the next but also practically all the future crops were very disappointing. Then an agriculturist friend said - no doubt you have done all that your host had asked you to do. But then do you realize that the soil composition there and here are different and the water could be of a different compoisition; finally the climate and the atmosphere could be different; with so many varying factors how to expect an identical fruit as grown in the relative's place.

Well, where does the above take us. A plant could bear the same name at various places in the world. But the same plant will be different in some way or other. If or they may not be identical with the extract from the extract that was proved for the proving. The difference will be very subtle. So always procure the one that was proved originally. Fincke recognized this fact when he procured substances that Dr. Herring had proved.

To recapture, the medicine should be well known; its history should be well known, with all steps and details. The potentization should be considered, the different hands it has passed through - all the little particulars of our high potencies should also be well known. This point is very important and hence potencies must be secured only from well-known sources. It will be wise to collect these from the headquarters, whenever possible.

We now proceed to the paragraph 144 of the Organon.

"From such a Materia Medica everything that is conjectural, all that is mere assertion or imaginary should be strictly excluded; everything should be the pure language of nature carefully and honestly interrogated."

The gist of the above is: the Materia Medica should not be from any imaginary or conjectural material. It should contain only the pure symptoms, in the most natural language and after the details have been honestly interrogated.

It is once again elaborated in different terms.

"A Materia Medica of this nature shall be free from all conjecture, fiction or gratuitous assertion - it shall contain nothing but the pure language of nature, the results of a careful and faithful research."

Go back and think a little as to how Dr. Hahnemann built his Materia Medica. It was by the proving on healthy individuals. Observations made were pure and un-adulterated. The provers gave out or recorded the symptoms very honestly.

To end the lecture we shall see pargraph 145 of Organon.

"Of a truth, it is only by a very considerable store of medicines accurately known in respect of these their pure modes of action in altering the health of man, that we can be placed in a position to discover a homoeopathic remedy, a suitable artificial (curative) morbific analogue for each of the infinitely numerous morbid states in nature, for every malady in the world. In the mean time, even now - thanks to the truthful character of the symptoms and to the abundance of disease elements which every one of the powerful medicinal substances has already shown in its action on the healthy body — but few diseases remain for which a tolerably suitable homoeopathic remedy may not be met with among those now proved as to their pure action, which without much disturbance, restores health in gentle, sure and permanent manner - infinitely more surely and safely than can be effected by all the general and special therapeutics of the old allopathic medical art with its unknown composite remedies, which do but alter and aggravate but cannot cure chronic diseases and rather retard than promote recovery from acute diseases."

We shall see the gist of the above paragraph.

We have in our Materia Medica a large number of proven drugs with which we can cure every natural malady in the universe. Certain drugs which were taken accidentally were also monitored helped us collect the morbid symptoms these drugs produced on healthy humans. So these also were proved and added to the Materia Medica. We still do not have suitable drugs for certain ailments. Homoeopathic medicines cure safely and permanently and surely. Allopathic medicines do not cure chronic disease; on the contrary they complicate and aggravate the conditions.

To put it in other words: "we ought certainly to be acquainted with the pure action of a vast number of medicines upon the healthy body, to be able to find homoeopathic remedies against each of the innumerable forms of disease that besiege mankind that is to say, to find out artificial morbific powers that resemble them." We have a remedy for every fully developed disease in the Materia Medica. Only mixed cases, which are not fully developed pose problem to us.

Summary

1. Homoeopathy is both an art and science.
2. It is also individualization through and through.
3. No two people are alike - so also their diseases.
4. No two remedies are similar.
5. Only one remedy can match the disease picture. So one remedy cannot substitute for the other.
6. A homoeopath must be able to individualize things that are widely dissimilar in one way, yet similar in many other ways.
7. Two remedies may be similar - but there will be some subtle differences between both. A homoeopath will have to learn to observe these subtle differences. This is individualization.
8. The generals help us to individualize and observe the distinctions.

9. Between two similar remedies one strong general rules out the other and helps pick up another.
10. Homoeopathic physicians must perfect their questioning skills with the idea of individualization.
11. Materia Medica helps to individualize the remedies. When we study the Materia Medica carefully we observe that the generals of one remedy differ from the other.
12. Though the remedies have never known to produce a symptom it may still be able to cure the disease because most of its generals are most suitable to generals of the case than any other.
13. One sick man is to be treated - not the disease.
14. The symptoms are not apart from the patient.
15. Each medicine produces particular actions on the human body. No other medicinal substance can create the similar identical effect on the same human body.
16. In homoeopathy alone healthy human individuals prove the drugs or remedies.
17. Homoeopathy is an applied science based on solid laws and doctrines and only facts.
18. Proven remedies are to be pure - kept unmodified - preserved and properly maintained so that it retains its full energy.
19. We should use the remedy from the proven samples. Otherwise we may not obtain the same results as was got at the time of proving.
20. Always procure potencies only from reliable sources.
21. Materia Medica is free from any imaginary or conjectural material. It should contain only pure symptoms in the natural

language. The recordings must be done after each remedy is properly and honestly proven.

22. Our Materia Medica consists of a large number of remedies for almost all the natural diseases.
23. Homeopathic medicines cure permanently surely and safely.
24. Allopathic medicines do not cure chronic diseases. They complicate the case and also aggregate the conditions.
25. It is imperative that we know both the disease picture and the drug picture well enough to select the appropriate remedy.
26. In Materia Medica we do have a remedy for every fully developed disease.
27. Mixed cases, which are not fully developed, pose problems to treat.

Aphorisms & Precepts

1. The wisest will make mistakes in perception, but the aim must ever be to find the most similar of any medicines proved, and to recognize that there is one most similar of all.
2. One remedy must be more similar than the other. It is true that one not conversant with the subject will be unable to see the finer shades of difference. Some are color blind, yet others can pick out colors.
3. Never leave a remedy until you have tested it in a higher potency if it has benefited the patient.
4. All susceptible provers will bring out the image of the remedy. The prover catches the drug disease from one or two doses just as people do the Scarlet Fever or the Grippe.
5. It is known that old-fashioned medicine of all sorts fails to recognize that there are principles of plain and intelligible

governing the practice of medicine. They regard it as a mere matter of "experience".

6. The most villainous doctors are always hunting for something strange and peculiar. Those out of the way symptoms and strange pains are not what we prescribe on and will seldom serve you. The generals are ruling symptoms and are what the patient says, the individual himself.

7. The more you cultivate Homoeopathic methods, and the finer you discriminate, the better you see, and the more you can understand.

8. There is much more to be learned about disease from the medicines, because disease is more obscured by the culminations.

9. It is only after a careful and complete study of the finer points proving of drug and the same of the finer features of the disease that a law can be demonstrated.

10. The modern provers note down only the common symptoms and the morbid anatomy which the remedy produces, and have left out the generals and peculiar symptoms.

11. There are general, common, and peculiar symptoms. The general is used in the sense of the general of an army, and the generals command all other symptoms, and really control the patient.

12. The increase of conditions show increase of sickness; the increase of symptoms often shows the diminution of disease.

13. The remedy pervades the economy silently and completely with its prodromal period, then comes the evolution of disease, which runs its course.

14. The one who understands best the nature of his remedies will remember most about their peculiarities.

Lecture - XXX

15. Two sick people are more unlike than two well ones.
16. No two remedies are absolutely equal in their similitude.
17. With the true physician, discrimination is not with eye alone; the consciousness of discrimination seems to occupy his entire economy.
18. Individualization is blocked by this inability to distinguish between the finer features of sickness, and of medicines.
19. It would seem as if the Old School would have asked long ago, "What are the effects of drugs upon healthy people?" Their experiments on animals do not answer this.
20. A prejudiced mind, decides without wisdom the way he wants to have it.
21. Homoeopathy is an applied science, not a theory.
22. Meteria Medica never inspires perception. The physician must have the love of its use, and he becomes wise in proportion as he loves his use and in proportion as he lives uprightly with his patients; that is desired to heal them; beautify their souls. Can the physician, who does not love his neighbor as himself, get into this position?

Lecture - XXXI

Characteristics

We now take up paragraph 147 of Organon. It reads as:

"Whichever of these medicines that have been investigated as to their power of altering man's health we find to contain in the symptoms observed from its use the greatest similarity to the totality of the symptoms of a given natural disease, this medicine will and must be the most suitable, the most certain homoeopathic remedy for the disease; in it is found the specific remedy for this case of disease."

The gist of the above paragraph is: where the totality of symptoms of any remedy has a greatest similarity to the totality of symptoms of any particular natural disease, that remedy could be taken as the specific remedy to that disease. This remedy will surely cure the disease under question.

We shall go into the lecture. "Of all these medicines that one whose symptoms bear greatest resemblance to the totality of those which characterize any particular natural disease ought to be the most appropriate and certain homoeopathic remedy that can be employed; it is the specific remedy in this case of disease."

Now-a-days we do read about specific remedies for this or for that. The old school affirms that there are only three or four specifics. But every offshoot starting at something for himself thinks a lot of specifics.

The quack physicians talk and advertise specific remedies for headache, diarrhea, this ailment, that ailment, etc. Homoeopathy does not recommend this at all. Don't you see this has become like allopathy? No rules, no laws.

Homoeopathy has only a few specifics. But then what is the specific? It is a remedy, which has a special power in a particular disease or an infallible remedy. The homoeopathic principle is — there is only one similitude. It cannot be substituted. If this be so and according to the Organon paragraph quoted above, every remedy is a specific for that disease for that person. For that person because the totality of symptoms were collected from that person. It may be said that the medicine, which is found to be similar to the symptoms, which characterizes this disease is specific.

This is to elaborate what we said above. Look at the word 'characterize' in the above. Organon has shown us in our earlier lectures that diseases make their existence known by symptoms. The complete and clear picture of the disease is given out by the totality of the symptoms. It cannot be taken blindly. The totality of symptoms must be studied carefully. We must ascertain among all the symptoms what characterizes the disease, or make the symptoms as peculiar.

Dr. Hahnemann gives us company and guides us to analyze the totality of symptoms, for the purpose of giving it a character. We have in our earlier lectures, impressed the need to do it. It has to be done. The information that makes or leads up to characterizing is really the information that makes the homoeopath wise. This will clearly indicate to the physician what he has got to treat in this specific case. The most apt medicine is the most similar. In homoeopathy we do not go by the experience as in allopathy. The medicine's homoeopathicity can be proved only after it cures

Lecture - XXXI

the disease. Hence it cannot be labeled as a specific beforehand. One can get an idea only after the examination of all the symptoms and finally proceed to find out what characterizes.

Always see what is there in that particular case, which makes it an individual, what is there in it that makes it. So unlike any that ever existed? What makes it to stand off from the rest? Similarly in the case of the remedy also ascertain the point that characterizes it.

When the physician thinks this way and approaches the case he also realizes that there is one remedy, which is the most similar of all the remedies in the Materia Medica. He also knows for certain this is the one remedy that will cure once administered. Its homoeopathicity is sustained; the similitude has proved itself as a cure.

We know that we cannot call a remedy homoeopathic until it cures the sick. Till its homoeopathicity is proved we can only presume that it is homoeopathic. We also say that it appears to us that which is characteristic of the disease are also the most similar of all other things to that which is characteristic of that remedy or *vice-versa*.

Our reasonable assumption that the remedy is the specific may be acceptable only theoretically. The homoeopathicity can only be proved after the cure. Homoeopathic remedies do not become specifics because a homoeopath uses them, or because they have been potentized, or attenuated or prepared as per fashion of our school.

In lecture XXIX we have spoken about homoeopathicity. We shall take the opportunity to look into it now, once again. We have also spoken earlier about a medicine being homoeopathic where the remedy has demonstrated its curative relation to the patient; after having been administered to the patient in accordance with the symptoms he has, the recovery must take place according to law. He must be cured from above downward, from within out, and in the reverse order of the symptoms. Such a qualification renders the remedy homoeopathic. Then it becomes the specific remedy. Under no other circumstances can it be a specific remedy.

In paragraph 148 of Organon Dr. Hahnemann gives out his theory of cure. Note the word theory — he says it is only theoretical. The choice to accept it or not is left to you. You are not compelled to accept it or to adapt it says the master. He says he offers it simply as the best in view not binding upon to accept it. Dr. C.A. Baldwin, M.D., comments as follows on this paragraph:

"Here is stated the theoretic technique of a cure with proper remedy and proper dose properly repeated. Stated concisely as brevity requires; the indicated remedy excites an artificial disease, of distinct similarity to the disease to be treated, by virtue of the remedy's similitude of pathogenesis and great certainty of action which liberates the organism from natural malady. The artificial disease soon terminates and leaves the organism free. It is fair to permit this explanation to be questioned, since an explanation is not necessary to the action of the remedy."

Here an aphorism comes to my mind. "How is it that bread and meat nourish the human body? We cannot say. How the homeopathic remedy cures the disease will never been known, but the direction, in which life flows into the body and the direction of cure can be known."

We shall now go to paragraph 149 of Organon. It reads as:

"When the suitable homoeopathic remedy has been thus selected and rightly employed, the acute disease we wish to cure, even though it be of a grave character and attended by many sufferings subsides insensibly, in a few hours if it be of recent date, in a few days if it be of somewhat longer standing, along with all traces of indisposition, and nothing or almost nothing more of the artificial medicinal disease is perceived; there occurs, by rapid,

Lecture - XXXI 407

imperceptible transitions, nothing but restored health, recovery. Disease of long standing (and especially such as are of a complicated character) require for their cure a proportionately longer time. More especially do the chronic medicinal dyscrasia so often produced by allopathic bungling, along with the natural disease left uncured by it, require a much longer time for their recovery; often indeed are they incurable in consequence of the shameful robbery of the patient's strength and juices, the principal fact performed by allopathy in its so-called methods of treatment."

Let us now analyze the paragraph in our usual way:

(a) We shall take up an acute disease case, with a grave character, attended by many sufferings.

(b) With a suitable selected homoeopathic remedy it subsides insensibly.

(c) When and how long does it take? It subsides in a few hours if it be of a recent date; subsides in a few days time if it be of a somewhat longer duration.

(d) All traces of indisposition vanish, and nothing or almost nothing more of the medicine induced artificial disease is observed.

(e) That means by rapid, imperceptible transitions the body is restored to health and a complete recovery is achieved.

(f) Do diseases of long standing and complicated nature also gets cured this way? Yes, but they take proportionately a longer time to get cured.

(g) What happens to natural disease where allopathic medicine interference was there? In such a condition also, the uncured portion of the natural disease, which was left so with the allopathic medicine uncured and the effect left behind by the allopathic medicine/s requires a much longer period to cure. But often we see such a condition is incurable. It is because the patient is drained off his strength and juices. This is a shameful robbery and a principal feat performed by allopathic treatment.

Dr. Hahnemann has also given a very nice footnote about the selection of the homoeopathic remedy — sometimes very laborious to search. We do have several books to guide us - yet some cases demand a deep study in spite of this availability of printed knowledge. Here he speaks of the mongrel cures - their cures are not permanent. It is antipathy and suppresses all the symptoms that disappear. Homoeopathy is a salutary art.

At this point another aphorism — " the greatest comfort on earth to man in incurable disease is homoeopathy."

We shall see the gist of the Organon paragraph 149.

"Suitable selected homoeopathic remedies administered in acute of diseases of grave character of recent origin get cured in a few hours. Where it is of somewhat longer duration the recovery also takes a longer time to get cured. They are sometimes incurable or are difficult to get cured. Where patients have consumed large quantities of allopathic medicines refuse to respond since the patient has lost his strength and juices."

Now we shall enter the realm of lectures. Earlier we have spoken about truth. An aphorism says, "Throw aside all theories and matters of belief and opinion, and dwell on simple fact." The simple fact in the aphorism is truth. Homoeopathy is a true science. It is based on truth. It is built on true laws and doctrines. Hence the science cannot be a pseudo science. They say truth always stands on two legs. With all this knowledge we have to accept the contents of paragraph 149 of Organon, since it is true. This paragraph is a general statement of the results of the homoeopathic remedy in the cure of disease. In case of a group or sect of people rejecting the paragraph it will amount to one group in believing and the other not believing it.

We go back to the paragraph: "when a proper application of the homoeopathic remedy has been made, the acute disease which is to be cured, however painful it may be, subsides in a few hours, if recent, in a few days if it is older, etc." This is an elaboration of item 'c' in our analysis.

Think for a minute. What do you surmise of the above? It very plainly says that under proper selected remedy the disease secured, where it does not get cured, it is obvious that the remedy was not right. Hence the homoeopathic physician is compelled to find the correct or most suitable remedy. Due to our false step it is not fair to blame the science. At this juncture an aphorism comes to my mind: "Those who say they have tested homoeopathy and it is a failure have only exposed their own ignorance". Homoeopathy is based on true law and order. The science is not to be blamed. The failure is due to the physician's wrong judgment and hence the blame is squarely on the physician's shoulder.

Let us consider a child with scarlet fever. We are able to choose the correct remedy and when it is administered the fever decreases and the child improves. The rash will remain, but the malignancy of the fever vanishes, in case of an ordinary scarlet fever. The child is alright and is able to go and attend the school. Here we have treated the child and not the fever. There is an aphorism, which comes to my mind: "One sick man is to be treated not the disease."

Here is the physician who thinks of the rash of scarlet fever or measles as the component to be cured, God help the physician, for the disease will not subside as quickly as in the earlier instance. It is the duty of the physician to prescribe for the patient on that which characterizes the disease, even though it is called as a self-limiting disease.

Next we go to paragraph 150 of Organon. It reads as:

"If a patient complains of one or more trivial symptoms, that have been only observed a short time previously, the physician should not regard this as a fully developed disease that requires serious medical aid. A slight alteration in the diet and regimen will usually suffice to dispel such an indisposition."

The above paragraph is self-explanatory. To word it briefly "Light indispositions are cured by a change of diet and regimen. They do not need serious medical treatment."

So when a patient complains of accessory symptoms which have just appeared, the physician ought not take this state of things for a perfect malady that seriously demands medicinal aid.

When your patients are under constitutional treatment, if they are affected by serious troubles it is alright to prescribe for it. That means slight indispositions are not to be treated. Patients will come to you at the slightest pretext - like every change of the wind, when the baby has the slightest snuffle, every little pain and even the lightest headache. In case you change your remedies often for the slightest problems, this will create confusion. Under this circumstance either you can tell the patient no treatment is required or give them a few doses of placebo. The indisposition will pass off by itself. Sometimes it may develop into a constitutional manifestation. On the other hand where there is a severe acute disease, which is decisive with a strong manifestation of the symptoms, symptoms prominent, there can be no confusion and it can be treated. Ignore indispositions that are non- descript. Placebo will be the best way to deal. We have also spoken in our earlier lecture about how placebo comes to the physician's help.

We close this lecture with the paragraph 150 of the Organon. The paragraph is not quoted here, but the gist of the paragraph is given.

"Where the few symptoms that the patient gives are really violent the physician can observe him carefully. He will generally find many other under developed symptoms. Such symptoms will furnish to the physician a perfect picture of the patient's malady."

Summary

1. This lecture deals with characteristics. This is a very important subject to be studied in depth by any ardent homoeopath.
2. First paragraph 147 of Organon is taken up. It is a basic conception of homoeopathy. It is, wherever the totality of the symptoms of any remedy bears the greatest similarity to the totality of the natural disease, under consideration, that remedy could be taken as the specific remedy for that particular natural disease.
3. In homoeopathy there are only three or four specific remedies.
4. There can be only one similitude. It cannot be substituted.
5. In homoeopathy every thing is individualized. We should remember ' no two persons are alike in sickness or in well being.' The same disease (when we go by names for convenience - again in homoeopathy we do not go by name of disease) does not produce identical symptoms in two different individuals.
6. Each medicine and each disease has its own drug and disease picture. We should study the totality of symptoms carefully. Consider only the symptoms that characterize the drug or the disease. See what makes this individualistic and helps it stand apart from the rest.
7. We also observe that which is characteristic also happen to be the most similar either in the disease picture or the drug picture.

8. The homoeopathicity alone can prove the efficacy of a remedy in the particular disease. The remedy must be from a genuine dealer, potentized properly as per instructions of our school.

9. The particular remedy must cure from above downward, from within out and in the reverse order of the symptoms. This is cure according to the law. Only under such circumstance can it be called a specific for those symptoms the patient suffered from.

10. In paragraph 148 of Organon Dr. Hahnemann gives out his theory of cure. It is up to us to accept it or not since it is only theoretical.

11. Next we go into paragraph 149 of Organon. This has got to be accepted. It says that a properly selected remedy will cure a recent disease in a few hours and those with a longer duration will take a few days. Those, which are complicated with allopathic drugs, may be curable or incurable.

12. Mongrel cures are not permanent. They only suppress the symptoms.

13. Homoeopathy dwells on truth and facts. Facts are truths. So truth and only the truth.

14. The physician alone is responsible for the consequences arising out of a wrong selection of remedy. The science cannot be blamed.

15. Light indispositions are cured by a change of diet and regimen. No serious medication is necessary. So ignore symptoms that are non-descript. Deal with placebo where necessary.

16. The lecture is ended with paragraph 150 of Organon. When a patient gives out symptoms that are violent a careful observing physician will notice several other underdeveloped

symptoms, which may bring out a clear picture of the patient's malady.

Aphorisms & Precepts

1. Those who say have tested homoeopathy and have found it a failure have only exposed their own ignorance.
2. Anything, which looks away from exactitude, is unscientific. The physician must be classical. Everything must be methodical. Science ceases to be scientific when disorderly application of law is made.
3. Man's unbelief and opinion do not affect truth. The experience, which the homoeopath has is experience under law and confirms the law and by this order is maintained.
4. Now when a person becomes sick, he becomes susceptible to a certain remedy, which will affect him in its highest potency while upon healthy person it will have no effect.
5. A remedy is not known simply because it has been used upon the sick. That is confirmation only and gives more ripened knowledge.
6. Homoeopathy is an applied science, not a theory.
7. When you look at morbid anatomy from the symptamotology, you are looking at it from the interior. Morbid anatomy must not be studied as a basis for prescription making.
8. No two remedies are absolutely equal in their similitude.
9. The symptoms themselves, point to the things, which the individual is sensitive to, and every one is susceptible in just this way to the remedy that will cure. That which he most wants, is that which nature has provided him with the means of reaching out after by the symptoms.

10. Diseases themselves cannot be suppressed, but symptoms can. The totality of the symptoms must disappear in an orderly manner in order to constitute a cure.

11. You see homoeopathy is a superficial way only when you see the similarity of the symptoms to the remedy. It looms up before you know it as a physician of experience knows measles or scarlet fever.

12. Only a few drugs will be similar enough to cure, there will be only one similimum.

13. Mongrel cures are by this method, and their cures are not permanent. It is antipathy and suppresses all symptoms that disappear.

14. We cannot even see all the symptoms in a disease. We can see the expression of the face but cannot know what that represents. There is nothing in the outer man that does not have its beginning in the inner man.

15. The more violent you see, and the more necessity for haste, and the more severe and the greater suffering of the patient; the more harm can you do by a false and foolish prescription.

16. How is that bread and meat nourish the human body? We cannot say. How the homoeopathic remedy cures the disease the disease will never be known, but the direction in which life flows into body and the direction of cure can be known.

17. The physician must penetrate the inner recesses of symptomatology. The very life of the patient must be opened. Learn the fears, instincts, desires, and the aversions of the patient. The remedy often crops out through the affections.

18. Belief has no place in the study of homoeopathy. The inductive method of Hahnemann is the only way.

Lecture - XXXI

19. It is inconsistent to say, "I gave a homoeopathic remedy and it did not cure". The administration of homoeopathic remedies is an applied science.

20. The limit of drug action is symptomatology.

21. In cases without any symptoms, the patient must be kept on Saclac. Until you can discern something in general such as aggravation of symptoms in the morning or at mid-night. If the patient is only 'tired' without guiding symptoms, you may know that is liable to terminate in some grave disorder - consumption, bright's disease, cancer or the like.

22. The homoeopathic physician must continue to study in the science and in the act before he can become expert. This will grow in him until he becomes increasingly astute and he will grow stronger and wiser in his selections for sick people.

23. That which we call disease is but a change in the vital force expressed by the totality of the symptoms.

Lecture - XXXII

The Value of Symptoms

Homoeopathy is a science of symptomatology. It is the only natural science to cure an individual completely, both internally and externally. The symptoms are the language of the nature to prove the existence of a malady, in body and the mind. The matter of health, disease and cure are all in a dynamic plane. It is so subtle that it cannot be seen, touched or felt. Even the very finest and costliest microscope is not able to see this dynamism through it.

A few words about the microscope and microscopist may not be irrelevant here. The microscopist has failed to show there is no vital force, no simple substance and no dynamism is seen. How can we expect him to foretell when the substance cannot be seen? A microscopist can be useful to homoeopathy when he can examine a grain of wheat and tell whether it will grow if planted in favorable soil. When he can examine a smallpox crust and tell whether it is still contagious, or whether its power has been destroyed by heat then he may be of use. Much belongs to man and the outer world, which the microscope is yet to reveal. The microscope cannot demonstrate any vital problem. The microscope is only suitable to demonstrate the most concrete of matter. The microscope, only furnishes us a field of results. It is not able to reveal the cause; we are only able to see the results. What can be said about the microscopist under our context will also hold good for the various other sensitive instruments used in the present day investigative diagnosis also. They all can only present us with the various parameters they are designed to give. They do not give out the cause. So they are of not much use in our symptomatology. After all the examinations the doctor declares all the parameters shown by the various instruments and machines have indicated the parameters as within the limit and everything is normal. But then the patient is suffering. The cause for the suffering is not indicated or known. Then what is the use?

We have already talked about indispositions. Disorder first in vital force, sickness and cure on dynamic plane and the removal of the totality of symptoms mean the removal of the cause in lectures VII, IX, XI and XII. It will be a good suggestion to rush through the above lectures and refresh yourself what is mentioned therein.

In homoeopathy a stress is made on symptoms because it is one of the pillars to prescribe upon. In our lectures XXIII to XXVI four lectures have been dealt with on the examination of the patient. This shows the importance of case taking or noting down the symptoms of the patient on paper and carefully studied, grouped properly and a suitable similimum drawn out. We spoke of homoeopathic remedies being specific to each case on individualization — even though only three or four remedies could be literally called as specifics in homoeopathy. We spoke of the characteristics. All discussions were about the disease as well as the cure. We also saw how proving were effected.

We shall now go into details of the value of symptoms. First of all we should know the classification of various symptoms.

Classification of Symptoms:

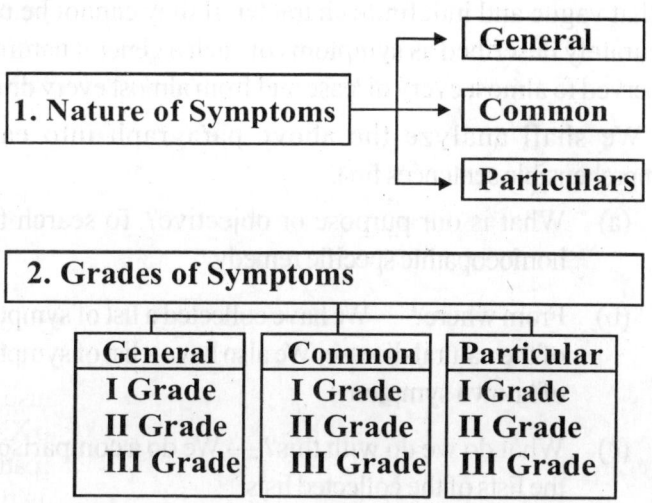

There are three symptoms — general, common, and particular.

Each of the symptoms is again subdivided into first, second and third grades, according to their value or importance.

We go to paragraph 153 of Organon. We reproduce it below:

"In this search for a homoeopathic remedy, that is to say, in this comparison of the collective symptoms of the natural disease with the list of symptoms of known medicines, in order to find among these an artificial morbific agent corresponding by similarity to the disease to be cured, the more striking, singular, uncommon and peculiar (characteristic) signs and symptoms of the case of disease are chiefly and most solely to be kept in view; for it is more particularly these that very similar ones in that list of symptoms of the selected medicine must correspond to, in order to constitute it the most suitable for effecting the cure. The more general and undefined symptoms; loss of appetite, headache, debility, restless sleep, discomfort, and so forth, demand but little attention when of that vague and indefinite character, if they cannot be more accurately described as symptoms of such a general nature are observed to almost every disease and from almost every drug."

We shall analyze the above paragraph into easily comprehensible sentences first.

(a) What is our purpose or objective? To search for a homoeopathic specific remedy.

(b) From where? — We have collected a list of symptoms of the natural disease. We also have a list of symptoms of known symptoms.

(c) What do we do with this? — We do a comparison of the lists of the collected lists.

(d) For what? — To find from the lists a morbific agent corresponding in every way by similarity to the disease to be cured.

(e) How do we do it? — We choose the more striking, singular uncommon and peculiar (characteristic) sings and symptoms, of the case. We keep in mind the above while doing the comparison.

(f) Why should we do this? — For, only when these symptoms which are more particularly and the very similar ones in the list of the symptoms of the selected medicine list correspond to the foretold symptoms of case, can the medicine - thus selected will be the most suitable to effect a cure.

There will be still some undefined symptoms left out. What are they? Loss of appetite, headache, debility, restless sleep, discomfort and so forth. They demand very little attention. They are vague and indefinite, cannot be described more accurately.

Lecture - XXXII

These symptoms of a general nature can be observed almost in any disease and from almost any drug.

We shall now make a gist of the above points:

For prescribing we should select the prominent (more striking singular), uncommon and peculiar (characteristic) symptoms into consideration. The common symptoms present in certain type of case does not help us to write down a prescription and so, useless, for this purpose. Vague and undefined symptoms may not guide us to select an appropriate remedy.

Homoeopathy is a science and an art. We have stated earlier in our lectures that homoeopathy is well founded on the principle of individualization. We need not stress it further, but to individualize a lot of discrimination has to be done. Individualization can be carried out only when we know of characteristics and grades of the symptoms. The sole purpose of this paragraph is to guide the physician, without any confusion to master the art of case taking and arrive at the proper similimum. What is the use of having sheats of paper full of symptoms, if one does not know what to do with it.

In our part of the world, we have a story. A coconut merchant had a small shop set up on the pavement to sell his coconuts. Every day a dog used to come and sit in front of his shop for some time and will run off. One day the coconut merchant took pity on the animal and threw a full-unbroken coconut at the dog. The dog first got frightened, but not for long. Then came over to the coconut and sniffed at it. The coconut rolled a little. The dog took it to be a plaything and played with it. Seeing this, the merchant got annoyed and hit the dog with stick shouting, " I gave it to you for eating and you rascal, you are playing with it." The dog howled. Just then an old person came along and stopped the merchant from being cruel to the animal. The old man said to the merchant how could a dog eat a full-unbroken coconut? You should break it and remove the pulp form the shell for it to eat - do not hit the dog again. The merchant saw the light and whenever the dog came again he used to give it some pieces of coconut, which the dog gobbled up happily. So the story goes. There is no need to elaborate the moral — it is self explanatory for our context.

If the physician takes the sheets of paper to a master, he may go through the list. The master will say 'son, this list looks like any other list to me. You cannot build your case on this and target the similimum. Further you have not taken your case properly. Your list contains no image of the disease. You have failed to get any symptom that characterizes the disease. Sorry we can do nothing with it.' The master gives the papers and refreshes the physician what we have spoken about in paragraph 153 of Organon.

Armed with this knowledge the physician will be more mature and bring out a more effective and useful list. He himself will know that he has taken down the case properly and has something concrete to show to the master.

We have heard people saying that homoeopathy has failed. Let us see what or why is it for a few minutes.

Throughout the world certain things are uniformly accepted. They all have become accepted. Chemistry, physics, mathematics, science etc. are such accepted things. Let us see how? Two parts of hydrogen and one part of oxygen can make only water anywhere in the world. Its composition is universal. Newton's laws of motion are universal. Multiplication, subtraction, division or addition all is universal. 2+2 in Congo will be 4. Similarly 2+2 in Timbkutu will also be 4. It cannot and will not vary. They may call it by different names, but the same all over the world.

We call homoeopathy a science. Science is universal. Science is universal because its principles are universal. So, when we call homoeopathy a science its principles are also universal. We recall here a few words about homoeopathy.

'Homoeopathy is an applied science not a theory. Those who say they have tested homoeopathy and it is a failure have only exposed their own ignorance.'

Lecture - XXXII

'When you make failures you may be sure that they are well within yourself. If you think the failure is in homoeopathy you will begin your corrections on the wrong side of ledger.'

'The whole homoeopathy is to cure. Homoeopathy is a God given natural science. The greatest comfort on earth to man in incurable disease is homoeopathy.'

Please note the second and third statements above. So it is clear that whenever there is a false understanding, a miscomprehension or wrong application, combined or individually, science only provides the user a wrong result. This is also universal and now you know due to what reason homoeopathy fails. In addition to the above when the physician is even very slightly prejudiced and full of ego and pride and lost all humility his approach to the science will most definitely give a very mistaken interpretation. So the fault lies not with the science but on the part of the physician. Remember once you call something a science it has been brought out into this world by many people who have most properly examined its principles, experience of those who have used it over and over and above all highly intuitive people who aimed to do good to the world by each and every action of theirs. This has come into the world from generation to generation and we have reached this level. We should be thankful to the innumerable noble souls who have toiled for the benefit of the universe, non-existing and existing presently. We can show our gratitude to these great people by correct interpretation of what they presented to us. We must not go headstrong with half-baked knowledge committing errors, and defame their noble pains. At this point I salute our great master, Dr. Hahnemann and wish to share one point with all of you about him.

'Hahnemann was always in a state of humility, he never attributed anything to himself.'

Many homoeopaths like the one we mentioned earlier are ignorant about characteristics. They keep on nibbling at their bunch of case records unable to dispose them properly. They may even ask whether there is any one peculiar thing, which can guide one to a remedy. Many minds hit at keynotes.

In lecture XXXI we spoke of characteristics. Here we continue. Think what helps us (1) to classify that which is available (2) to perceive the value of symptoms and (3) when you have two or three remedies, out of which you have got to decide upon one remedy to zoom in on that remedy. Contemplate how you could individualize in the absence of a characteristic - it is absolutely essential to individualize.

The things that make you hesitate and meditate are a characteristic. So this is what solves all the above problems. Here we have a very brief but very clear definition for characteristic - yes, what makes you hesitate, meditate.

Let us take a case of whooping cough. We have handled several cases of whooping cough earlier. But in this case we find a peculiar symptom that puzzles us, which we have not hitherto confronted. Now we hesitate and then we meditate upon this and realize that it is strange, rare and peculiar. With this symptom on hand we refer to our Materia Medica. This seems to be a very strong feature, and a high-grade symptom and to the remedy similar to that in the patient. This is peculiar to the patient and not to the disease. This peculiarity will open up the case completely to the remedy.

Where you observe, that the remedy has that symptom, along with the other symptoms it is important and cannot be ignored. Sometimes we may have two or three of such peculiar symptoms. They form the characteristic features.

We have talked earlier about common symptoms. We shall see here what constitute a common symptom. The common symptom appears in all cases. In high fevers people would have thirst. See, this is common.

Lecture - XXXII

In case the patient has high fever and no thirst, it is strange. In such a case, hunt will be for thirstless medicines.

From the above we are able to observe that the absence of a striking feature of the disease indicates a peculiarity in that patient.

When does a remedy be a specific for the patient and will be the similimum?

That which is pathognomonic is common since it is common to the disease, but an absence of the pathognomonic characterize that particular disease, in that patient; and in proportion as you have that class of symptoms, just in that proportion that you have things that characterize the patient the specific remedy will prove to be a specific for that patient and will be the similimum. It is absolutely necessary to know the sickness. We cannot consider the pathological or physical diagnosis for this purpose whatever their importance might be. It should be done from the symptoms only because it is the language of the nature.

How is a true homoeopathic prescription made out? Is it based on pathology or on the morbid anatomy? It is based on neither. Why? The proving in homoeopathy is not made in that direction. Hence we cannot do it that way. Let us collect some more details about this. Pathology can only yield us the results of the disease. It cannot convey to us the malady in nature's own language. Homoeopathy is a natural God given science. Symptomatology is the true subject to know, and it is the nature's way to indicate the malady inside. Hence pathognomonic or morbid anatomy symptoms cannot help us make a prescription of homoeopathy. Further the homoeopathic physician alone is trained to use his knowledge and well acquainted with the manner of expression of each and every disease. He alone knows how each disease expresses itself in language, appearance and sensations.

The physician must also know how each remedy affects exactly the mankind in memory, understanding and will. That is because there are no other things that remedy can act upon as to the mind.

He also must know how the remedy affects functions, because there is no other way in which the remedy affects the man.

When a physician knows how disease declare its signs and symptoms, then he knows what makes a disease unique from the rest. We have spoken about two persons not being alike either in well-being or in sickness. The same disease affects different patients in different peculiar ways — the difference is the symptoms each one exhibits. They make the symptoms strange, peculiar and rare. The pathognomonic nature in the remedy is what the physician will spend most time to study since it is related to the patient; the physician must always keep his mind tuned to this study. Once the thinking is bent this way the physician can then study the symptoms of the disease for gradation purposes.

The symptoms of the remedies must always be studied keeping in mind the order on their grade. If read from looking at the symptoms just like that, distinctions cannot be made. In fact symptoms to a great extent, are on a sliding scale. We find that a peculiar symptom in a remedy is not in any degree peculiar to another remedy. We find that many symptoms in a chronic disease may be true. But the same may not be so, and even diagonally the opposite in acute disease.

The physician must know and also keep in mind that the chronic miasms are the very opposite in their character and order to the acute miasms.

We have a case of inflammation of the parotid gland. When the physician examines this patient, the patient shouts out a caution. He asks the physician not to press upon the inflammation, as it is very sore. Now would you classify this as common or strange? It would be a strange thing for such an inflammated gland not to be sore. Hence here we must not prescribe for the soreness. Something is to be known in the general view of the case. The indicated remedy should have indicated the inflammation and soreness of the gland. But then there is nothing striking in that.

Lecture - XXXII

From the Materia Medica we can collect a few remedies or a group of remedies capable of producing artificial hardness and soreness of gland. It may be one of those or the one of those things, which has not, produced these things, which the patient has, and this is a characteristic of the patient.

In sickness there are symptoms which cannot be explained. They are often very peculiar. Remember that things that which can be accounted for are not so often peculiar. Peculiar things are less known to man.

We see a person sitting always with his feet elevated — say puts his legs on the table and sits or keeping his legs on a low shelf where the top is elevated than his chair and he always prefers sitting this way. Think for a minute here. Why does this man sit like this? He ought to be a great sufferer, if his legs hang down. That is the reason why he puts up his legs. How will you word this symptom? 'Worse from putting the feet down or worse from letting the legs hang down'. Let us see how we could interpret this in a better way. You ask the patient to put some light on 'worse' he explains 'when I bring my nates down upon the chair there is a sore place.' The patient is an old man. He has an enlarged prostate gland, which is painful and sore. When the patient lets his feet hang down, more so on his sitting the sore gland comes into contact with the chair. The gland is sensitive to touch and this is a common symptom. There are symptoms where letting the feet ameliorates the patient or legs hang down. We can never tell why that handing down relieves limbs. In a case of periostitis, we observe the patient lying across the cot with legs hanging down. No one can figure out why he lies this way and why he cannot lie on his back. Refer *Conium* in Materia Medica and you have these symptoms in *Conium*. It also happens to have relief 'putting feet on chair relieves pain.' We find in *Conium* all the symptoms the patient has. Other, than the above, perhaps are common.

This is a specialized way of thinking. Once followed ardently it will not take a long time for one to master the technique. This will put in a habit of estimating among the symptoms that appear in a record - things that are common, things that you would expect and the things that are strange.

We have to take certain types of symptoms of the remedies, which are general. The general symptoms will also have to be taken into consideration while examining any record. All the symptoms that are predicated of the patient himself are to be taken as general. All the symptoms that are predicated of any organ are things in particular.

So from the above we see three things - how things are in general, things in common and things in particular. Sometimes it may be a condition or state or sometimes it may be a symptom.

We have said above that what the patient predicates himself would at once appear to be something in general. Where the patient says 'I am thirsty' where is the symptom - it is in the mouth, consider for a minute. Though the sensation might be in the mouth, the fact is that the entire economy needs water.

Wherever the patient says 'I feel' are apt to be generals. As an example the patient says 'I have so much burning' you question and examine him. You will observe that his head is burning, the skin burns, there is burning in the anus, the urine burns and the affected regions also burn. The word 'burning is a general feature. This feature modifies all the patient's sickness. Where and when the burning is on a particular region or organ this would have been a particular but when it refers to the whole of the man are things in general.

Normally, if you study your cases, you will observe that patient tells things that affected him - these are what are most general. Collect data, during the examination of the patient. He will be speaking of his desires and aversions. He is speaking of very closely related things about the patient himself. The changes in these things will be marked by the changes in his very ultimate. The aversion is a general symptom. It completely permeates his entire economy. This symptom qualifies all the patient's symptoms and is the very center of all his states and conditions. A patient may state that he has a desire to commit suicide. This is the loss of the love of his life — i.e., he has lost his love to exist. Think where this thought could come from. It can come from only one point - the innermost of that individual.

How do medicines affect a man? Medicines affect man primarily by disturbing his affection, by disturbing his aversions and desires. I remember an aphorism here — 'man is known by his affections'. Things that he loved to do are changed and now he craves for strange things. Sometimes the remedy may change the patient's ability to comprehend and turns his life into a state of contention and disturbance. His will may be changed. This can result in troublesome dreams in his sleep. That is really a mental state. Those that lie close to the patient and his life, and his vital force are strictly general.

We said things that are closest to man's life are strictly general. As these generals become lesser and lesser general, they become particular.

Now let us take a female. She menstruates. This period gives us a state that we may call general. When she says 'I menstruate', so and so. This she does not attribute to her ovaries or to her uterus. When a female is menstruating her state is, as a rule, different from her normalcy. So here again things that are predicated of self, of the ego, the things 'I do so and so', 'Dr. I feel so and so', I have much thirst', 'I am chilly in every change of weather', 'I suffocate in a warm room', and many other similar statements by the patient are all general.

After the collection of the above, the physician makes a tour, organ by organ. He thereby states what is true in every organ. Many times we can observe that the modalities of each organ conforms to generals. Sometimes we do come across cases where there may be modalities of the organs that are opposed to the general. This is why we find remedies that appear to have in one subject one thing and in another subject the very opposite of that thing. Where it will be a general in one thing the same becomes a particular in another.

In this lecture, we have seen the three symptoms to some wide extent. This subject is a pillar of homoeopathy. We deal with this subject in our next lecture also. We suggest you carefully go through your notes on these two lectures till you master and understand what is told here and in the next lecture.

Summary

1. Homoeopathy is a science of symptomatology.
2. The symptoms are the nature's language of saying that a disease or sickness exists inside the body.
3. We cannot see the dynamism through even the most powerful of the microscope. The microscope cannot demonstrate any vital problem.
4. There are only three or four specifics in homoeopathy.
5. The symptoms are classified as (1) general, (2) common (3) particulars. These again are chosen according to their importance as first, second and third grades.
6. To write out a homoeopathic prescription we should select the prominent uncommon and peculiar symptoms.
7. Vague and undefined symptoms may not guide us to select an appropriate remedy.
8. Homeopathy is both a science and an art.
9. Homeopathy is based on individualization.
10. Individualization can be carried out only when we know and understand characteristics and grades of the symptoms.

Lecture - XXXII

11. Case taking should be done attentively, systematically and carefully.
12. The symptoms taken down must be able to provide us with a image of the disease, patient's aversions and desires.
13. If someone says homoeopathy failed it must be due to that person's ignorance.
14. Homeopathy is an applied science, not a theory.
15. The greatest comfort on earth to man in incurable disease is homoeopathy.
16. Homeopathy can fail only due to human failure, or human inadequacy.
17. The characteristic alone helps us to classify that which is available, to perceive the value of symptoms, and to select one appropriate remedy from two or three nearly identical remedies and thereby individualize.
18. That is what makes you think, hesitate and meditate upon, is the characteristics.
19. Sometimes you have two or three symptoms that cannot be ignored. Such are referred to as characteristic features.
20. A common symptom is that which appears in all cases.
21. In some cases where a striking feature might be absent in the patient. That is the peculiarity of that patient.
22. Under what condition will a remedy be the specific for the patient? The remedy must be:
(a) Pathognomically common since it is common to that disease.
(b) An absence of pathognomic in the patient being a peculiar or characteristic of the patient.
(c) Have certain class of symptoms in the same proportion as that characteristic of the patient.

23. A homoeopathic prescription is not made upon pathology or morbid anatomy.

24. Symptomatology is the true subject to know.

25. The physician must also know the pathognomonic nature in the remedy, as it will be related to the patient.

26. The symptoms of the remedies must be studied keeping in mind the grades.

27. The chronic miasm symptoms may not be identical with acute miasm symptoms. They may be even diagonally opposite.

28. While preparing a prescription we should weigh the symptoms and the grades properly. They may lead to questioning the patient further and also for confirmations of the symptoms already recorded. We must also study each symptom deeper than what it appears to be — must find out whether the symptom is as plain as it looks or the consequence of some other symptom.

29. In sickness there might be some symptoms, which might be unexplainable. Such symptoms often are peculiar.

30. Prod all the angles of every symptom. Do not take it on its face value.

31. All symptoms that are predicated of the patient himself are general. All symptoms that are predicated of any organ are particular.

32. Sometimes the symptoms could be a condition or state, or could be the symptom itself.

33. Wherever the patient says 'I have or feel so and so' is all general. This refers to the whole economy - not the territory alone to which it is related.

Lecture - XXXII

34. Desires and aversions are very close to the patient himself. Changes in these things will be marked by the changes in his very ultimate.
35. Aversions are a general symptom. It completely permeates the patient's entire economy. This symptom qualifies all the patient's symptoms and is the very center of all his states and conditions.
36. The generals become lesser and lesser related to the self and ultimately become particular.
37. Many times we do come across cases where there may be modalities that are opposed to the general.
38. Where a symptom will be a general one in one thing becomes a peculiar in another.

Aphorisms & Precepts

1. The external man is but an outward expression of the internal. So the results of disease and symptoms are but the outward expression of the internal sickness.
2. Those who say they have tested homoeopathy and it is a failure have only exposed their ignorance.
3. The affections make the man.
4. Understand the remedy first, the keynotes last.
5. The disease is not to be named, but to be perceived; not to be classified but to be viewed, that very nature of it may be discovered.
6. You must be able to recognize every ambassador of the internal man.
7. The signs are visible but the *esse* is invisible.

8. The personal stamp is upon every disease and upon every proving and the individual must be permitted to stamp himself upon the disease as well as upon the proving.
9. Homoeopathy is an applied science, not a theory.
10. One sick man is to be treated, not the disease.
11. When you make failures you may be sure that they are within yourself. If you think the failure is in homoeopathy you will begin your correction on the wrong side of the ledger.
12. A prejudiced mind, decides without wisdom the way he wants to have it.
13. When we conceive that innumerable causes may give rise to the same pathological conditions, we see that the pathological condition in itself, cannot furnish us with the slightest idea of the remedy.
14. When you look at morbid anatomy from symptomatology you are looking at it from the interior. Morbid anatomy must not be studied as a basis for prescription making.
15. With a true physician, discrimination is not with the eye alone; the consciousness of discrimination seems to occupy his entire economy.
16. The whole aim of homoeopathy is to cure.
17. Only a few drugs will be similar enough to cure, and there will be only one similimum.

Lecture - XXXIII

The Value of Symptoms (Contd.)

This lecture is in continuation of the previous lecture. It is very important to know well the various symptoms like general, common and peculiar ones. We shall go through these at a quick pace.

The generals are made up of particulars, sometimes. When we are studying the symptoms of any individual part or organ we are looking up at the particulars. If our attention is drawn towards the symptoms of any part alone, we are examining the particulars. For e.g., if we examine the liver symptoms alone, we are after particulars. We can put this in another way - when and where we are considering the part or region apart from the whole man, we are examining particulars.

Now we have examined all the regions one by one and collected their symptoms, also one by one, we have particulars. Now carefully examine the symptoms of each region, group by group. On examination we do find that certain symptoms run through in all the particulars; now those symptoms have become generals and at the same time they are particulars as well.

Symptoms, which apply to all the organs, may be predicated to the individual himself. Those things, which modify all parts of the organism are those, that relate to the general state. Whatever the individual predicates of himself is also general. The patient may state the symptoms relating to only one of his organs that become a particular. But most of the things that the man predicates of himself are general.

Now let us take up the symptoms of sleep. Sleep is not related to brain for the brain does not sleep any more than the individual. When an individual states ' I was wakeful last night' how do you look at it? Since the patient is predicating something of himself it is a general, when he says 'I dreamed' the entire man must have really dreamed. When we attribute the sleep, here, to the mind we should not forget the mind is the man. We are able to observe the sleep and dreams are very important factors in the history of a case. Are you able to draw out what we are talking about, yet, it is the importance of these symptoms in a case.

We shall take up a case of menstruation. Look at how closely menstruation is linked up to the woman. It relates to the entire woman. This makes it the most important. Similarly, you cannot separate the special sense of the patient from the patient, the entire patient. These cannot be separated and identified. Take the case of smell. It is again the entire man who is very closely related to the smells - smells that are agreeable and the smells that are so disagreeable. Just because the smell is disagreeable to the individual one cannot ignore it or say that it is not closely related to the patient. Here the symptom becomes general.

Yet there are smells, which relate more close to the nose itself. This may be because of some pathological reasons or conditions of the nose. So here the symptom pertains to the organ and its conditions. Hence is a particular symptom. Note how the logic relating to particulars we spoke about in the last chapter is easily put into use.

We will see another case of smell. A hungry man accepts the food smell as agreeable. It relates to the whole man, as

Lecture - XXXIII

demonstrated earlier. Now consider one who has a vicious catarrh of the nose; there is much local disturbance. His olfactory senses are totally perverted due to the catarrhal condition. Here the symptom relates to the organ, the nose. Hence this is a particular, in this case.

An individual says 'I see' so and so, without seeing him. Can you categorize this symptom? Note the words within the inverted comas. That leads you to the category of the symptom. Whenever a patient tells a symptom in the first case — uses 'I' then that becomes a general symptom. See the last paragraph of lecture XXXII — it will refresh your memory. Remember, the more the symptoms relate to the internals, which involve the whole man the more they become generals.

What do we understand from these lectures so far? What do we do with this? We understand that the things that relate to the man are the ones that have to be singled out and marked first in our anamnesis.

After gathering all the symptoms of a patient, the physician must single out for study each and every symptom that can be predicated to the man. Everything where the individual says 'I feel' so and so or 'I suffer' from so and so, sit with your anamnesis thus collected and individualize. With the help of Materia Medica choose out what remedies relate to these symptoms first. Do not be callouse at the job. We may be about to get three remedies of the anamnesis or may be one remedy. In ninety-nine out of every hundred cases you can leave out the particulars since particulars are usually contained in the generals themselves.

When we have pitched upon one remedy having numerous generals, and it cover those generals absolutely, clearly and strongly that will be the remedy, which will cure the disease. You may find several little particulars that may appear to contraindicate - but they cannot because nothing in the particulars can contraindicate generals. Sometimes one strong general can over-rule all the particulars you can gather up. 'Aggravation from heat' will throw out *Arsenicum* altogether from being considered in this case.

We shall now take up common symptoms. Sometimes we find in female cases prolapsus, which is common to the ladies. It is common for them to say 'Dr. I have such a dragging down in my bowels as if my inside were coming out'. This is a common feature among ladies and is a common symptom. There is nothing about that alone which can help you picking up a remedy. But for these common symptoms we do have a class of remedies. When you see a rubric containing a dozen fifteen or twenty remedies you can often know it is a common symptom.

Earlier we mentioned that all women having prolapsus having to a great extent the dragging down feeling, as if the uterus would come out. When we take up this symptom and follow it up we can see that it works in various directions. We will see that it runs into generals and particulars. How can we decide when to give *Sepia*, when *Lil-tig.*, when *Murex*, when *Belladonna*, when *Puls.*, when *Nux* and when *Nat. mur.*? To pick out the remedy that will cure, we have to study both the generals and particulars of the patient — the generals always the first.

In case the patient was to be given *Nux vomica* on what basis will we select it? What will she say of herself that *Nux* is indicated? She would be chilly; full of coryza with stuffing up of the nose even in a warm room. She would be very irritable, snappish, and want to kill somebody, want to throw her child into the fire, want to kill her husband. She would have constipation and every pain she had with it would make her run to the stool, urging to pass stool, but only a little quantity is passed and she wants to relieve herself frequently. These all pertain to *Nux vomica* and are indicated as generals in the patients as well. So we see that we go from generals to particulars. Always when following up symptoms go from generals to particulars. That is the right approach.

Lecture - XXXIII

Well, if *Sepia* is the indicated remedy for that patient. There we will observe the common symptom, what no other patient has. What is it? She will have the dragging down symptom. This is common. But the patient will have an all gone sinking feeling in the stomach. She will get relief only when she sits with her legs crossed. The other generals of *Sepia*, she will have. She has a constant feeling of lump in the rectum that makes her go to the stool, but she goes for days without any urge at all. She is sallow and sickly, speaks about bilious symptoms. *Sepia's* tell-tale indication of yellow saddle over the nose. She tells us she has an aversion to her own children and feels very sad at the thought of her not loving her husband as she ought to. See how the generals are good indicators of the remedy. In addition to these symptoms she has two symptoms in particular, yet peculiar. Can you identify them in the above symptoms? Go through the above once or even twice. The particular, yet peculiar will loom up in front of you. We shall explain them. Yet sir, she made a statement about her stomach and rectum - she has a feeling of constant lump in the rectum and an all gone sinking feeling in her stomach. They are those particulars, yet peculiars, wherever a symptom indicates an individual organ it is a particular, remember it? The dragging down feeling is common to prolapses. So, in this case we have all the categories of symptoms — viz. generals, particulars and common and also peculiar.

We repeat once again that when the symptoms are indicative of any region they are particulars. Common indicate a state of condition in all similar cases.

We shall take scarlet fever, for instance. First we will group all the striking symptoms that indicate scarlet fever - the rash, the appearance of the mucous membranes, the sore throat, the fever, the history, its period of prodrom, etc. The remedies for scarlet fever must also possess the same symptoms in common if it was to cure the fever.

The appearance of the scarlet fever is among the common features of B*elladonna*; *Ailanthus* also has in its common things the appearance of scarlet fever. *Rhus* has a rough scarlet fever appearance. *Sulphur* and *Phosphorous* have rashes similar to scarlet fever. So to make a rubric for the repertory we have to put in the name of all the above remedies in the common group and call it by the name scarlet fever. Here is a beautiful example of particulars indicative of region of the body and also commons as it indicates and describes a state.

Then the question comes up as to when you will administer one remedy and when another. Sometimes we can figure out from the local manifestations things in general. We shall take up an example in an *Arum. triph.* patient. The most striking symptom here is the patient picks his nose and his lips till they bleed. When we study the case carefully we can ascertain that these parts and the fingers and toes tingle. The circulation will be feeble about the extremities. Here the nerves are in abundance - in the fingers and the toes. In these areas there is an unusual tingling like the ants creeping. So the patient picks at these parts. This is a state marking almost all the whole economy. We can, on the closer observation, see that a liquid oozes from these parts. The skin is denuded in these parts. Now this becomes a part of the general state.

Earlier while we were speaking out of scarlet fever we were talking about *Phosphorous*. *Sulphur* and *Phosphorous* have rash similar to scarlet fever, where we have a case that is putrid, the rash looks very dusky and the skin mottled and purplish and there are places in the body with a tendency to suppurate. Swellings are noticed about the neck, hands and fingers. These are inclined to suppurate. Where suppurated there is an oozing round about them — it is so putrid and has an offensive stench completely drenching the room. The patient is not getting sufficient water. The countenance is sunken eyes, puffed and swollen and red. Blotches of a specific character intermingled with scarlet fever blotches.

Lecture - XXXIII 441

Now this is the drug picture of *Phosphorous*, and *Phosphorous* will stop this torture to the patient curing this disease. The general state of the body and we are having our hands full of generals clearly indicating towards *Phosphorous*. We see putridity and a zymotic state. We may have to face several types of malignant scarlet fever; we can manage all with our marvelous remedies.

In our lecture XXXII we spoke of the categories of the three symptoms; general, common and particulars. We also said that each of the above is graded as first grade, second and third grade. In Boenninghausen he has included a fourth grade. But these are only probationary remedies. They require demonstration by reproving and clinical confirmation.

How is this gradation of the symptoms done? We have three grades for common, generals, and particulars. Here we should go back to proving. We have told that proving of each remedy is done by a group of provers. All the provers are healthy individuals. The group contains both male and female volunteers. Each volunteer in each group is given the same potency of medicine and the same doses. The volunteers sincerely and carefully note down the reactions brought about by that medicine. The volunteers do not consult notes. They do not know what remedy has been given to them. They handover their lists of reactions to their leader who is aware of the remedy which was taken up for proving. At the most the leader informs the group whether the medicine is short or long acting. This is done to enable the volunteers as to when reactions would or could start. The leader then makes a list of the reactions and the group reaction is taken as reactions on a single healthy individual and the drug picture is drawn according to the Schema as it appears in our Materia Medica. The drug is again put up for reproving and finally sent for a clinical confirmation. Well, this is how each medicine is proved.

Let us take the group consists of forty healthy individuals. When they turn in their list of symptoms the leader does his homework. Where all or the majority come up with a same particular symptom it is marked as first grade.

We shall take *Apis* — a symptom emerges as suffocation in a warm room. This symptom is found with all the provers or the majority of provers. Now this becomes a first grade symptom.

All the provers of *Pulsatillla* were worse in a warm room. This symptom is found with all the provers or the majority of provers. Now this becomes a first grade symptom.

All the provers of *Pulsatilla* were worse in a warm room. *Kal. hyd.*, *Pulsatilla* and *Apis* have this in the first grade - worse in a warm room. These symptoms existing as generals among the provers come into the experience of the practitioner. He cures extensively such states wherever administered and are confirmed. Then after the clinical confirmation these remedies are fully and completely entitled to get its first grade stamp. Note this confirmation is got where several provers proved the same reaction. By the use of the physician it is further clinically confirmed, and said to have been verified.

So the steps are (1) the symptoms are recorded (2) confirmed by reproving and (3) verified upon the sick.

When *Pulsatilla* was observed to have worse in a warm room, other provers confirm it and then verified upon the sick; it immediately places *Pulsatilla* in the first grade of that general state. Similarly *Pulsatilla* was studied with relation to the bladder. The provers, a majority has a symptom of frequent urination. Here the reference of proving is a particular region. So it is a particular symptom. Hence it is classified as a particular. Now when all or the majority of the provers had an irritable bladder on taking *Pulsatilla* that would be a confirmation. If it cures that condition for years and also experience confirms it, this symptom of *Pulsatilla* is placed under the particulars. It gets its place or is ranked as in the highest grade. Similarly symptom that is bearing down coming under *Pulsatilla* will be a common symptom. Here since it is a common symptom this is placed under the first grade.

Invariably there will be many more symptoms, which have been brought out by a few or a small quantity of the provers. But these symptoms have been verified occasionally after occasional confirmation. Then they do not get the merit of first grade. They are not entitled to so much consideration and importance as the first grade symptom. Now what do we do with it and where do we classify and record it? This case or symptom gets a second grade. This is because that symptom has not produced these symptoms, have not reacted identically with all or nearly all the provers. This is free to all the three symptoms - generals, common and particulars.

A prover brings out a symptom. This is very strong. Yet others do not bring it out. This has not been, say, confirmed for want of support from other provers. It has not been reproved. Thus not getting the requisite confirmation. But then it has proved its efficacy by verification and cure of the sick people at clinical level and hence admitted as a clinical symptom only. This is placed in the third grade in the symptoms, whatever category it might be in from an overall view. Let us take a certain symptom was not in the proving. Yet yielded to certain remedy. Others have also confirmed its clinical values. Such symptoms are labeled as third grade. We do not shift it to any higher grades. Boenninghausen was very cautious with such symptoms that were never verified. This fourth grade remedies are those which after slight marginal consideration were included from what he had gathered from his clinical experiences. He was so doubtful and cautious not to include these even in the third grade. Such symptoms that occurred in the provers, and having no proper confirmation were the ones not verified. Then were passed on to the future generations to prove and brought into the realm of gradations.

We have brought out the classification and how grades were allotted to the symptoms, be it common, general or particular. One need not break his head to grade out the symptoms. This, our grand masters have already done and have offered to us on golden platter. All the gradations are in the Materia Medica. Since this is so readily available for us it must not mean that we should not know how to allot grades. This lecture should drive us to prove new remedies or prove the hitherto unproven remedies and present it to the homoeopathic world. That is the least gratitude we can show our masters who must have toiled day and night with these things to make the world more comfortable place for the posterity. What are you waiting for - brace yourself and shovel in your portion for the sake of future generation. God bless you.

Summary

1. This lecture is the continuation of the previous lecture, the value of SYMPTOMS.
2. It is important to learn how the three symptoms; common, general and peculiar are categorized.
3. The generals are made up by particulars. When we look at the symptoms of an organ it becomes a particular symptom. There are some symptoms that run through in all particulars. They are both generals and particulars.
4. Whenever a patient says, "I am" so and so, it is general.
5. Things that relate to the individual are to be considered in our case histories.
6. Particulars are contained in the generals themselves. So keep out a watchful eye.
7. Ladies may complain in their ailment, "I have such a dragging". Almost every lady will mention such a statement. Such a symptom is a common symptom.

8. Further, in the Materia Medica where several medicines, twelve, fifteen or twenty remedies have the same symptom you can often know it is a common symptom.
9. Where several remedies are there how to select one among them which is the most appropriate. Here, we should study each remedy in relation to the patient's symptoms and select that one medicine which corresponds with the patient's symptom absolutely. You must know to identify the peculiar among the particulars that suits the patient like a "T".

Aphorisms & Precepts

1. The upright man, whose desires are good, wants the truth. His perceptions are intensified.
2. Man today, is destroyed to his interiors, so that truth looks as black as smoke, and false philosophy as bright as the Sun.
3. When we conceive that innumerable causes may give rise to the same pathological conditions we see that the pathological condition itself, cannot furnish us with the slightest idea of the remedy.
4. All quick prescribing depends upon the ability to grasp comparatively the symptoms.
5. Irregular action expressed in signs and symptoms is the disease. The disturbance in Vital Substance has no other means by which it can make itself known to the intelligent physician. This is in accordance with the law. This leaves morbid anatomy out of the question.
6. Individualization is blocked by this inability to distinguish between the finer features of sickness, and of medicines.
7. That which we call disease, is but a change in the Vital Force expressed by the totality of the symptoms.

8. The quiet, silent manner of perception is to be cultivated.

9. The prejudiced mind is not content to write down a few simple facts and symptoms but says, "I will examine the organs and parts and see if congested or inflamed, then I shall know what to do".

10. We must think what makes the patient sick; not what causes changes in his liver, his kidneys and his other organs.

11. When you give a remedy be sure that the nature of the remedy and the nature of the disease (as well as the symptoms) agree.

12. The physician must penetrate the inner recesses of symptomatology. The very life of the patient must be opened. Learn the fears, instincts, desires and aversions of the patient. The remedy often crops out through the affections.

13. There are general, common and peculiar symptoms. The general is used in the sense of the general of an army, and generals command all other symptoms and really control the patient.

14. The limit of drug action is symptomatology.

Lecture – XXXIV

The Homoeopathic Aggravation

We shall see Paragraph 154 of the Organon. It reads as under:

"If the antitype constructed from the list of symptoms of the most suitable medicine contains those peculiar, uncommon, singular and distinguishing (characteristic) symptoms which are to be met with the disease to be cured in the greatest number and in general similarity, this medicine is the most appropriate homoeopathic specific remedy for this morbid state; the disease, if it not be one of very long standing, will generally be removed and extinguished by the first dose of it, without any considerable disturbance."

Let us straight away go to the gist of this paragraph.

In an acute disease, where the drug or remedy covers

(1) The uncommon
(2) Singular and
(3) Characteristic symptoms

Corresponding to the disease symptoms, then this remedy will surely remove and cure the disease by

(a) One single dose
(b) That being the minimal dose

(c) With the least inconvenience to the patient

The homoeopathic law and principle is to cure the patient with a single dose, minimum dose, rapidly and gently forever. To achieve this purpose, the physician must find out a remedy or drug that suits the conditions mentioned in the 153rd paragraph of the Organon mentioned above.

In our two lectures earlier we have deliberated the three categories of the symptoms in their order of importance and how to relate them to the drug picture. The previous two lectures are very important and those of you who feel to refresh the points therein mentioned are hereby encouraged to do so. Remember the more thorough you are with the laws and doctrines you will be a successful homoeopath, when you adhere to them.

In acute diseases we do not see the patient driven to the death's threshold. It is neither severe, unless it has lasted many days thereby threatening to breakdown the blood and tissues. When the disease is driven to this state we see sharp aggravations, great prostration, violent sweating, exhaustion vomiting and purging after the administration of the remedy. The most severe reactions have been observed and these are necessary to put the patient back on the road to recovery.

Where the acute disease has lasted many days without a remedy and with great threatening present will be the same to an acute disease what will be to a chronic disease of long standing. We can understand this better if interpret it as a matter of progress where we say a disease of much progress, or of considerable ultimate. We have spoken of ultimate earlier. Ultimate is not the disease; it is only the result of the disease. So, in an acute disease where ultimate are observed it is an indication that the disease has been in existence for some time. Where such ultimate have set in, there we notice striking aggravations. Aggravations may be so severe where recovery is not possible. We find this in advanced form of tissue change. We see such things where the kidneys are

Lecture - XXXIV

damaged and destroyed, liver destroyed etc.; in pthisis we see the lungs are destroyed.

We should always consider and determine whether a disease is acute or chronic. Where you observe no tissue changes or no ultimate present, under such circumstances the remedy will cure the patient. Then there can be no serious aggravation or any sharp inconvenience to the patient. This is because there is no necessity of any reaction due to any structural changes.

We shall now look into a deep-seated septic condition. With pyemia sometimes we observe vomiting and purging. Let us see why this should be so. When the order of the human economy is set in order, when there is a reaction, there is a process of house cleaning. The drug does not do it. It does it by itself. That is how nature protects us. We can understand a crude drug acting as above — but, when the same is potentized the power of potentization can only turn the economy into order. That is how it is with chronic disease.

In a chronic disease let us assume that ultimate has not set in and tissue changes have not occurred yet. Under this circumstance we cannot expect an aggravation. Perhaps there will be a very slight exacerbation of the symptoms. This will be of a different character.

We have seen earlier that a homoeopathic remedy is capable of inducing an artificial disease in proportion to its strength or intensity due to the potentization. This means that it establishes a new disease upon the economy. We saw above that when there is a reaction there is a house cleaning. This has taken place in this instance. In this case all these have been suppressed and hence a house cleaning could not take place.

Let us now take a case of a patient having been affected by a paralysis of a limb due to neuritis. This has been in existence for some years now. When you critically look at this in the above scenario this entire thing may appear like an aggravation. By administering an appropriate remedy, which is in the highest sense homoeopathic, certain things occur in the paralyzed limb. It may commence to tingle and feel like crawling of the ants, etc. resulting in the patient having sleepless nights. This is definitely due to the reactions of the nerves in that part. Now a new life of activity comes into existence. This can be observed in paralysis.

Now let us consider a child that has lain in a stupor for a long time. There has been no action of the brain. The tingling feeling that happens in the scalp, in the fingers, and toes is dreadful. This results in the child turning and twisting, screeching and crying. At this misery to this child its mother cannot bear the child's torture and will be the first one to hold down the child. It takes really an iron hand on the part of the doctor to keep the mother away from the child. The child turning, twisting, screeching and crying are all natural and that is the way nature wants it to be. By all these, the child will ultimately feel a little better. On the contrary due to the mother's intervention if this natural process is restricted the child will die. We shall now see the reason for the child's restlessness.

This is nothing but a reaction. The blood starts flowing all over the benumbed parts where the circulation has been feeble, the nerves which had lost the sensations are slowly made sensitive now, etc. So we now have a reaction, which is the result of things being turned orderly. The distress occurs because that portion which had been benumbed is getting its circulation back and the body repairs that part to order - its tissues have a reaction and what else can you expect except the present distress. Think about this.

Here the homoeopath must be cautious. He cannot afford to be hasty in thinking the present situation calls for another remedy. He must not rush to his medicine chest in search of another medicine, for if he administers another medicine the case will be spoilt and the homoeopath will be in trouble.

Right from the beginning of these lectures off and on we have

Lecture - XXXIV

been insisting on the various qualities of the homoeopathic physician. One such important quality we have been repeatedly hammering is that the homoeopathic physician must learn to discriminate. Here is one more opportunity to use his discriminatory prowess.

A homoeopathic physician must use his discriminative power to distinguish which is a reaction and which needs to be medicated. Only in homoeopathy can we have these observations. We do not see them in any other practice. Dealing with reactions is a very tricky affair and sometimes drives the physician to his wit's end. In the mother and child involvement mentioned earlier the mother and the child's relatives would literally drive away the physician. But then the physician will have to be firm. He must be patient and deal with the mother's and her relatives' or friends' ignorance squarely and educate them the need to leave the child to his care. The physician cannot afford the violation of the principles even once, for he may not have a second chance.

Sometimes a very longstanding disease does not yield to this aggravation resulting in distress and turmoil to the patient. The deeper it is the more is the tissue changes. With more tissue changes the reaction is also more and more distressing. Pain is also more.

Let us assume a patient comes back to you after every dose of medicine. Every time he has a violent reaction with violent aggravations of the disease, with violent aggravations of the symptoms. Now there is some deep-seated trouble, as otherwise this cannot occur.

There is a clear-cut difference between the ultimate of the disease and the vital force. There happens to be a state as weakness of the economy and there is also a state as activity of the economy, with much tissue change. Where a feeble individual is concerned the reactions would only be feeble. We have spoken about this earlier. In feeble patients, there may even be no reaction at all after the administration of the remedy. But then in feeble patients there may be a few symptoms. There you cannot find a remedy that is truly specific to that case.

We shall take an example here. We have on our hands a patient. We suspect he has an attack of consumption. A remedy is administered and the patient exhibits a violent reaction. What does this tell us? What is the conclusion we can surmise of this situation? This is a trailer of what is going to happen several years later from now, if the remedy does not cure him.

Such a patient will be shocked. The patient may be frightened by the violence of the reaction. He may come back to tell that the medicine was an awful one perhaps poisoning him, etc. Stop to look at this situation and see what you can draw or learn out of this.

We have spoken much of drug induced artificial disease. Every drug is capable of creating an artificial disease - that is what we call a drug picture, the symptom it can bring out.

In the present condition the drug or the remedy has brought about a violent reaction. What prompted this to happen? A remedy was administered. It brought out some symptoms now. This is exactly a forerunner of the future of the patient. Today the patient received a remedy that was not similar enough to him. It could not do such things to him due to the similitude of his state. So, whatever he exhibited was actually in shadow.

A remedy cannot throw out symptoms the patient does not have. It cannot give him symptoms, which are not related to him, except in cases that are oversensitive. We have spoken a lot about oversensitive patients in our Lecture XVI. You may refresh your thoughts by going through it again.

We should know whether the patient is oversensitive. Oversensitive individuals are capable of proving everything that comes along their way. The homoeopathic physician must be able to know whether the individual is oversensitive and because of this he is proving the remedy or whether he has a vigorous constitution wherein the patient gets an aggravation. As we have said above the remedy could be exaggerated in the oversensitive patient and sometimes in feeble constitution persons. People with a receding chin, sunken eyed persons and those with senility in their eyes can also be oversensitive.

Paragraph 155 of Organon goes further on this.

Paragraph 155 of Organon reads as:

"I say without any considerable disturbance. For in the employment of this most appropriate homoeopathic remedy it is only the symptoms of the medicine that correspond to the symptom of the disease that are called into play, the former occupying the place of the later (weaker) in the organism (i.e., in the sensation of the life's principle in the sixth edition) and there by annihilating them by overpowering them; but the other symptoms of the homoeopathic medicine, which are very numerous, being in no way applicable to the case of disease in question, are not called into play at all. The patient growing hourly better, feels almost nothing of them at all, because the excessively minute dose requisite for homoeopathic use is much too weak to produce the other symptoms of medicine that are not homoeopathic to the case, in those parts of the body that are free from disease, and consequently can allow only the homoeopathic symptoms to act on the parts of the organism that are already most irritated and excited by the similar symptoms of the disease, (in order that the sick life principle may react only to a similar but stronger medicinal disease, whereby the original malady is extinguished in the sixth edition) thus changing the morbid affection of the vital force into a similar but stronger medicinal disease, whereby the original malady is extinguished."

Though this paragraph is long, the main point is, "I say without any degree of suffering, because when a homoeopathic remedy acts upon the body it is nothing more than the symptoms analogous to those of the disease laboring to surmount and annihilate these latter by usurping their place."

Well, the above is the law, principle and doctrine of homoeopathy. We have said several times that the cure should be effected by minimal dose, permanently and rapidly without any discomfort to the patient. The cure must have the identical symptoms of the disease with sufficient power to combat and surmount the existing symptoms and restoring the economy to order - all these without any degree of suffering to the patient. That is the perfect homoeopathic remedy. This is what we have experienced also.

We have taken up an acute disease for treatment. We administer a homoeopathic remedy selected as per the law. After a few minutes, a slight aggravation is there. You will hardly even think of giving another dose of the medicine. We said above "a homoeopathic remedy selected as per the law". This means that the medicine is having an extremely similar picture as that of the disease. Hence this medicine does not leave any stone unturned. It is not necessary to repeat since you can be sure that the remedy will do its work.

In many places we have repeated several times "wait and see". This patience is absolutely an essential quality of a classical homoeopath. Under the present situation also he must wait and watch. He must not be hasty and repeat the dose. He should watch the effects of the medicine already administered. So give a single dose and wait, watch its effects.

Typhoid is a continuous fever. The way to administer medicine in such cases is to give the medicine in water. Then it is better to sit back and watch for several days. The moment you are able to sight the slightest sign of the action of the remedy stop administering the medicine. Observe this as a rule. *In fever conditions, particularly where the patient is feeble never, never attempt to gain an immediate reaction. This should never be done.*

We have been repeatedly hammering on single dose and cure. We have to speak about it once again here. In case of remittent fevers the cardinal rule must be one single dose. In cases of typhoid the reaction may not come in a few hours. It is a matter of few days. Here repetition is permitted. In typhoids that are somewhat delicate never repeat the medicine. Where you find the patient possessing more vigor in his constitution the remedy can co-operate more with that vigor and hence bring about a safer and quick reaction.

Where the patient is feeble the physician must be extremely cautious, about using the smallest dose that can be administered. In several chronic cases it is possible to bring about a reaction in the first night. There is a danger of repeating the remedy. Remember that when you observe that the delirium has subsided, or moisture appearing on the skin surface and you find the patient slumbering peacefully, do not give any further medicine. That state is the limit, there are times in diphtherial conditions the repetition of a remedy will cause death to the patient. There are also conditions where repetition of the remedy has saved lives. But these principles are yet to be discovered.

From here, we proceed to paragraph 158 of Organon. It reads as:

"This slight homoeopathic aggravation during the first hours - a very good prognostic that the acute disease will most probably yield to their first dose — is quite as it ought to be, as the medicinal disease must naturally be somewhat stronger than the malady to be cured if it is to overpower and extinguish another one similar to it only when it is stronger than the latter (paras 43-48)."

The mild aggravation after the administration of the remedy is a very good sign. This heralds that the disease will soon be cured because the greater proportion of the disease will yield to the very first dose. The mild aggravation will become obvious in the first few hours.

A natural disease can destroy another by exceeding it in both power and intensity. Above everything the remedy's similarity to the disease symptoms is the main factor and the truth. Keeping this in the mind now look at the problem. It is clear that there is no need for a repetition of the dose of remedy in an acute disease.

We shall consider another proposition related to the above. In this case of acute disease the remedy has been administered. We find no aggravation as in the previous case, here. Now, where is the snag? There is no aggravation but the patient feels gradually better after administration of the medicine. We have seen the aggravation heralds the cure - but then what has happened which has not given the expected reaction. Stop here and think of the alternatives, which could have brought about this situation?

According to the homoeopathic principle the symptoms of the disease must correspond to the symptoms of the drug. When these tally, the remedy cures. But then the remedy must also possess the power and intensity to combat the disease. This is the foremost and the first consideration. When the parameters given above do not agree the medicine cannot and will not bring in the desired result. So this is one proposition.

The second proposition could be that the remedy selected is not appropriate. Then the case would be totally a different one. Fresh symptoms may crop up instead of the expected aggravation.

The third proportion could be that a complete picture of the drug symptoms have not been properly collected and listed. Thereby it was mutilated.

Of course the other proposition could be the human error. But then a good homoeopathic physician cannot afford to be lax and, by and large he is aware of what he is doing. So, this factor can be conveniently forgotten.

For the present we shall ignore the second and third factors given above. We shall take the first factor only. So from it we are able to see that the remedy chosen and administered was not exact or close to the disease symptoms. The remedy fitted the situation reasonably close. Hence it did not bring in the expected results. But then the patient felt better because of the closeness of the remedy to the disease. It has not been able to penetrate deep enough. The relief may cease after some time in an acute disease. When the relief ceases there can be no reaction either. You have waited and watched this. So you have afforded sufficient time in this case for the medicine to take its course of action, and cease its activity. This is the right time to give another dose of medicine and this modus operandi is 100% correct to follow.

Where you find relief beginning to set in, without aggravation, does not last for long, in an acute disease. But then when there is an aggravation after the remedy the relief lasts long. We have said several times that when an aggravation is slight it is a good omen for cure.

We talked about oversensitive patients a few minutes back. We are back with them once again. You have an oversensitive patient, you select the remedy - say it does not correspond to the disease symptoms like a 't' — but all the same is a near similar. The oversensitive patient is given that remedy. Think what happens now? The medicine plays its role according to the similarity with the disease picture. Since it is not a perfect match or similimum there is an aggravation in an oversensitive patient. With a normal patient the aggravation will not be there. Now in the oversensitive patient what has brought in the aggravation? Of course it is the medicine — so this is a case of medicinal aggravation.

We have also spoken of vigorous constitutioned patients, a little while earlier in this lecture. We repeat what we said there. A good vigorous constitution patient is in. We take down all his symptoms and find or select a remedy. Again in this case also, the remedy is just similar, not perfectly similar to the disease picture. Here the constitution is good and vigorous. What do you find in this instance? The remedy does not act fully as it is only partially similar and by virtue of the strong and vigorous constitution there is no aggravation. What does the physician do now? The answer is clear — symptoms have been eliminated partially and there are some symptoms left behind without attention or care. Now all these partial symptoms hanging behind have to be eliminated - so a few more partially similar remedies are required here to conclude the case.

We do find many homoeopathic physicians flouting the most basic rule or law of homoeopathy. It is a single remedy, minimal dose principle. We do see many physicians giving two or three remedies at a time to their patients. This does not go by the law. A master physician sticks to a single remedy. Here again we have to insist on the homework to be done by the physician towards a single remedy. When cure is sought with a single remedy homoeopathy becomes a science and an art. We wish all the physicians start thinking on these lines and do honor to our great master, Dr. Hahnemann, and Homoeopathy.

Now let us see what paragraph 159 of Organon teaches us. We reproduce the paragraph:

"The smaller the dose of the homoeopathic remedy is, (in the treatment of acute diseases in the sixth edition) so much the slighter and shorter is the apparent increase of the disease during the first hours."

A little while ago, we saw about aggravation. We spoke about trifling homoeopathic aggravation of the malady in the first few hours, in paragraph 158 of the Organon. Now, here is an extension to it. Here in this paragraph Dr. Hahnemann says, that in acute diseases when we administer a remedy, which is a very small dose, and then the aggravation will also be of a shorter duration. *The smaller the dose the shorter the aggravation.*

Now what do we mean by a smaller the dose? Is it the quantity of the medicine or is it the quality of the medicine? What is it? The 30th potency could be called a lower potency. Dr. Hahnemann

Lecture - XXXIV

tried several medicines with 30th potency. So he had ample experience with this potency. He also tried the 60th potency and there were tremendous turmoil with the highest attenuations.

It can be more understandable when this is read as "the smaller the dose is of the homoeopathic remedy the lesser and shorter is the aggravation in the first hours." This might be understood as an apparent aggravation or an apparent aggravation of the sickness or disease.

The disease itself is actually intensified and made worse by the remedy, where the remedy is found to be precisely similar. When a crude drug is potentized to the 30th potency we have a milder action — but it does have a deeper penetrative curative action and thus we arrive at this conclusion. We also make a note of the words "there is an aggravation in the first four hours." Dr. Hahnemann talks about this aggravation.

Sometimes we do find that *Belladonna* after the third or fourth potency creates a violent congestion of the brain. The aggravation is as we said violent. We have to stop the medication or else the child will die. Here, the disease itself may appear to be aggravated. The child seems to be susceptible to *Belladonna*. Now this appears, as it were, to be added to the disease. According to Dr.Hahnemann in 30th potency the aggravation is *slight* and *short-lived*. In our example we had used 3rd or 4th potency. In this the proportion of the medicine is comparatively more than the 30th potency. Our axiom is that the smaller the dose of the medicine the aggravation will be milder and shorter in the first few hours. In our present case the aggravation has been from outside, i.e., the aggravation has been caused by a drug that was administered by the mouth. Now what has happened? Think well.

There has been susceptibility in the body. We also know that a drug can induce a disease - an artificial one. All the more so when the susceptibility is also present. There has been a natural disease present and added to it is the artificial disease with the same phenomena. In some cases we do see a patient under similar circumstances may say, "I feel better, somehow", in spite of the aggravation.

With reference to these types of aggravation, too low a potency remedy may prolong the aggravation, unnecessarily. Similarly when a further dose of medicine is administered under these situations the aggravation is prolonged as well. Note these two points. It has always been our advice to wait and watch.

A repetition of the dose has to be administered in a carefully studied manner. A physician cannot be hasty in this baecause the repercussion could become serious. Anyway we have spoken about this earlier as well.

A dose of *Bryonia* was sent to a robust young woman. The instruction was to take the medicine - a dose on the tongue. The patient however mixed the medicine in water and developed pneumonia. She had contracted a harsh dry cough. What has happened here? The young woman was proving *Bryonia*. On stopping *Bryonia*, she recuperated, by next morning. This has been observed in several cases, where the medicine was similar.

We have seen what a very similar medicine will do. Now let us consider a slight deviation. The drug picture does not totally correspond to the disease symptom, but is partially similar. Yet it could be similar enough to cure. So here we see the need to make out correct and accurate prescriptions. We do have all the tools in our hand, so we have no excuse to make out either a wrong prescription or prescribe a remedy that is partially corresponding to the disease symptoms. By doing this the physician will be doing very best work and we can observe this in the very best constitutions.

The patient is sensitive to the medicine that will cure as well as to the disease that the patient has. Diseased state can be made worse by unnecessary repetition and also where the dose of

Lecture - XXXIV

medicine is not small enough the medicine in such potency is as good as a crude drug. Always remember that third, fourth and sixth potencies are dangerous ones to play with. A good prescriber will remember this. A slip-shod prescriber however demonstrates little of everything. You will naturally go to higher and higher potencies since you want to keep away from the poisonous dose.

This action is different from the aggravation of a very high potency of a CM dose. In this the patient will feel very much better. It is short and decisive and only the characteristics of the disease symptoms will be aggravated. Please note that the disease itself is not aggravated - but the symptoms of the disease stand out sharply. The disease itself is not added to. Here the patient will always say, "I feel better."

In homoeopathy we always say that there is an internal and external man. Whenever the disease occurs it hits in the dynamic plane. This is because the disease also is in a dynamic plane. So always the internal man is affected first and the external man after that. So, when a higher potency medicine is administered it always easily reaches the depth and works in the higher plane. The higher potency medicine as mentioned above does not add to the disease itself. It is able to create an aggravation alright. But in spite of the fact it works in higher plane, characteristic of the disease is brought to more sharply and the patient also feels better.

Now let us proceed to paragraph 160 of Organon. It reads as:

"But as the dose of a homoeopathic remedy can scarcely ever be made so small that it shall not be able to relieve, overpower indeed completely cure case of acute diseases, we do not allow this first dose to exhaust its action, nor leave the patient to the full duration of action of remedy, but we investigate afresh the morbid state in its now altered condition, and add the remainder of the original symptoms to those newly developed in tracing a new picture of the disease."

From this paragraph, we see that as we climb the ladder in very high potencies the medicinal dose is extremely small, but the same is capable of combating the disease. Here we see an altered condition of the disease in addition to the remainder of the original symptoms. Now a new picture emanates totally. What can we understand from this? Dr. Hahnemann has repeatedly told that 30th potency is a good platform to start with in an acute disease. We are able to observe any reaction in the first few hours. Let us stick to the master. He also speaks about various potencies. We shall see the other alternatives available and the comments that have been made, and consider them as well.

There is a general comment that we have departed from Dr. Hahnemann. In his period he worked out that 30th potency was sufficiently high to give an aggravation in the first few hours and sufficiently low in danger range. Dr. Hahnemann has remarked that potentizing must stop at some limit, during his investigations. A little contemplation of the general comment will lead to the reason for this. The present day physicians give different doses going away from Dr. Hahnemann's suggestions. Hence this comment. But is this really so? We shall presently see it is not so.

Please read paragraph 279 of Organon for this purpose - we reproduce the relevant portion here for a quick reference:

"It has been fully proved by pure experiments that when a disease does not evidently depend upon the impaired state of an important organ the dose of the homoeopathic remedy can never be sufficiently small so as to be inferior to the power of the natural disease which it can at least partially extinguish and cure, provided it be capable of producing only a small increase of symptoms immediately after it is administered."

Assume we give a 200th potency to the patient. We find it will aggravate. If we go to the 50M, CM, or MM we find all these will aggravate. Yet all these powers are capable of intensifying the symptoms, since the remedy does still have the capacity to cure.

Lecture - XXXIV

We can be sure that when it is not capable of giving out an aggravation of the symptoms, there is no medicinal power left in it. To put it in other words if there is no aggravation of symptoms after administration of a very high potency, the so-called drug is void of its medicinal power. It is as good as taking a few Saclac globules. In the lab tests, the homeopathic forerunners have gone up to 13 MM potentisation and at this level they found the medicinal effect was still present. But still they have not found the end.

We have also seen in our earlier lectures that one should choose a potency that will just be enough to combat the disease symptoms, based on the intensity of the disease and the state of the patient. At no place we have made a claim that every potency will be suitable to every individual.

If at all we do find a patient who will have aggravation of his symptoms in the most positive and definite fashion, that potency will be verified. So, where have we diverted from Dr. Hahnemann? We have only acted in accordance with the master's doctrines.

We shall now read what is said in paragaraph 280 of Organon.

"This incontrovertible axiom of experience is the standard of measurement by which the doses of all homoeopathic medicines, without exception, are to be reduced to such an extent that after their ingestion, they shall excite the scarcely observable homoeopathic aggravation, let the diminution of the dose go ever so far, and appear even so incredible to the materialistic ideas of ordinary physicians; their idle declamations must cease before the verdict of un-erring experience."

Dr. C.A. Baldwin gives the gist of the above paragraph as:

"This incontrovertible principle, founded on experience furnishes a standard by which the homoeopathic dose may be gauged. Do not be deterred from its use by reason of its ratification. Any argument against it will be silenced by the verdict of infallible experience."

Everything is clear here. We can have no doubts of what Dr. Hahnemann meant when he spoke of the smallest dose. He has clearly said that attenuation may go to a limit beyond which the remedy cannot be further potentized since it would have lost the medicinal properties at that limit. But as we saw earlier, we have gone up to 13 MM potency and still we have not found the end. To make it clearer still our master says the potency has reached a state of inactive medical power when it is not able to provide the aggravation thereby having lost its medicinal capacity.

Paragraph 249 has a note. Therein it is said, "All experience teaches us that scarcely any homoeopathic medicine can be prepared in too minute a dose to produce a perceptible benefit in a disease to which it is adapted. Hence, it would be an improper and an injurious practice when the medicine produces no good effect or an inconsiderable aggravation of the symptoms, after the manner of the old school to repeat or increase the dose under the idea that it cannot prove serviceable on account of its minuteness."

For an explanation: Experience does teach us that a correctly chosen homoeopathic remedy in its most minute dose will be capable of producing some good effect when it matches the disease symptoms. However, when this does not happen or take place, one can be very sure and certain that the remedy could affect the disease symptoms adversely. Having known this, the physician must, the moment he sees that the remedy is working adversely, immediately antidote the remedy and quickly go to the correct or possibly the next remedy close to the appropriate remedy.

The physician instead of doing this must not think of either repeating or increasing the dosage of the damaging medicine. It will prove disastrous.

So, till now what is it that we have tried to prove? Even the minutest dose is capable of working wonders. We cannot afford to think the dose being 'micro', it may not work or function. It is clear that the senses have no relation whatsoever to the minuteness of the dose. The medical personnel have a tendency to measure the dose from the standard of a poisonous dose. He usually measures off a little less than that which would poison and he would call that a dose. For him it must be visible and seen. In homoeopathy the doctrines teach us otherwise. We say the *'esse'* is invisible. We have spoken about the high cost highly sensitive instruments in an earlier lecture. Therein we said the costliest and the most sensitive instrument cannot 'see' such a subtle form.

To recall what the master has said, the test of the dose as, one capable of producing a slight aggravation of the symptoms. He has not limited the attenuation in any place. It is unlimited and no one has ever found the end, yet.

We now come to the material dose. Barring the strict followers of homoeopathy or Hahnemann, some physicians feel that the dose of medicine is too small to cure — that for the people of Hahnemann's period it could have been alright. This may not be suitable for the current population. Well this thought is irrelevant and a fatal error.

An increase of the dose cannot make it more homoeopathic. The principles are very clearly laid before us. The first and the foremost point for consideration in any homoeopathic treatment is the similarity — a very close one — between the disease symptoms and the drug symptoms. The second point that we have to consider is the dose. These are fixed law and principles, which have been repeatedly tried and success attained. In addition to the doctrines our experience also confirms this. So, to say that the dose suggested by Dr. Hahnemann is too little or insufficient is a fatal error. The above law holds good under all circumstances and is suitable to all the periods. No doubt we have in our hands the wide range of dosages possible. Hence the point of dose is kept flexible.

We have spoken earlier about homoeopathy and individualization. In homoeopathy individualization plays a very important role. Where there is time to analyze and fix up the potency it is always good to fix up the potency keeping the patient's state in mind.

But from experience and the teachings of various doyens of homoeopathy, 30th potency is ideal to start with, in any acute diseases, or chronic diseases. No mortal can see the higher limit. You can only go for an ideal potency suitable to the individual and you cannot have a fixed rule by which you can proceed.

We want to follow up the series, so that we may get the very internal states that exist in the degrees of the medicine. Each potency is distinctly different from the other, we must remember these. Some may be far apart, yet invariably they are connected. We again repeat that it will be a mistake on the part of the homoeopath if he feels the idea of medicine laid down by Dr. Hahnemann is too small to cure. This clearly shows the individual who thinks on these lines is of the material mould. He is non-flexible and cannot yield to higher observations. He is not capable of observing and following higher and higher as the true experience would lead. A homoeopath must be true and truth must be in his mind. Only then his experiences will also be true. Otherwise it will be false. Truth in mind gives good experience and where the mind is in a state of truth his experiences also will be true. It cannot be otherwise.

We can never trust the experiences of men who are ignorant of what is true. They cannot be lead into truth by these fallacious experiences.

Summary

1. This lecture deals with the homoeopathic aggravation. Several paragraphs of Organon have been explained in this lecture.

2. In any acute disease the uncommon, singular and characteristic symptoms of the remedy tallies with the disease symptoms, the remedy will surely remove and cure the disease. It will be according to the homoeopathic law, one single dose, that is minimal will cure with the least inconvenience to the patient.

3. By and large the acute diseases do not drive the patient to the death's door.

4. If the acute disease has existed many days, it may threaten to breakdown the blood and tissues. In this state sharp aggravations, great prostration, violent sweating, exhaustion, vomiting and purging after the administration of the remedy. These reactions are necessary to cure the patient.

5. In an acute disease where ultimate are observed it goes to mean that the disease has existed in that body for some time. Ultimate cannot crop overnight.

6. Where ultimate have set-in in acute disease we notice striking aggravation. It may be so severe that recovery becomes impossible. In certain advance conditions important organs like liver, lungs and / or kidneys are damaged and destroyed.

7. We must always determine whether a case is acute or chronic. In acute diseases where there are no ultimate set in, there is no necessity for any strong reactions due to the structural changes.

8. Where there is a deep-seated pyemia we notice vomiting and purging. Whenever the deranged harmony or economy is brought back to order there is always a house cleaning. Hence the vomiting and purging. This is the nature's way of protecting us. The body does this by itself.

9. In a chronic disease where the ultimate have not set in there might not be any severe aggravation - but there might be a

very slight exacerbation of the symptoms - this will be of a different character.

10. In such a case due to the remedy administration and the reaction it sets in, all the excretory organs get suppressed and here the house cleaning becomes impossible.

11. In case of a paralyzed limb due to neuritis, which has been in existence for some time, with the administration of an appropriate remedy, there is a reaction. The blood circulation in the affected part is regulated, the numb nerves become sensitive again. This causes the patient to twist and turn - screech and cry. Never ever attempt to resist this twisting and turning, etc. It is the nature's way of bringing back things to order. If resisted, the patient can die.

12. The homoeopath cannot afford to change the medicine thinking that the above situation calls for another remedy. He has to wait and watch. Administration of another remedy can bring in a different reaction and is capable of causing confusion.

13. A homoeopathic physician must be capable of good and correct discrimination. He must be able to differentiate between a reaction and what needs a medication.

14. The homeopathic physician cannot afford to violate the principles at any stage ever. If he is careless or indifferent at the first opportunity, he may not have a second chance.

15. In a longstanding disease it may not yield to the aggravation. Then the distress is more and so is the turmoil. The deeper it is the more is the tissue changes. With more tissue changes the reaction becomes more and more distressing, pain is also more.

16. When a patient comes in with violent reaction every time a medicine is administered - there is violent aggravation of the

disease and the symptoms. This indicates that there is a deep-seated trouble.

17. In feeble patients the reactions may be only feeble, sometimes no reaction at all after the remedy. But then there may be a few symptoms. Under these conditions a true specific cannot be found.

18. When a remedy is administered in a case of suspected consumption case the patient exhibits a violent reaction this is a forerunner of what will happen several years later, in case he is not cured now.

19. Oversensitive patients prove everything that comes along. So, the physician must be able to stamp the patient oversensitive or otherwise.

20. The remedy could be exaggerated in the oversensitive patients. This can occur in feeble constitution persons.

21. Persons with a receding chin, sunken eyed persons and people with senility in their eyes are more viable to be oversensitive.

22. The patient must be treated in such a manner that the cure is effected without any suffering.

23. The homoeopathic remedy is chosen which corresponds in its nature with the disease symptoms. This or such a remedy will not leave any stone unturned in curing the disease completely.

24. *Wait and see* must always be your guideline. In cases where the physician cannot wait to watch the progress due to the intensity of a case he must discriminate and do what is best for the patient under the circumstances.

25. In a continuous fever like typhoid the best way to give the medicine will be to give it dissolved in water.

26. In fever conditions we have to wait. Never, never try to gain an immediate reaction.
27. In case of remittent fevers always stick to one single dose. In typhoid fever, etc., we have to wait a few days. Under that condition, repetition of the dose is permitted.
28. In certain delicate types of typhoid fever it is better never to repeat the medicine. In a vigorous constitution, here, there can be a quick and safe reaction.
29. Be cautious with feeble constitution patients. In such cases wait — do not repeat the medicine. A repetition may become a fatal error. But in some cases the repetition has saved the situation. How, no one is able to explain.
30. The slight homoeopathic aggravation in the first few hours after the remedy is given is a good omen. This indicates a cure is around.
31. The mild aggravation will always become obvious in the first few hours.
32. A natural disease can destroy another by exceeding it in both power and intensity.
33. The medicine's similarity to the disease symptoms is the first point of consideration, in homoeopathic treatment.
34. We saw above that the drug symptoms must totally tally with the disease symptoms. The second point is that the medicine should be powerful enough to combat the disease.
35. When the drug symptoms do not correspond fully or very closely with the disease symptoms there can be no aggravation. But the patient may feel better, since the remedy is capable of dealing with most of the disease symptoms. It is also possible that the case has not been properly taken. We cannot overlook the possibility of human error. But this

is unexpected of a homoeopathic physician. He is supposed to be alert always.

36. The solution in such a case will be to wait sufficiently for the medicine to act and then cease its action. Then a dose of the correct appropriate remedy is to be administered.

37. We shall consider a case of over-sensitiveness. Where the drug does not fit perfectly we cannot lookout for the aggravation. Due to the drug's partial correspondence with the disease symptoms the medicine is unable to penetrate deep enough. Here also after waiting we can administer the proper remedy once more.

38. Since the drug is only partially corresponding with the disease symptoms, in an oversensitive patient there will be an aggravation. This will not be there in a vigorous constitution or normal person. In the oversensitive patient the drug has brought about the aggravation and hence this is a medicinal aggravation or a homoeopathic aggravation.

39. In a vigorous constitution a partially matched remedy to the disease may cause no aggravation. Here due to the partial match certain disease symptoms could have been eradicated. There is a residue left. To eliminate this residue we have to select remedies that will suit the residual symptoms and throw them out. Thus we have to conclude that case.

40. A master homoeopathic physician will administer only a single dose of a single remedy. We should not give several or two or three remedies to meet a case. It is not homoeopathic ethics.

41. The smaller the dose the shorter the aggravation.

42. After an aggravation, the relief lasts long.

43. We have on our hands a wide range of potencies. Then what is the smaller dose? Dr. Hahnemann has suggested

30th potency. In this potency we have milder aggravations in the first five hours after administration.

44. Where Dr. Hahnemann tried the 60th potency the patient underwent great turmoil and distress due to the aggravation.

45. The disease is actually intensified and made worse by the remedy where it is similar to the disease symptom.

46. A 4th potency *Belladonna* dose created a violent congestion of the brain. The aggravation as said was violent. The susceptibility has also its role in this drama.

47. Remember always the smaller the dose of medicine the milder the aggravation.

48. Too low a potency will prolong the aggravation unnecessarily. Similarly a repetition can also prolong the aggravation.

49. A dose of *Bryonia* was sent to a robust young woman with instructions to take the medicine on the tongue. She dissolved the medicine in water and took it till the end of next day. She contracted symptoms of pneumonia. The moment the medicine was stopped the symptoms also vanished. She was proving the drug *Bryonia!* Similar proving of various medicines has been observed when taken like this. Proving, proving, proving!

50. Diseased state can be made worse by repetition of the medicine.

51. In very high potencies, the reaction is different. The characteristic of the disease will be brought out sharper. The patient will feel definitely better. The disease itself will not be aggravated, the symptoms stand out sharp. The patient will say, "I feel better".

52. Whatever the potency, the remedy is capable of curing. Even where the potency is very high the trace of medicine is very

very low. Yet it has within it a wonderful curative power.
53. Dr. Hahnemann has said that this potentizing should have a limit. Our masters have gone up to potentization 13 MM. Still they found the drug possessing curative or medicinal power.
54. Each potency will have its own range of action though they may stand apart.
55. The criterion for choosing the potency is that it will be just enough to combat the disease symptoms and cure it.
56. The homoeopathic physician must know when to antidote a remedy already given.
57. It is wrong to think that micro level of medicine in higher potencies may not be sufficient to meet a disease head on or the dose might be too small.
58. We repeat that the two considerations in homoeopathic treatment is (1) drug symptoms must totally tally with the disease symptoms if we want a cure and (2) the dose according to the state of the patient.
59. Homoeopathic medicines work on the dynamic plane and not on physical plane.
60. A homoeopath must be true.

Aphorisms & Precepts

1. The wisest will make mistakes in perception, but the aim must ever be to find the most similar of any medicines proved, and to recognize that there is one most similar of all.
2. One remedy must be more similar than the other. It is true that one not conversant with the subject will be unable to

see the finer shades of difference. Some are color blind, yet others can pick out colors.

3. Never leave a remedy until you have tested it in a higher potency if it has benefited the patient.

4. The expressions by which we know that he has been sick for a long time we know by our study of pathology and anatomy. These are the results of disease but the primitive disease if evidenced by the symptoms, the morbid sensations.

5. These are degrees within degrees to infinity. All may be made sensitive or become so to certain things and with differing degrees of susceptibility; hence what folly to lay down the rule for a fixed dose beyond which the result would be fatal, and beyond which if a physician should go he would be responsible in case of death.

6. When a case comes back in a few days with all the symptoms changed, unless they are old symptoms, the prescription was inaccurate and unfortunate.

7. All things that change the aspect of a case should be avoided.

8. Unless the inner nature of the remedy corresponds with the inner nature of the disease the remedy will not cure the disease but simply remove the symptoms, which it covers; that is, suppress them.

9. It is worse than useless to give a second dose until the effects of the first dose have ceased.

10. The increase of conditions shows increase of sickness; the increase of symptoms often shows diminution of sickness.

11. Confusion comes from losing one's head, prescribing on few indications and giving medicine when no medicine should be given.

Lecture - XXXIV

12. Anything that exhausts makes manifestations internal.

13. Low potencies can cure acute diseases because acute diseases act upon the outer most degree of the simple substance and the body. In chronic diseases the trouble is deeper seated, and the degrees are finer, hence the remedy must be reduced to finer or higher degrees so as to be similar to the degrees of the chronic disease.

14. Sickness exists on varying planes. Acute diseases occupy an outer plane and do not take so great a hold upon the life. The chronic disease reaches what we may call the innermost potency of man.

15. The lower potency corresponds to a series of outer degrees less fine and less interior than the higher.

16. When the third potency cures, there is something higher in it. No substance permeates the vital force when it is coarse enough to be seen.

17. Power comes in the direction of similitude, not of intensity and gains power only in proportion, as it is similar.

18. When you give a remedy be sure that the nature of the remedy and the nature of the disease (as well as the symptoms) agree.

19. An inappropriate prescription may be the stepping-stone to breaking down.

20. Crude drugs aggravate the disease, while high potencies aggravate the symptoms of the disease and do not engraft upon the economy a drug disease, provided the remedy is not repeated.

21. The action of the remedy is mild, the medicine does not act violently, but the reaction of the economy in throwing off the disease may be violent. As soon as order is restored a tumultuous action may begin.

22. Avoid unnecessary aggravation of symptoms by adjusting the potency of the patient.
23. Homoeopathy causes aggravations; it touches the very secret. It relates to the patient. All disease causes exist in this realm.
24. Note the difference between the aggravation of the disease, and that belonging to the remedy. Large doses really aggravate the disease; high potencies aggravate the symptoms of the disease.
25. The physician is not called upon to cure the results of disease, but the disease itself. All pathological changes must be regarded as the results of disease since all disease are dynamic.
26. The result of disease never form the image of the nature of the disease, the symptoms alone do this.
27. When a man takes a remedy in too large a dose, he feels worse and his symptoms are worse; with a higher potency, he feels better though his symptoms may be aggravated.
28. Power, then, is due to degrees of similitude. It is true that as it is more similar the remedy is more powerful and *vice versa*.
29. Nature never cures except by similar. Year by year you will gain respect for this similar.
30. If you have an idea of the nature of sickness, you will know about the action of the remedies.

Lecture - XXXV

Prognosis After Observing the Action of the Remedy

Prognosis — what is the meaning of this term? We shall see presently.

Prognosis: —

(1) Foreknowledge — the act or the art of foretelling the course of a disease from the symptoms.

— **Twentieth Century Chambers Dictionary**

(2) The foretelling of the probable course of the disease - a forecast of the outcome of a disease.

— **Steadman's Pocket Medical Dictionary**

(3) A forecast as to the probable result of an attack of a disease.

— **Dr. P.S. Rawat**

(4) Medical name for the outlook of a disease.

— **Webster's Medical Dictionary**

(5) Prediction of course and end of a disease.

— **Gould**

We shall take the meaning of Prognosis as the prediction of course and end of a disease.

So, now we know exactly what we mean by prognosis. No one can have any doubts about it.

Let us mentally visualize the drama after we find the physician having administered a remedy. After his prescription has been made, the physician starts his observations. The whole future of the individual may depend upon the physician's conclusion. He draws his conclusions from his observations. His entire action now depends totally on his observations. A homoeopath's top most interest has to be his patient. Whatever he chooses to do must be in the interest of improving his patient's condition. If his observations are not proper the physician may take a wrong step and that may prove detrimental to the patient's condition.

The only way to do the correct thing is the intelligent way.

If you discuss this activity with a few physicians a majority of them will say "once the prescription is made that is all there is to it - what do you expect after that". They see nothing beyond making the prescription.

In several lectures we have been repeatedly shouting from rooftops 'wait and watch'. Here is one more situation to use this axiom. This will bring in lot of dividends if practiced sincerely.

What we are saying about this is from the practical experience. The physician must be patient - *wait and watch* for long time. The physician should be an excellent observer. Otherwise his long wait and watch will prove useless and the entire purpose will be lost. If he is not an accurate observer his observations will be indefinite, his prescription will also be indefinite. As simple as that. At this juncture we would suggest the ardent followers of homoeopathy go back a few lectures and refresh themselves of the nature and quality of the physician we had narrated in the form of a list therein.

Lecture - XXXV

Let us take up a case. We have made a prescription. The prescription is the most appropriate one that suits the disease symptoms like a 't'. Now what is going to happen? The remedy is the ideal one. So it will act. As soon the remedy starts acting there are immediate changes in the patient. How do we recognize this? Again it is the symptoms and signs, which happen to be the language of nature, which indicate the change.

The physician understands that a person suffers a malady by or through the symptoms exhibited. The physician has to wait and watch. He cannot be in a hurry as far as this is concerned. He has to sit back, wait and watch observing the patient. Only when he does this, the physician can judge by the changes he had observed. His next step has to be based on this. He will understand and know what to do in his next step in this particular case. He also will be guided as what not to do. He quickly ascertains what not to do for an index that will guide him as what not to do.

We have always repeatedly said that a homoeopathic physician has to be constantly alert and observant. When he is a sharp vigilant observer, the physician will be able to see the index of every case.

When a remedy or a prescription does not relate to the case it can effect no change. Where that is the case, it will not take long to see what to do. There you cannot go according to the axiom wait and watch. It can only be wastage of time. Here the symptoms also will not be of any value. Where a remedy is sufficiently related to the case it brings in some changes in the symptoms. These symptoms are those of value.

What are the observations to be made and studied by the homoeopathic physician in respect of case, after administration of the remedy? We shall enumerate them one by one. This will also show us what are the changes that a properly chosen remedy will bring about.

1. On administering the remedy, some changes will begin. The homoeopathic physician should be alert to watch out for this beginning. Then he should

    (a) Observe what are these changes like?

    (b) What do these changes try to convey?

    (c) What do they amount to?

2. The physician must listen carefully to the patient's narration and reports. He must make note of the patient's words - the words that the patient uses could mean a lot more than what is observed. Nevertheless do not underestimate the value of observation. If the physician is alert, by listening to the patient, he will know what is going on.

3. When the remedy starts working, there will be changes in the symptoms. We shall see what changes are possible

    (a) The disappearance of a symptoms or

    (b) The increase of symptoms or

    (c) The amelioration of the symptoms

    (d) The order of the symptoms.

These happen because of the administration of the remedy. All these changes due to the remedy will have to be observed and studied.

We shall see things in more detail now. We have learnt that the medicines either aggravate or ameliorate. In our earlier lecture (Lecture XXXIV) we have seen about the homoeopathic aggravation. The aggravations are of two types.

1. An aggravation when the disease is aggravated and the patient becomes worse.

Lecture - XXXV

2. The other aggravation is the aggravation of the symptoms. Here the patient actually grows better.

We will now see the result of the aggravation of disease. In such a case the patient grows weaker. The symptoms grow stronger.

In the true homoeopathic aggravation of the symptoms, actually the patient grows stronger and better. The homoeopathic physician can observe this after the true homoeopathic prescription. In such cases, the patient will say he is better or 'I feel better'.

When we observe a patient carefully we find certain things. We shall take one aspect, which plays an important role. It concerns the particulars related to the states as to the time and place, as to how the aggravation occurs, as to how the amelioration takes place and its duration, etc., even the moon-phase has its own part to play.

We have been repeatedly telling that homoeopathy is individualization. The aggravations and ameliorations, the directions of the symptoms and many other things related to the disease will have to be observed. All these things are to be considered carefully and then the judgment passed upon them.

The homoeopathic physician has as his topmost mission to cure the patient. He can do so only when he is alert and discriminates the situation carefully. By this we mean the physician's total attention must be centered on the patient. The physician must gather whether the patient is improving or deteriorating. What guides the physician to settle this? (i) He can take the word of the patient if he is known to be totally reliable and co-operative. Where this is doubtful or we are certain it is totally wrong to accept the patient's version, homoeopathy has taught us to be after facts. How do we work our way to the facts in this case? We have learnt so much about the art of questioning a patient and observing him. (ii) So, by studying the symptoms after the medicine is administered and the changes in the symptoms are collected and analyzed, we are thus able to reach at this fact. After all, our mission is to cure the patient and we can afford not to turn every stone on the way. Only by such a persistent habit we can accomplish our mission. Why we have mentioned this here is because a patient actually feeling better may say he is worse. Only on investigating all the symptoms, we may understand that the patient is really getting better. Now think for a moment - had you taken the patient's word for granted and then where would you stand as a physician? So it is always better to study the symptoms and judging the case.

The symptoms also can guide us to inform that the patient has really become weaker. What do we mean by the patient is really becoming weaker or worser? In homoeopathy we say the cure is from within out. So obviously if the disease is worsening the symptoms will go inwards, from outwards. When this occurs the patient is going from bad to worse. The symptoms speak volumes about the disease. When properly interpreted we can depend totally upon the symptoms.

In the old school only the information of the patient was available. This does not help the homoeopathic physician in any way. The symptoms the homoeopathic physician observes must be corroborated. The patient's true opinion must also be corroborated with the symptoms. In most of the cases the symptoms do corroborate with the statements of the patient in many instances. Now you know why we said above the 'true opinion of the patient'. All said and done the symptoms are only of real value. These are what which decide the case and are the physician's most satisfactory evidence.

We have been consistently saying that symptoms are the main guiding factor in any case. We shall presently see how the symptoms guide to assess the disease. The homoeopathic physician observes that the changes are occurring in the exterior, by this the

Lecture - XXXV

physician will understand whether the disease is being healed from the innermost or the symptoms have changed to their superficial nature.

We will speak of palliatives and palliation in our later lecture. Incurable diseases are often to be palliated by mild medicines. These medicines act only superficially, act upon the sensorium, act upon the senses. But all the time the disease, which is hidden and deep-seated trouble, goes on and progresses - sometimes made worse. Yet the patient feels more comfortable.

See, how symptoms help us. We can know the depth of the disease. This will help us to know whether the patient will recover. The direction that the symptoms are moving will be sufficient to inform us the exact progress or declining of the disease, especially in chronic cases.

We shall now consider a case of aggravation. How the progress has been in steps.

A patient visits the clinic. He is somewhat stoop-shouldered. Has a hacking cough. This hacking cough has tortured the patient for several years. He has been sick for a good while - he looks sickly. He looks emaciated and anxious; he is care-worn suffering from poverty, poor clothing and scanty food. Now you have an idea of the patient's over-all appearance.

Next we shall go into his symptoms. Form the symptoms we find that the patient must be given an anti-psoric medicine. Studying the patient's history we are able to understand that he had been in need for the anti-psoric, in your mind it is re-inforced. On examining his chest we find that there is no sufficient chest expansion. The patient has tuberculosis. This is ascertained by the patient's feeble pulse and so many other corroborating symptoms. We are also able to understand that the patient's condition is slowly going from bad to worse.

The next obvious step here is to administer the appropriate remedy. We have taught to wait and watch after the administration.

So, we do just that. But, in the mean time in about a week's time the patient comes to the clinic. We notice a sharp aggravation of the symptoms. The cough has increased — there is nocturnal sweating. The patient feels feebler. In homoeopathy we all welcome an aggravation — for when there is aggravation after the administration of a suitable remedy. The patient is sent back after suitably being advised. But see what happens now. The patient returns after another week. We notice the aggravation is still present - now it has only increased. The patient's cough is worse now. The expectoration is all the more difficult now. The night sweat still present. The next visit also shows that the patient's health is now definitely on the decline. The patient has become worse than the previous week. He has gone from bad to worse since taking that medicine. Before the medicine's introduction the patient was comparatively better and more comfortable. Four weeks after taking the medicine the patient has become worse - his sickness having progressed. Generally after the initial aggravation, where human meddling is not there normally there must be an amelioration. Only then we are on the road to cure. Here, in this case, we had not amelioration, only aggravation through and through. It is evident that the patient is sinking. Now he has become so weak that he cannot even come to the clinic. This is what you call aggravation of the disease and declination.

We shall enumerate the few observations that a homoeopathic physician has to observe in the course of his work.

(1) **First Observation: A Prolonged Aggravation and a Final Decline of the Patient**

Let us consider the above case. Think what we have done to drive the patient to this condition? Think we gave an anti-psoric. What did this do? Chronic miasmatic cases have to be treated gently and thoughtfully. These anti-miasmatic remedies go deep into the system and work violently when carelessly handled. In this present case the remedy has gone deep — perhaps to the core and established the destruction.

In this case, the vital reaction was impossible, he was incurable. The next logical question that pops into our mind is what are we to do in such a situation? The patient is steadily declining. Are we not going to administer the homoeopathic remedy in such a case? Here the homoeopathic physician should be very clear in his mind and action. He must not panic. He must be aiming at doing only well to the patient.

In such a serious case always think of 30th potency and 200th potencies. After this potency being given, watch. Observe how the aggravation is going to be—whether it is going to be deep or prolonged.

There are many signs in the chest in such cases. The physician may doubt whether he will give a deep remedy where an organic disease is present. This does not apply where things are only threatening, when we have the fear of their coming, but when we are sure of their being present.

In our present case we shall see how this has all happened? We said that the patient required the anti-psoric for quiet some time. Well, there is a clue here. Can you guess it? The probability is that the remedy has been given too late. The remedy has worked out to arouse the patient's economy. But this must have turned towards the destruction of the whole organism.

What do we learn from this? Always in these cases, start with a low potency. Dr. Hahnemann has suggested 30th potency, which he found most practical in many cases. So, let us follow our master. Let us stick to 30th

potency in such cases. *Remember that 30th potency is low enough for anybody at any time, for anything.*

Let us see it from another angle. Let us assume the patient contacted us a little earlier when he was comparatively better and not in such a bad condition when he came to us. We had given a high potency. We make a second observation. Now there will also be an aggravation. This might last a long time - but there is a final reaction. We see light there. The final reaction brings in amelioration. The aggravation could be lasting for many weeks. The patient's feeble economy appears to react. Now there is a slow but sure improvement. What can you surmise here compared to the earlier situation?

In the present consideration we can easily understand one thing. The disease has not progressed so far; the changes have not become quite so marked. Well, let us wait for another three months. *By then the patient could be ready for the next dose of medicine. This time also we see a repetition of the same thing. Then we must understand that the patient is in a borderland and had gone further. Cure would have been impossible.*

It is always well in doubtful cases to go to the lower potencies. *In this way we proceed very cautiously; always prepared and ready to clamp down the action of the remedy by antidoting the medicine if it takes a wrong course.*

(2) **Second Obsrvation: The Long Aggravation but Final and Slow Improvement.**

Here let us assume that the patient gets a little better

Lecture - XXXV

after a few weeks of administering the remedy. His symptoms are a little better than when he took the dose of the medicine. Then there is some hope that finally the symptoms may have an outward manifestation. This is an indication he will finally recover - but the aggravation may prolong for many years. In such a patient we will find in the patient some very marked tissue change in some organ at the beginning. We may always know by observing the action of a remedy what state the tissues are in. We will also know definitely something about the prognosis for the patient.

(3) **Third Observation: Aggravation is Quick Short and Strong with Rapid Improvement of the Patient.**

Whenever and wherever an aggravation comes quickly, is short lived and that aggravation is more or less vigorous then we can be sure that the patient will improve. This improvement will be well marked and the reaction of the economy is vigorous. There is no structural change or a tendency to structural change in the vital organs. Whatever structural change is found will be on the surface, in such organs that are not vital. Abscesses will form; often glands that can be done without will suppurate in regions that are not important to the patient's life.

These organic changes are only surface changes. These are not similar to the changes that occur in the liver, kidney, heart and brain. We should understand well and be clear on the organic changes, which occur, in the vital organs, which carry out the work of the economy, and those, which happen in structures of the body, that are not vital to the life or essential to the life.

An aggravation, which is quick, short and strong is what should be desired and wished for. It is ideal because this is followed by quick improvement. Such slight aggravation of the symptoms appears in the first few hours after the administration of the medicine in an acute disease. In a chronic disease this aggravation sets in a few days' time.

(4) **Fourth Observation: No Aggravation is Noticed After the Administration of the Medicine.**

We do notice this in a class of cases. there will be satisfactory cures in these cases but following the remedy we can observe no aggravation, whatsoever. There is not organic disease or no tendency to organic disease.

The remedy is given to take care of the chronic disease or conditions. But the remedy is such that it will not penetrate deep. It will act on the nerves functions. It will not act on the threatened changes in the tissue.

We must realize here that the changes in the tissues are so marked. This is bound to disturb the vital force flowing through the economy. This is so slight that no high precision costly equipment can detect them.

In these circumstances we may have sharp sufferings but the cure will come by without any aggravation.

We have talked about potency in our earlier lectures. When the potency matches the patient's state it is the most ideal situation. We also know that when there is no aggravation the potency is exactly fitted to the case. But then under these situations we need not expect it always.

When the potency is not suitable say, either crude or too high for that particular patient then we will have the symptoms aggravated. So do not adjust or fit the potency to the patient - avoid aggravations that are unnecessary.

In cases where there has been no aggravation we know that the potency is most suitable to the patient's state. We also know that the remedy was the most appropriate since the patient's symptoms will be driven away and the patient returns to health. He returns to health in the most orderly way.

This form of cure is of highest order in any acute conditions. But always any homoeopathic physician will be happy to see the mild aggravation. He will be greatly satisfied about it. This aggravation must be in the beginning soon after taking the remedy. This is just a satisfaction he seeks to know that he is on the right road.

So, the fourth observation is we have no aggravation but accompanied by the recovery of the patient.

(5) Fifth Observation: Here the Amelioration Comes First and the Aggravation Comes Afterwards.

At times we see very sickly patients in the clinic. We make a long study of the case then finalize the remedy. This is given to the patient. The patient comes in a few days later for a review and also reporting his condition. He comes in and says he became better almost immediately after taking the medicine. He also reports he is getting better and talks about the decided improvement. But wait for a few more days. Say, about a week at the maximum. In severe cases there is a very common thing. Quite many symptoms get ameliorated as soon the remedy is taken. But all said and done such a condition is unfavorable.

Here the remedy was only a superficial one. Hence it could only act as a palliative dose or the patient was incurable though the remedy was somewhat suitable. One of these of the two conclusions, which we can arrive at in this situation. This can be done by the re-examination of the patient and also re-checking the remedy to see whether the symptoms related to that remedy.

Sometimes we do find that the choice of the remedy was erroneous. Continued examination of the case also proved that the remedy was only partially similar to the case — similar to the most grievous symptoms - it did not cover the entire case fully nor did the remedy fit patient. Then we can see that the patient is incurable and the choice of medicine was unsuitable.

The highest choice is the return of the symptoms - reappear exactly as they were. Then the original picture of the disease is not changed. But often they do come back in a very much-changed manner. Under that situation we have only one choice. We have to wait through the patient's suffering for the picture. The patient will also co-operate if informed of the fact that the choice of the remedy was not proper and we will do it better the next time.

When the physician accepts his mistake and takes the patient into his confidence and tells the truth, patient's confidence in the doctor increases multifold. Always the physician's acknowledgement of his wrong selection or wrong judgment begets a lot of confidence in the patient.

We shall now see about potencies. We shall take the higher and the highest potencies. These potencies act in curable disease for considerably a long time.

The remedy in these potencies act immediately and puts everything in order. This action can continue for a long time, even for several months. We have always said 'wait'. During this action of the remedy the patient is better off without any of this medicine that was given. While it is already in the system if a dose is repeated it will be chaos.

In curable diseases, whose prospects are good these remedy action will go for a long time. The patient will be relieved of their symptoms and feel healthy.

A patient may feel bad after a dose of CM *Sulphur.* But here the patient may be so for the first, second or third weeks. But the patient professes to be doing well all along. After the fourth week he comes with a dog's look and says, 'doctor, I have been running down — but I was feeling better the last few weeks.' Now the physician has to take a decision.

The physician must find the answers for a few questions for sudden decline. The physician must find out:

(1) Has the patient done something, which might have spoilt the action of the medicine?

(2) Has he used alcoholic drinks?

(3) Has he been handling any chemicals of late?

(4) Was he exposed to the fumes of ammonia for any reason?

(5) Have any of his friends wrongly influenced him?

The physician gets an emphatic 'No' for all these queries. Then what has gone wrong here?

The overall picture is an unfavorable one now. Any CM dose medicine, we all know will work and be active for months together. If there has been no interference of any sorts with this remedy in economy we may be suspicious of this case.

(6) **Sixth Observation: Too Short a Relief of Symptoms.**

We give a constitutional remedy to a patient. We expect it to work in the patient for some time. For some reason it does not act long enough as it ought to. In the third observation we saw that there will be a quick aggravation followed by a long amelioration. Here in the sixth observation we find short-lived amelioration. This amelioration is of too short a duration. Where we see an aggravation immediately after the administration of the remedy followed by a quick rebound we will *positively never* see too short an amelioration of that medicine. Wherever there is a quick rebound that amelioration should definitely last. If we notice it otherwise it can be only because of some condition, which intervenes with the action of the remedy. It may be unconscious on the side of the patient or it may even be intentional.

Wherever and whenever there is a quick rebound it means only two things. The remedy is well chosen, and the vital economy is in a good state. If every thing goes well, the recovery will most certainly take place. In acute cases we may see short amelioration of the symptoms. We have on our hand a case of most violent inflammation of the brain. A dose of medicine is administered. This remedy totally removes all the symptoms, but for just one hour. So the remedy is repeated at the end of one hour. Again the symptoms disappear — this time for just thirty minutes. We see that the pa-

Lecture - XXXV

tient is in a desperate condition; the ameliorations are too short.

We shall take *Belladonna* as an example to cite here. This remedy is very good and result oriented in some very acute red-faced conditions. Its action in these conditions is almost instantaneous. We can find the amelioration in five minutes.

But, we know there exists a slow and steady amelioration that is the best. Such amelioration comes in about an hour or two. This is likely to remain.

Where the amelioration is too short in acute cases it indicates there is such a high-grade inflammatory action present in the remedy. Such an explosive action is harmful to the organs. This rapid process that goes on at a high speed threatens them.

In *chronic cases* let us assume we see such a short-lived amelioration. What does it mean here? Here *there are structural changes in the organs and they are destroyed or they are being in the process of destruction or the organs are in a very precarious condition.*

Such changes cannot always be diagnosed in life. All said and done there is no denial of this occurrence. A really sharp and acute observer/homoeopathic physician with a long experience will very often be able to diagnose these conditions. He has been trained to see such maladies by his own persistent practice and development of this trait. He is capable of diagnosing the meanings of the symptoms even without examining the patient. He can prophesy as to the patient like a soothsayer.

This is a very very valuable experience on the part of an intelligent physician and his family will consider him a wise person. He knows well about the constitution of the family members.

How is this capacity earned? We have mentioned earlier that every homoeopathic physician has to toil hard, intelligently. This is acquired by hard work only.

He has to study the patient's symptoms with great concentration; then must know the action of the remedies upon them. He also must know what to expect after the medicine is administered. This knowledge enables him to conclude the reaction of a patient, whether to expect it slowly or quickly. For all this he must know his patient also well. All these have been hammered into an experienced and elderly physician. For a neophyte he has to learn it the hard way. There is no short cut for this knowledge.

(7) **Seventh Observation: We See a Full Time Amelioration of the Symptoms Yet No Special Relief of the Patient.**

Certain patients have a limit. Any further goading will show no further improvement. That is all. Such patients can gain only so much. There are latent conditions, or latent existing organic conditions. In such patients the above conditions prevent the improvement beyond a certain stage.

Let us take an individual with one kidney failure. The other kidney is functioning. When we try to improve the condition what can we expect? We can expect only a limited improvement.

Individuals with fibrinous structural changes in certain places, tubercles that have become encysted and lungs capable of doing only limited work will have symptoms. These symptoms will be ameliorated from time to time with medicines. We will see the individual cannot get any improvement or cure beyond a certain level.

Several medicines have been administered. Amelioration has existed often the full length of time of the remedies. With all this the patient's condition has not improved above his own pitch in this length of time. With all this the individual is not cured. Unfortunately he can never be cured. All this while the patient has only been palliated. This palliation is suitable for the homoeopathic remedies.

(8) **Eigth Observation: Some Patients Prove Every Remedy They Get.**

In our earlier lectures we have been talking about over-sensitive patients (Lecture XVI). Here we suggest you go back to your notes on this lecture for a refreshing.

Patients who are inclined to be hysterical, over-wrought, and over-sensitive to all things belong to one category. They are all over-sensitive to all things. The patient is said to have an idiosyncrasy to all things. These over-sensitive patients are often incurable. When we administer a dose of a drug of high potency they will prove that medicine. Remember we talked about *Bryonia* — a patient who was suggested to take a mouth dose dissolved the medicine in water and she went on to prove *Bryonia*, mentioned in that lecture?

These over-sensitive people when they come under the influence of that medicine, they will be totally under the influence of that medicine only. They cannot be influenced by anything else at that time.

The medicine takes complete possession of such people and acts on them as disease does. We had already suggested in the earlier lecture of the ideal potencies suitable to these people. It is 30th or 200th potencies.

In such over-sensitive people the drug takes over. As we said above, it acts in them as a disease does. The medicine takes over such patients — the remedy has a prodromal period, a period of decline. We had explained this of acute diseases in our earlier lectures. It was even illustrated by a chart. Go back to your notes and locate it.

These over-sensitive patients are most annoying; we can often cure their acute diseases by the 30th or 200th potency medicines. We can handle and manage their chronic diseases by 30th, 200th or 500th potency. Be cautious - never approach them with higher potencies.

Such people are congenitally sensitive. The sensitiveness can only die with them. These over-sensitive patients can never rise beyond this over-sensitive or over-irritable and over-wrought state.

Such persons after getting out of one proving will be ready to go into another proving or repeating the earlier one.

(9) **Ninth Observation: It is the Action of the Medicine Upon Provers.**

We have mentioned that provers must be healthy individuals. All healthy provers always benefit from the proving, when the proving is conducted properly. We have mentioned about all these things in our lecture XXVIII. If you desire to refresh your knowledge pull out your notes on the above lecture and read it.

We should always carefully observe the constitutional state of the prover to be. We must note them and subtract them from the proving. Thus we can be precise to the point. Normally the symptoms will not very commonly appear when the proving is underway. If they do appear, we must make a note of the change in the symptom.

(10) Tenth Observation: The New Symptoms That Appear After the Administration of the Remedy.

We administer a remedy to a patient when the remedy fits the symptoms of the patient. This point must always be in the physician's mind. We will forget this for a moment now. A remedy has been administered. Now assume several symptoms crop up after the remedy is given. We all know why this should be so. Guess? It goes to prove that the remedy was an unfavorable one. So simple.

Occasionally a new symptom may come up. The patient might not have observed this properly and chances are that he might be thinking that this is a new symptom.

Whenever we do get an array of new symptoms we should doubt our remedy more and more.

After all the new symptoms pass away the old symptoms will still remain. We are in square one. The patient has not been cured. So we know that the true homoeopathic relationship was not sustained between the remedy and the symptoms.

(11) Eleventh Observation: The Old Symptoms Reappear.

The old symptoms do appear after administration of our remedy. What is to be gathered out of it? We should understand under this condition one thing. Old symptoms, which were long been away - in the same proportion of their return, the disease are also curable.

The old symptoms had only disappeared because of the newer symptoms that cropped up.

Commonly we see old symptoms do re-appear after the aggravation has come. Hence we see the symptoms disappearing in the reverse order of their coming up. This indicates to the physician that the patient is on the road to recovery. We can say this to the patient and encourage him.

We have been hammering almost in every lecture that the cure is a cure only when it is from above downward, etc. Old symptoms often come back and go off by themselves. No medicine need be given. This shows that the medicine must be left alone and we should not muddle up the situation. But then when the old symptoms do come back and stay, then a repetition of the medicine becomes necessary, often. So until we are very sure that repetition of the dose is necessary, do not give it, but WAIT.

(12) Twelth Observation: Sometimes the Symptoms Take a Wrong Direction.

Let us take a case of rheumatism. Rheumatism of the hands, feet or knees. We administer a remedy. Now the remedy being a suitable one the patient is relieved of the same. So far, so good. But then the patient is taken down with a violent internal distress. This distress settles in centers in the region of the heart, or centers in the spine. Now what do we see here?

From the extremities the disease has been transferred to the center. In homoeopathy we always say the disease spreads from circumference to center. For the cure it is from the center to the circumference. That is, the disease goes from the circumference to center - that is from minor organs to major organs - from skin to internal major organs like kidneys, lungs and heart.

Now you can imagine the havoc that is created in this present case. Do you need any explanation? What are we to do now? There is only one way. Antidote is the remedy without any further delay.

If immediate antidoting is not done structural changes will start in that new site.

When the disease travels from center to circumference, going out from centers of life, out from the heart, lungs, brain and spine - out from the interiors to, upon the extremities it is a good sign. This is why we see many gouty patients seem well when their fingers and toes are in the worst condition. When we give a remedy for the gouty condition and observe that the heart symptoms get worse it is a very sad state of condition.

It is always a very good sign to have skin eruptions and the extremities affected. This shows the disease is in the circumference.

Be very cautious when dealing with the management of external symptoms on the skin. We must always take the totality of the symptoms - not only the skin symptoms. We should not ignore the whole economy as well as the patient's state.

Of course the remedy will act and cause the skin conditions to travel inside and disappear. But we must not take it to be a cure because the patient here is not really cured. Such a patient will remain sick till the eruption does come back. This eruption may re-locate itself in another place.

We have so far seen twelve observations that we have to learn well. All these must become a part of the homoeopathic physician and it must be automatic in his part. This will help the physician to become a successful practitioner to a great extent.

The physician will have to be alert to the case. He must definitely know to judge every situation before and after the administration of the remedy. This is an important lesson. Learn it well and above all practice what has been given in this lecture. We wish you all good luck following the instructions given here in this lecture.

Summary

1. Prognosis means the prediction of the course and end of a disease.
2. Prognosis can be made by proper observation of the case after the administration of a remedy.
3. Prognosis helps the physician to calculate his next step in the case.
4. In prognosis, 'wait and watch' will pay a lot of dividends, when practiced sincerely and deligently.
5. The physician should be always alert and an excellent observer. He must be capable of good judgment.
6. On administering a remedy as soon as it starts acting, we will be able to see some symptoms.
7. The symptoms alone are of value.
8. There are three things that a physician should observe in a case after the administration of a remedy. They are:

    (1) (a) What are the changes like?

(b) What do these changes try to convey?

(c) What do they amount to?

(2) The physician must carefully listen to the patient's narrations and reports - without interruption preferably. He can obtain clarifications wherever necessary. Beyond that he must be 'all ears' to the patient's narrations. He should note the expressive words as used by the patient. Later on he can interpret it properly. He must watch the facial expression, any peculiar movements and the patient's conduct in the clinic.

(3) When the remedy starts acting there will be changes in the symptoms.

(a) The disappearance of a symptom,

(b) The increase of symptoms or

(c) The amelioration of the symptoms

(d) The order of the symptoms' appearance.

9. Aggravations are of two types:

(i) Aggravation of the disease where the patient becomes worse.

(ii) Aggravation of the symptoms. Here the patient actually grows better.

10. In aggravation of the disease the patient grows weaker and the symptoms stronger. In a true homoeopathic aggravation there is an aggravation of the symptoms. But actually the patient feels better and stronger.

11. Things that the physician must observe in addition to the above: He must note down the time and place of aggravation, its duration, how the changes in the weather affect the above conditions, etc.

12. In both the above even the moon-phase plays a role.

13. The direction of the movements of the symptoms must be noted. From center to circumference, from above downwards will be a good sign.

14. All the above points will have to be carefully studied and then the next step for the patient's welfare ought to be decided. The homoeopathic physician must be always alert and observant to plan his next step intelligently.

15. By and large never ever accept your patient's version. Note what he has to say and you make your own observation and take a decision of your step after considering very carefully all the symptoms, way of conduct of the patient, etc. A homoeopathic physician must make up his work to only fact finding and nothing else.

16. When we say the disease are growing stronger and the patient weaker we mean that the disease is traveling from outward to center. The symptoms will go inwards. See the value of symptoms? They help you to judge the patient's condition. Proper interpretation of the symptoms is totally reliable.

17. For palliation in incurable disease conditions, use mild medicines not the deep acting ones. Such mild medicines act only superficially; act upon the sensorium and on the senses. Though the disease is all the time progressing these palliatives keeps the patients comfortable.

18. The homoeopathic physician must be well versed on the patterns of ameliorations and aggravations after the administration of a remedy. He must be absolutely alert and sensitive to even a subtle change and interpret it properly for the benefit of the patient. These are listed below. Learn them well.

(1) **A prolonged aggravation followed by a final decline of the patient.**

Reason

The patient might have needed a deep acting remedy for quite some time. Here the needed remedy has been given a bit too late. As the remedy tried to act and correct the economy the patient's condition was too fragile to contain the reaction. As a result the remedy took a destructive direction and affected him beyond cure and blasted him internally. Hence, the prolonged aggravation and finally the patient's decline.

Solution

We can start with a 30 or 200th potency.

Again wait and watch - see and check the action of the remedy. This would prove less dangerous. In these types of cases abstain from using a deep acting remedy.

When we take this line of action, the patient's feeble economy can co-operate and respond favorably.

(2) **There is a long aggravation followed by final and slow improvement.**

Reason

When the patient came to us there must have been some marked tissue change in some organ. When we administered the remedy it was able to help the vital force to bring back the economy to order. To accomplish this the remedy would need a lot of time. Hence the long aggravation.

As soon as the economy was set in order there was a slow improvement.

Solution

Here again the physician must wait. The long aggravation must not influence the physician to change the remedy and administer it. However since the improvement sets in we can leave it at that and wait.

N.B.: How will we know the tissue change in the patient? A proper analysis of the symptoms can indicate the malfunction of the organ due to the tissue change. *Investigate the particulars here.*

(3) **Aggravation is quick, short and strong with rapid improvement of the patient's condition.**

Reason

The drug picture synchronizes perfectly with the disease picture. The potency is also just right to combat the disease successfully.

The medicine as soon as it is administered starts acting. In its action it is able to wipe out the disease symptoms. As the order is re-established the aggravation is also rapid. Then the improvement starts.

We can always find this aggravation in the first few hours in acute disease. In chronic diseases where there is no structural changes of the vital organs this aggravation can be seen in the first few days or in about a week.

Solution

Here no further attention is needed since the patient is well on his road to recovery.

(4) **No aggravation is noticed after the administration of the medicine. The patient's recovery is also there.**

Reason

Here the potency of the medicine is most suitable to the patient's state. The medicine is also very appropriate. All the symptoms are driven away. The patient's recovery is most orderly.

This form of cure is the highest order in any acute conditions.

Solution

No further action is needed since the patient recovers.

(5) Here the amelioration comes first and the aggravation follows it.

Reason

The remedy chosen could have been partially suited to the disease. So wherever the symptoms and medicine symptoms coincided they were wiped out. So initially there appeared an apparent amelioration. After the amelioration aggravation followed.

So here the medicine is partially suitable or it has been erroneous. The remedy also did not fit the constitutional conditions of the patient.

Then we can see the patient is incurable as well.

Solution

When there has been no interference of any sorts and the aggravation severe the physician has to act in the best interest of the patient's welfare with particular attention to the situation.

(6) Too short a relief of symptoms.

Reason

There is a high-grade inflammatory action present in the remedy.

In chronic cases the remedy's explosive action will create structural changes in the organs or they are destroyed or a process of destruction of the organ is set.

This can be found out by the symptoms and a careful observation by any diligent homoeopathic physician.

Solution

The case has to be handled by an experienced and intelligent physician who can judge the serious situation of the patient and act in the patient's best interest according to the circumstances and situation.

(7) **We observe a full-time amelioration of the symptoms yet no special relief of the patient.**

Reason

In a cup of coffee or tea, you can go on adding sugar. After a certain limit of sugar there will be no further sweetening. Any more adding of the sugar will make no more sweetening of the brew.

Similarly for some patients they can improve only to a particular level. Beyond that we can never improve the situation or condition of the patient. This is because there are latent conditions in the organs.

Solution

These patients may get ameliorated now and then by the medicines. But they cannot have any real relief.

(8) **Some patients prove every remedy they get.**

Reason

Hysterical patients, over-wrought and over-sensitive patients are so sensitive they automatically prove every medicine they get.

Solution

A safe procedure here is to start with either 30th or 200th potency.

Never, never approach an over-sensitive person with any higher potency lest he becomes a prover.

(9) The action of the medicine upon the provers.

Reason

We see a medicine in Materia Medica. There are several provings. The proving of a group of several healthy individuals is noted therein. At this point we must remember one thing. Each prover though healthy will be of different constitutional states. Now in each person's proving we have to consider the individual's constitutional state. This must be subtracted from that individual's proving. Only then the precise proving will be realized.

Normally fresh symptoms will not very commonly appear during the proving. If they do, we have to note the change in the symptom.

Solution

The physician must recognize the above point, and use this knowledge in his practice.

(10) The new symptoms appear after the administration of the remedy.

Reason

The remedy was an unfavorable one, or perhaps the patient might not have recognized the symptom and now felt it as a new symptom. This does occur occasionally.

But when we do get an array of new symptoms the remedy administered must be the culprit.

A true homoeopathic relationship was not sustained between the remedy and the symptoms.

Solution

Wait for the new symptoms to disappear and the old symptoms will emerge.

(11) The old symptoms re-appear.

Reason

In the administration of a medicine we should expect a cure. Sometimes very old symptoms may re-appear. This will be after the initial aggravation. This old symptoms disappeared because the newer symptoms appeared. The disappearance of the old symptoms in the reverse order will show us that the patient will soon recover.

Solution

Old symptoms come back and go off by their own accord. Here we must not interfere with the process and must abstain from administering any new medicine at this stage. But there may be the necessity of a repetition of the old medicine. So if you are sure that a repetition of the old medicine is necessary then administer that dose.

(12) Sometimes the symptoms take a wrong direction.

Reason

The remedy appears to have gone berserk and shot up

the wrong direction. If it is from circumference to center this must cause a great concern to the patient and the physician. The disease has worsened.

Solution

Immediately antidote the medicine which caused this havoc. Start treatment afresh.

Be very cautious when you are dealing with skin problems. The disease might be driven inside, from external to internal, from the non-vital to vital organs.

The knowledge we have been taught here is to be learnt well and followed in the daily practice. In the main lecture almost for every observation a case has been presented. This will cover almost all probable cases after the administration of the remedy. So whenever you meet a similar case you must know what to do. So, learn all the above twelve probabilities to become successful and effective.

Aphorisms & Precepts

1. Everything is working harmoniously in the well man. Consider the man, heal the sick.
2. If you lose the attitude of mind, which seeks the good of the patient you will lose your homoeopathy.
3. You cannot depend on lucky shots and guess work; everything depends on long study of each individual case.
4. Anything, which looks away from exactitude, is unscientific. The physician must be classical; everything must be methodical. Science ceases to be scientific when disorderly application of law is made.
5. The sick are entitled to exact knowledge, not to guess work.

6. You must be able to recognize every ambassador of internal man.

7. A disease may be suppressed by a medicine as well as by a stronger dissimilar disease.

8. Homoeopathy is an applied science not a theory.

9. When old symptoms return, there is hope. That is the road to cure land there is none other.

10. The outer world is the world of results. The inner world is not discoverable by the senses but by the understanding.

11. You need not expect great things when you have only pathological symptoms.

12. The whole aim of homoeopathy is to cure.

13. It is inconsistent and irrational to think that there are several active diseases in the body at the same time.

14. All prescriptions that change the image of a case cause suppression.

15. Diseases themselves cannot be suppressed, but symptoms can. The totality of the symptoms must disappear in an orderly manner in order to constitute a cure.

16. Perception comes with use.

17. A piano tuner has restored harmony to a piano; has added nothing and taken nothing from it, yet has restored it to harmony.

18. If you have an idea of the nature of sickness, you will know about the action of the remedies.

19. Increasing the dose cannot increase the homoeopathicity. If it is right at all, you increase its homoeopathicity by elevating its quality towards its interior nature so that it corresponds more perfectly with the vital force.

20. When a man takes a remedy in too large a dose, *he* feels worse and his symptoms are worse; with a higher potency, *he* feels *better* though his symptoms may be aggravated.

21. One who thinks from the material, thinks disease is drawn in from without, but it is drawn out from within.

22. Homoeopathy causes aggravations; it touches the very secret. It relates to the patient. All disease causes exist in this realm.

23. Note the difference between aggravation of the disease, and that belonging to the remedy. *Large doses really aggravate the disease; high potencies aggravate the symptoms of the disease.*

24. Avoid unnecessary aggravation of the symptoms by adjusting the potency to the patient.

25. The action of the remedy is mild. The medicine does not act violently, but the reaction of the economy in throwing off the disease may be violent. As soon as order is restored a tumultuous action may begin.

26. Crude drugs aggravate the disease, while high potencies aggravate the symptoms of the disease, do not engraft upon the economy a drug disease, provided the remedy is not repeated.

27. Do not change the slightest symptom, observe everything. Receive the message undisturbed and get it on paper, there is no other way for a physician to perform his function and do his duty.

28. When symptoms are removed by the reaction of the economy they are more likely to stay away than when removed by the action of the drugs. Crude drugs given on theory only suppress symptoms.

29. If a remedy whose superficial symptoms agree with the superficial symptoms of a disease, but whose nature is different be given, it will cause suppression if it acts at all.
30. An inappropriate prescription may be the stepping-stone to breaking down.
31. When you give a remedy be sure that the nature of the remedy and the nature of the disease (as well as the symptoms) agree.
32. Power comes in the direction of similitude, not of intensity, and gains power only in proportion, as it is similar.
33. It does not take any enormous quantity to cure people any more than do make them sick.
34. The word disease really means the signs or symptoms before organic disease has taken place.
35. Sickness exists on varying planes. Acute diseases occupy an outer plane and do not take so great a hold upon the life. The chronic diseases reach what we may call the innermost potency of man.
36. Low potencies can cure acute diseases because acute diseases are upon the outermost degree of the simple substance and the body. In chronic disease the trouble is deeply seated, and the degrees are finer, hence the remedy must be reduced to finer or higher degrees so as to be similar to the degrees of the chronic disease.
37. Every sensation has its correspondence to something within.
38. Every action in homoeopathy must be based on a positive principle.
39. Anything that exhausts makes manifestations internal.
40. Confusion comes from losing one's head, prescribing on few indications and giving medicine when no medicine should be given.

Lecture - XXXV

41. The finest degrees of sensation are to be perceived for these changes constitute the nature of the disease. If drugs could not produce these changes they could not cure. This is the foundation. If you would discover whether the law of similar is the law of cure you would need to draw upon this store of finer symptoms.

42. When a remedy has benefited a patient satisfactorily, never in your life, change your remedy, but repeat that remedy so long as you can benefit the patient. Do not regard the symptoms that have come up.

43. When we recognize the fact of the long years of existence of chronic cases, also that they are after inherited for several generations, if a cure is made in the course of two or three years it is indeed a speedy cure. It takes from two to five years to cure chronic diseases.

44. In incurable cases where there are extensive structural changes use short acting remedies and such anti-psorics as do not relate to the case as it was in the beginning. The remedy that fits the previous condition will tear the case down.

45. Unless the inner nature of the remedy corresponds with the inner nature of the disease the remedy will not cure the disease but simply remove the symptoms, which it covers, that is, suppress them.

46. Such anti-psorics which do not relate to the constitutional condition of the patient are comforting and palliative and act as short-acting remedies.

47. When a case comes back in a few days with all the symptoms changed, unless they are old symptoms, the prescription was inaccurate and unfortunate.

48. We see the difference between short and long-acting

remedies from this. Short-acting remedies are only capable of corresponding to the outer most degrees of man.

49. The expression by which we know that he has been sick for a long time we know by our study of pathology and anatomy. These are the results of disease, but the primitive disease is evidenced by the symptoms, the morbid sensations.

50. The physician cultivates his eye for everything that it is possible to pass judgment upon, must write down everything that is unnatural, everything that is expressive of illness.

51. In this section we have given you a number of Aphorisms and Precepts. If you go through each one you can know that it is very much related to this lecture. It has a great impact. Read them one by one and connect it to the lecture. Then you will see their connection and the great impact that you must feel. Read these in depth, and benefit from this section.

Lecture - XXXVI

The Second Prescription

What is this second prescription? The second prescription may be any of the following:-
 (i) A repetition of the first prescription.
 (ii) It could be an antidote.
 (iii) It could be a complement.

What preliminaries are to be observed before the second prescription? The case must be studied completely, again. The original symptoms, when the patient came in, the administration of the medicine at that time and the other changes in the symptoms that has since occurred should be studied. Only after this process the second prescription can be made out.

But then, is this always feasible? One main difficulty that the homoeopathic physician generally faces is the patient changes the doctor. Unless that doctor provides all the details about this patient when he was with him in the form of a report the new doctor has his own difficulties to deal with this case afresh. Remember, in an earlier lecture of ours we had mentioned that a good reliable and really service minded homoeopathic physician who is genuinely interested in his patients must send this record along with the patient. Then the present physician will know what to do and how to proceed. Lack of such records accompanying the patient is one reason why the patient does not do well. In the absence of the records the second doctor should advise the patient to go back to the old doctor himself, for he will know the complete case of the patient and also be aware of the next correct or appropriate step to be taken in his case. The homoeopathic physician's top-most priority is the welfare of the patient. So in directing the patient to go back to the old doctor will not be out of the way.

Very few physicians follow this procedure. To do this, the physician must be a strong willed person and not interested in building up his bank balance but has the patient's well being at the top of his mind. God provides everyone with his share - so there is no need for any physician to grab another physician's patient. Such a physician will be respected in the community and also have a great respect among his colleagues.

Some doctors may demean his colleagues when another physician's patient comes to them. They say "Oh doctor so and so? Well what does he know about this? Many of his patients with this ailment have come to me from him and got cured." Well, this is a very bad thing for the morale of the doctor. Sooner or later he will earn a very bad name as a mudslinger and go into ill fame. This is not befitting of a homoeopathic physician.

We have elaborated about the importance of record keeping and also the necessity of transfer of records to the second doctor when the patient leaves the first doctor in our lecture XXVII. You may please go through your notes on this lecture to refresh your mind.

If the patient leaves the town permanently he may seek the help of a new doctor in the place where he settles down. Unless there is a sound reason for the patient to go to another doctor he must be advised to stick on to his first doctor. This will make a lot of sense.

Lecture - XXXVI

We are not talking here of ethics. Most of the doctors are broad-minded to accept one doctor accepting a case, which has been earlier, attended by another doctor. Generally all can tolerate with good humor such 'fly-offs'. But then a partially cured case with a particular remedy is taken up by a new doctor without the patient's earlier record from the previous doctor, it is going to be an up-hill task for the next doctor to deal with the case. He has got to or is compelled to start from the beginning to the present date afresh. Secondly, this patient could have changed from one doctor to another somewhere in the middle. There might be no records for that. Thirdly, the doctor now has to study the patient for various sensations, desires and aversions, fears, etc., for the entire period of the patient's suffering. The patient may not be able to coherently narrate all these at one or two sittings. There will be spurts of memory now and then — then he will convey the events in bits and fragments. The doctor will really have to apply himself to all these things. By then it may be too late and the patient's disease or sickness may be progressing. Hence, with so many drawbacks should the new doctor take up the case of another doctor? That is why it is better for the patient to stick to the old doctor and not change from him, when he cannot produce his earlier records.

The homoeopathic physician's one and only goal must be acting for the benefit of the patient under all circumstances. Now let us proceed with the lecture.

It will be wise to follow a rule about making a second prescription. It is:

Once the first and appropriate correct homoeopathic prescription is made and the remedy administered, the striking features for which the remedy was given, has been removed, there is bound to be a change. The guiding symptoms have been wiped out and only common and the trivial symptoms remain.

In other words the administration of the appropriate first homoeopathic prescription will wipe out the guiding symptoms of the disease. Then only the common and trivial symptoms remain.

Here it is true that these symptoms will reappear after a long time. For this we have to wait. But in our haste we do not allow the proper time. A second prescription is made out on the symptoms left out. That is the greatest folly a homoeopathic physician can make. We have always insisted almost in all our lectures that a homoeopathic physician must *wait and watch*. We must sympathies with the patients who fall into the clutches of a homoeopathic physician who does not wait and watch the action of the medicine administered.

The first prescription itself, when appropriate, has brought relief to many patients. This fact cannot be denied. But some patients get a relief first and suffer a little later on. They complain, "initially it did benefit me, but then later on the medicine could not benefit me." Can you imagine why the patient got relief initially and suffered later on? The answer is the first prescription was the appropriate one. Hence the patient got relief.

It is the duty of the doctor to wait — wait till the first prescribed medicine exhausts its action. However, in this case, the physician acted a bit hastily. Waiting for the exhaustion of the remedy's action he must have administered another dose of medicine hastily and indiscriminately. This has prevented the cure of the case and hence nothing further was accomplishable. This was solely due to the physician's hasty action. He ought to have waited long enough. It would have been wise for the physician to provide a few doses of placebo or Sac-lac, as it is known. The patient would have been happy he got the medicine while the physician can be happy in getting the wanted results. So, both are happy - each one getting what he wanted.

Please remember — *An Early Repetition of the Remedy and Also Giving the Same Continuously will Prevent anything*

Like an Opportunity for Providing a Second Prescription.

You may ask why we lose the opportunity of making a second prescription in the above statement? The homoeopathic physician has made the first prescription. The remedy is very appropriate to the case. We have said this remedy must not be repeated too soon. What happens if it is repeated too soon? Once the appropriate well-chosen remedy is administered it will start its action immediately. The remedy being appropriate and well chosen it combats the disease and keeps on effectively working internally, for some time. If during its working period another dose of the same remedy is repeated this causes a block for the symptoms and prevent them from reappearing. So now the opportunity for a second prescription gets automatically prevented. The symptoms get intermingled with the drug symptoms. Hence the rational second prescription cannot be made.

Did you notice a repetition of a particular thing in the above paragraph? It is 'appropriate well-chosen' remedy. Why has this been done? — Is it due to inadvertency? No, no, no. A second prescription does pre-suppose that the first prescription has been a totally correct one. It has taken effect on administration and should be left alone.

For a second prescription there ought to be a second observation. A second observation can be made possible only when the first prescription has been left alone without interference. In addition where the first prescription has not acted curatively is also needed. Then only a second observation is possible.

The second prescription becomes possible when the second observation is made where the case has come to a stand still. It is because the symptoms come and go after the first remedy is administered. There are some changes also effected due to the drug. Remember that a rational observation is impossible when the symptoms appear and disappear. A second prescription made at this stage can only spoil the case.

It is advisable for the patient to take good complete rest and no further dose of remedy administered. Now we have an opportunity to make a real observation. Such a second prescription based on these observations will be sound and rational. This is because now we can see the original symptoms return. For a second prescription this is the first thing to be considered.

Where these old symptoms do return and they are not so marked the physician must make it a point to search for them. After the administration of the remedy at the first instance it tries and works for the restoration of the internal economy. Sometimes we do not see any return of the original symptoms even after several days, weeks or months. But where we do not see the return of the original symptoms at all, what is to be done?

Homoeopathy is symptomatology. Without symptoms, in the sea of homoeopathy the case is like a ship without compass or rudder. We have stressed the importance and value of the symptoms in all our lectures now and then. We have even made special efforts to convey this in our lectures XXXII and XXXIII. Two lectures have been devoted for this. Please go through your notes on these two lectures for refreshing your memory on this.

Symptoms, symptoms, symptoms - this is the language of the nature and every physician must recognize each ambassador of the internal condition of the patient. The ultimate are visible, so not much to worry about them - but they are the result of the internal condition.

With so much importance to the symptoms in homoeopathy treatment what can be done or accomplished without symptoms? Signs and symptoms are the only guideposts available for the homoeopath. Are you not able to realize the great importance of even a simple symptom? Don't you think that such VIPs are worth waiting for? Do you see the reason why we have been shouting from rooftops "WAIT

Lecture - XXXVI

AND WATCH"? Do you see the wisdom in this? Have you not started to think and realize that it is the sacred duty of every homoeopathic physician to wait for the return of the original symptoms?

We shall proceed further. We have seen that if the old or original symptoms do re-appear, slightly changed in their intensity, either increased or decreased it is an excellent sign. This conveys that the patient will recover. We bring to your mind the Aphorism on that *"when the old symptoms return, there is hope. This is the road to cure and there is none other."*

How do you know that your first prescription was a good and effective one? There are three things that point to the effectiveness of the drug on the patient. They are:

(i) Where the patient has not had these symptoms for some time.

(ii) Where the symptoms do reappear in their original form.

(iii) Where the symptom is slightly differing in intensity.

So, from the above we know that the first prescription is a good and effective one.

We have been repeatedly saying wait and watch. We have waited. We have watched. Now the old original symptoms return and the patient reports his case. We check the symptoms that are present now with the earlier records. We see from that these signs and symptoms that they are the old ones which we have noted down for the first prescription.

Now it is two or more months since we administered the first prescription drug. The symptoms now found were the original ones as we find from our records. Can you guess where we are moving towards in this case? You must have guessed, after all these lectures. Yes sir, the first remedy has exhausted its action. The disease or sickness was contained till the drug action in the body existed. Now the drug has exhausted its action and the original symptoms are now rearing their head. Nothing to worry. Our first remedy has been effective. That has contained the sickness though for a short time. There were no new symptoms due to the remedy. We know that the first remedy was effective and curative. It has a certain active period and now its active period is over, i.e., it has exhausted its drug action inside the body - but it has set the economy in order, temporarily though. *Now, yes now is the time to repeat the first prescription drug to the patient.* Do not change the remedy. Do not worry about the potency now. Hold on to the first prescription and repeat it in the same potency. We shall talk about the potency later on. Now do not worry about it.

At this point however we wish to tell you:

(1) Avoid unnecessary aggravation of the symptoms by adjusting the potency to the patient. You saw first prescription potency was satisfactory. So there is no need to alter it now.

Remember that we have to increase the homoeopathicity by elevating the quality of the drug towards the inner nature to correspond with the patient's vital force.

Even though this point on homoeopathicity is provided here do not make any alterations in the quality of the medicine just now.

(2) When a remedy has benefited the patient satisfactorily, never in your life change the remedy but repeat the remedy.

So, now you know when to repeat a second dose of the first remedy, i.e., make your second prescription under the above circumstances.

In some cases, after administration of the first prescription remedy we find several new symptoms crop up or appear. These new symptoms take the place of the old symptoms. Understand the situation well. Here, the symptoms are new; no old symptoms. The patient will say, ' well, doctor, the old symptoms have vanished, but now I have some new symptoms.' Now the physician checks up the new symptoms. He also checks the pathogenesis and finds these symptoms in the drug picture of the drug he had administered. Now it looks like proving of the drug, isn't it? The doctor checks up with the patient whether he had similar symptoms at any stage earlier. The patient says 'no'. Now it is the duty of the physician to carefully check up with the patient, event by event in his life, to get confirmation that the patient had not had these new symptoms at any stage in his earlier life. The doctor is convinced that the patient has not experienced the present symptoms at any stage, earlier.

Here is the click. Can you imagine the reason for the present symptoms? Think well. We have informed earlier that these symptoms were found in the drug. So what is it due to? It is obvious — the drug had no homoeopathicity to the disease and the prescription was an unfortunate one. The drug has caused the disease to progress in some other direction. Here it has developed the new symptoms causing distress to the patient.

Now we have known the cause of these new symptoms. What is our next step? We must take the route of safety here. We must antidote the erroneous drug that caused the new symptoms to crop up, if possible, immediately.

Think of the situation here. There were some original symptoms before the administration of the second prescription. To these symptoms the newly induced symptoms have added up. So, to combat the present condition, the drug that we may hunt for should be capable of wiping the old and the newly appeared symptoms. Such drug must be corresponding in a greater percentage to the new symptoms, than to the old. It will cause the new symptoms to disappear and also have a possible effect on the old symptoms.

This will be the modus operandi for the subsequent prescriptions as well. The same problems faced and surmounted in the second prescription will also have to be faced in the future prescriptions.

Where the first prescription was an unfortunate one all the subsequent prescriptions are to be made cautiously with great difficulty and dread.

Sometimes the case comes to a standstill. In such a case a new prescription is rarely necessary. Let us see how the first prescription worked its way through.

The first prescription has been made. The medicine starts acting. The symptoms change in a very orderly manner. They change and interchange and new symptoms appear. All said and done the symptoms return to their original state. But they do not have the original verocity. They are docile even to the extent of having no importance. The patient also does not suffer and the patient has reached a stand still state. The patient also says, 'I have no symptoms, yet I am NOT improving. I have reached a stand still state.' All this pertains to himself. They do not relate to the symptoms. It all comes down to the patient being in a state of stand still.

What does the homoeopathic physician do now? What will be his next step? We have mentioned earlier that it is the sacred duty of the physician to wait - wait for a long time if necessary. But then if after many months we see no outward symptoms. There is also no external tendency exhibited by the disease then we can repeat the earlier remedy. It will do no harm. In these and similar cases only the earlier remedy alone can be administered and none other.

A new remedy cannot be considered here. Since the symptoms are the guideposts of homoepathy and they being not available a new remedy cannot be considered.

Lecture - XXXVI

Since the conditions can only tolerate or receive only the earlier remedy, when this is administered as a repetition it will keep the patient 'going on' feeling better. But remember — do not be hasty about it. Waiting for a long time is the only solution.

Please remember that *"it is better to do nothing at all than to do something useless; it is better to watch and wait than do something wrong."*

We have covered two conditions here as to the repetition of the dose. They are:—

(1) The reappearance of the old symptoms.

(2) The patient comes to a stand still condition.

Do remember one thing - you have to wait for a considerable time and make sure the earlier remedy administration has ceased being active in the patient.

So far we have been talking and talking in this lecture about the first and second prescriptions. We will now give it all in a short and precise manner in which you can always remember it. This is not memorizing. Any principle that is perfectly understood can be retained and recalled just like that. We give it here.

The first prescription is that one which by its action has effected changes in the symptoms and subsequent to that; the next is the second prescription.

So, now you know what exactly is meant by the first and second prescriptions. We would like to tell you one thing. A dozen drugs could have been administered one after the other. But they may not have any effect what so ever on the economy. From what we have learnt above all, these remedies do not come under any prescription at all since they have not effected any changes. These remedies are not related to the case.

We are now to consider another important point. Upon now we have been speaking of the first and second prescriptions. So far, we dealt in the usage of the same remedy in both the first and second prescriptions. Now, we are going to see when and where we may have to change the first prescription remedy in the second prescription. We should also know why this change is needed. In homoeopathy we do not act on our opinions or whims and fancies. We go by the facts.

Earlier we said that a long lasting trouble has ceased and then after some time new symptoms do appear - and these new symptoms are striking ones. The complete base in the symptoms has changed, but the lasting trouble has ceased. We also find from the patient that he has not experienced such symptoms earlier in his life. Here and in circumstances like this, after the administration of the medicine a new group of symptoms have appeared somewhere in the body relative to the patient. The patient as said above has not experienced these groups of symptoms earlier. In these circumstances, we have to combat this new group of symptoms only with a new remedy. We know that each homoeopathic remedy has its own symptoms. Each one therefore can combat only the corresponding disease symptoms. In this case the first prescription remedy wiped out an old symptom. New symptoms now appeared. The old remedy had a circle of range and symptoms. Since the old symptom came within its radius it wiped it out. Now new symptoms have come in. These do not fall or correspond to the first prescription remedy's symptoms, hence it cannot be repeated. Necessity guides us to select a remedy that is different from the first prescription remedy. Hence herein the second prescription remedy has been changed.

When old symptom is wiped out and new symptoms appear which are totally different from the first prescription remedy a change of remedy in the second prescription is necessitated.

There are also other instances where the second prescription remedy has got to change and wherein the first remedy prescription is not valid. Its administration will only prove to be a futile

Lecture - XXXVI

experience. Do you know why I call this a futile experience? A repetition of the earlier remedy any number of times may not be able to bring about any change in the symptoms, because it now happens to be irrelevant here since it could bring in no further change. Only when a remedy is relevant to the case, it can bring in changes. Only when a remedy brings in a change we could call it first prescription, second prescription, etc. when it can bring in no changes then what else will you call it? It can only be a futile exercise.

Now, we shall consider the second reason where the remedy has got to be changed from the first prescription, necessarily.

We shall take a patient who has been under treatment for years. He is undergoing treatment for constitutional disorder. He has been administered the remedy in a wide range of potency, from the lowest to the highest. All have acted curatively in the patient. The complete range of potencies has been utilized. This remedy has been repeated many times on paucity of symptoms. In this case you cannot think of giving another remedy. It is simply because the remedy happened to be the constitutional remedy of the patient.

In the above paragraph, we have said a complete range of potencies of the remedy has been given to the patient. Pause a little here. Why was this so? Let us say, you started with a low potency. We have also said in the above paragraph that all the different potencies have acted curatively. Now, then why so many changes in the potency? Yes sir, the medicine at the lower potency did act curatively. But after some time it was observed that this potency failed to act. So the physician took the option of going to the next higher potency. After sometime, this was also found not working. So at various stages, each potency worked for some time and the physician increased the potency in steps till he went to the highest potency. He stuck on to the constitutional remedy only.

We have been saying so many things in these lectures. We have always supported our statements with homoeopathic law and justified our statements. Now it is so with the physician sticking with the remedy - stepping up the potencies. Can you connect any of our earlier statements to support the physician's action? Think and contemplate a few minutes. It is worth knowing why this has been done - on the patient's side and the drug's side. We have said that homoeopathic law or doctrine says one thing about any remedy. It is, "When a remedy has benefited a patient satisfactorily, never in your life, change the remedy, but repeat that remedy as long as it can benefit the patient. Do not regard the symptoms that have come up." In the present case the remedy has acted curatively. That is what we have said. So, you see that the statement is supported. When the patient has been continuously benefited and improved even if the symptoms have never changed, never change the remedy. Thus far, we have seen that the physician has taken the proper road. He has remembered "never leave a remedy until you have tested in a higher potency, if it has benefited the patient."

Let us put it in another way. The patient affirms he has improved continuously from the use of a particular remedy. The physician observes some symptoms in the patient. Actually according to the homoeopathic thinking and doctrines the present remedy could not combat the presently observed symptoms. Yet since the remedy is benefiting the patient take this above as the consideration and forget about the symptoms that have cropped up, stick on to that remedy till you are able to see the patient benefits.

Physicians may argue here. "When the symptoms change we have to change the remedy to combat them. How come you say stick on to the old remedy that benefits the patient when you find different symptoms present?" Here, the answer for the physician's question is in the question itself.

Note the word "benefits the patient". Yes, that is it. The

Lecture - XXXVI

physician's top most mission is to cure the patient, with minimum discomfort. Is this not tallying in the above condition? That is the patient is comfortable with the remedy and he is free from suffering. So, as long as the drug is making the patient comfortable with its curative action continue with it. Yes, keeping the patient comfortable is the only aim of the physician.

Let us see what will happen if the remedy is changed at this stage.

Till now the patient was getting improvement with a remedy. There are some symptoms observed by the physician. In spite of these symptoms the remedy is benefiting the patient. That is the scene now.

This remedy is stopped. The result is the patient may start feeling uncomfortable. The reason is the remedy has a time of activity inside the body. Once the action of the remedy's action ceases, the patient has to and will feel uncomfortable. We have said the continuation of the remedy is beneficial to the patient. Now, no medicine, no comfort or no benefit. Of course, as said in this lecture, as long as the medicine is active inside the body the patient will feel comfortable. But when the remedial action ceases patient will not be comfortable.

Secondly, there are symptoms observed. Now a remedy is chosen to combat this group of symptoms in the patient. Hitherto there were no old symptoms in the patient due to the old remedy. But the very fact that the physician has continued the old remedy and the patient benefited from each dose goes to prove that the disease is not completely cured in the patient. It may be latent and not showing its teeth due to the policing by the remedy. Now the old remedy is stopped.

There are already some symptoms existing plus the old symptoms, which have been under control. Now both these may join hands and cause a complexity. O.K., accepting that the symptoms that are present suppress the old original symptom you must still be worried that the original disease is inside the body and has not been completely cured. By trying to eradicate the new symptoms, the original disease is not going to be cured. So the patient is bound to feel unwell and uncomfortable at the change of a remedy. This will be so if the old remedy is still benefiting the patient. Understand this last point well. "Still benefiting" is the word.

So you see the wisdom in not changing the remedy if it is benefiting the patient as long as it benefits him.

Now we will go to the other side of this case. The patient has been 'drugged'. In homoeopathy, we say that any homoeopathic drug induces an artificial disease. The physician chose that remedy in the initial stages very carefully to cover the disease completely. Or in this case it has been a constitutional remedy. O.K., the patient has had it from the lowest to the highest potency. Each potency has improved the patient or benefited him. After a particular level we have a different problem. Now the patient will become a prover, proving the remedy he has been taking continuously and for so long. Thereby he starts exhibiting the drug symptoms.

Always keep in your mind that as long as the drug's curative action is *benefiting the patient* keep off from the very idea of changing the remedy. It is always a wise policy to wait, whenever in doubt. It is better not to do something that may prove harmful and stay put. At this place we would like you to make a note of the two points given below:—

(1) *All prescriptions that change the image of a case cause suppression.*

(2) *It is better to do nothing at all than to do something useless. It is better to watch and wait than to do wrong.*

You must have noticed one thing in this lecture. We said that the physician remembered his lesson; the lesson is:

Lecture - XXXVI

"Never leave a remedy until you have tested it in a higher potency, if it has benefited the patient."

The physician has gone to the highest potency and tested it here. It has brought in curative effect in every potency. But at one place the remedy fails to support the patient and does not act curatively. At this stage any one can say the remedy has not acted since the patient is not benefited. What do you do at this stage?

Yes, this is THE TIME you must consider of changing the drug that has been benefiting the patient till then, so long. It has done all the good to the patient.

So, you now know when and why to change from the first prescription to the second prescription, with a different remedy. This is the second reason.

At the beginning of this lecture we explained what is a second prescription and what makes a second prescription. To refresh your memory we shall call it back now.

A second prescription may be:—

(1) A repetition of the first prescription.

(2) An antidote or a complement.

We have dealt with, in detail, about repeating the first prescription. Why, when, etc., has been furnished then.

Here now we shall deal with an antidote or a complement used as a second prescription. We shall see about a complement now.

Homoeopathy says that a complement has to be given to the former remedy. Well, what is a 'complement'? Complement can be something that which can complete or fills up. We can also say supplement. But under our context we shall take the meaning of complement as one that which fills up or completes. Sometimes a second prescription becomes necessary to complement the first prescription remedy. It must be a complement to the first prescription remedy to complete the case. So this remedy in the first prescription is changed to its complementary remedy. Hence this becomes a second prescription, since there is a change in the first remedy.

Let us take an example case here. A child four to five years old, large-headed, blue eyed takes cold frequently. Every cold settles in his head. His face is flushed and has throbbing carotids, etc. *Belladonna* suits this case. *Belladonna* relieves but then it does not act as a constitutional remedy. The boy continues to suffer with his headaches. This is due to his psoric condition. A time does come when *Belladonna* cannot relieve him. We make a thorough study of the complete case. We do find that when his symptoms are not acute and when he does not have cold and fever he does not have the headache. We see a different remedy indicated here - different from *Belladonna*. We study the flabby muscles aspect and we find his glands are enlarged; he contacts a cold easily with every change in the weather; he craves for eggs. The case is calling for *Calcarea*. We note the point that *Belladonna* acted on the boy only as a palliative confirms *Calcarea*. We will loose time if we treat more than one or two acute paroxysm. *Calcarea* should not be administered during a paroxysm. *Belladonna* has already been given and the violence of the paroxysm has been pacified a little. *Calcarea* is a constitutional remedy and also a complementary to *Belladonna*.

When we go through our Materia Medica we do find many remedies associating with each other in the above manner.

Lycopodium, Sulphur, Calcarea is series of remedies. Always one remedy takes us to one of its own cognates. It has been our observation that the cognates are closely related to each other. *Sepia* and *Nux vomica* are related like that.

A billious fever in a *Sepia* constitution calls for *Nux vomica*, most likely. That billious fever or the remittent fever subsides.

Lecture - XXXVI

Sepia's symptoms come to the fore immediately. This shows the complementary relation between *Nux vomica* and *Sepia*. Suppose the patient has been under *Sepia's* influence. He is affected with some acute inflammatory attack. He will probably be cured by *Nux vomica* or may be any one of its cognates. As mentioned earlier Materia Media is full of the complementary and cognate relationships.

The second prescription takes care of the change of the plan of treatment. We should know that there is a psoric influence when the second prescription is to be made. We can see that there is a psoric history behind the patient's symptoms.

Sulphur happens to be THE remedy for psora. *Graphites* and many more anti-psoric remedies are available to us and are at our disposal.

In some cases we come across a complex situation - all the miasms, psora, syphilis and sycosis - may be involved and make the case a complex one. When the miasms are present the first step is to cure psora, then syphilis - Mercurial poisoning, etc. and then sycosis. In our book on Miasms and Their Effects on Human Organism we have given a detailed step-by-step treatment of these miasms.

The miasmatic affections may alternate with one another. When one miasm is prominent the other may be silent. Hence the plan of treatment has to be kept totally flexible to suit the patient's state.

Only after a very careful and proper prolonged study of any case, any prescription can be made. We must know properly the symptoms - or rather understand the symptoms properly- thereby clearly understanding the disease picture. That is the most important thing. It is wise always to study the cases in depth.

We must also know the constitution of the patient. Only then we can administer the proper remedies. If you do not understand all these things and start the treatment it may prove hazardous. It is an unwise thing to do.

In this lecture we have seen when the first prescription can be repeated; what is meant by a second prescription, why, when and under what circumstances it is made, etc. This lecture is an important one to get along famously with your practice.

Summary

1. A second prescription is

    (i) A repetition of the first prescription or

    (ii) A complementary or

    (iii) An antidote

    (iv) A change of the remedy, after first prescription.

2. When is the second prescription made?

    (i) Repetition of the First Prescription

    (a) The first prescription has been administered. The original symptoms have disappeared. The physician waits and watches. After some time the original symptoms appear in the patient, but in a changed intensity.

    Then the first prescription can be repeated in the second prescription.

    (b) The patient has been administered the first prescription. The symptoms have gone. The physician waits and watches. No more appearance of the symptoms is there. But the patient says, *"The symptoms have gone, but I do not feel better."* The case has come to a stand still. At this time the first prescription may be repeated as the second prescription.

(ii) **When change of the first prescription remedy is essential.**

    (a) The old symptoms of the patient are wiped out by the first prescription. The physician waits and watches. After some time a new group of symptoms appear. All the new symptoms are totally different from the old symptoms. The patient never had experienced them. This is the time to change the remedy.

    (b) The patient is administered the first prescription remedy. The patient improves with the low potency. After some time this fails to give any improvement to the patient. The physician uses the next potency. It works for some time, then no improvement. Similarly the physician runs up the potency ladder till he has used the highest potency. That is the stay. No more high potency is available. He cannot go higher. The patient stops improving. It proves that the drug had done all it could to benefit the patient. Its effects have stopped at a certain stage.

    This is the time to change the remedy.

    (c) First prescription is made out. The patient is benefited - only temporarily the remedy has acted more as a palliative rather than as a curative. So a closely related remedy that is a complementary to the first prescription is given.

    So here a change of remedy is effected.

    (d) When the tri-miasmatic complication is there, one miasm will be active while the other/others be silent. So at each step as each miasmatic manifestation comes up the remedy has to be suitable to the situation. So there will be a change in plan of treatment.

3. Always remember this rule — "the administration of the appropriate first homoeopathic prescription will wipe out the guiding symptoms of the disease. Only the common and trivial symptoms remain after that."

4. A second prescription is made out for combating the symptoms left out, after the physician makes sure that the first prescription has ceased to function.

5. In case the physician makes a second prescription without waiting and hastily, the patient will suffer, instead of getting cured.

6. An early repetition of the remedy and also its continuous administration will prevent the opportunity of providing a second prescription.

7. While the first prescription is active a repetition of the remedy will block the symptoms from re-appearing. So do not interfere.

8. A second prescription pre-supposes that the first prescription has been totally a correct one.

9. The re-appearance of the original symptoms may take a long time also.

10. Homoeopathy is symptomatology.

11. Symptoms are the language of nature. The physician must be able to recognize every ambassador of nature, or internal conditions.

12. Signs and symptoms are the only guideposts available for the homoeopathic physician.

13. Wait and watch. Do not do something in haste. Always think of the patient's cure first.

14. When old symptoms return there is hope for patient's recovery.

15. There are three things that point out to the effectiveness of the first prescription:—

    (i) Patient does not have the old or original symptoms for sometime.

    (ii) The symptoms reappear in their original form.

    (iii) The returned symptoms are modified in their intensity.

16. The first prescription has set the economy in order - may be temporarily — because its action has ceased. Then the symptoms reappear because the sickness has only partially been cured.

17. Always avoid any unnecessary aggravation by adjusting the drug potency to the patient.

18. When you see that a remedy has benefited a patient, do not change that remedy. Repeat it.

19. When a drug has no homoeopathicity to the disease, the drug can induce some new symptoms. The prescription will be an erroneous one. In such a case further prescriptions will have to be made with great care.

20. When a patient says that he has no symptoms and also feels no relief, the case has come to a stand still. After waiting and watching for a considerable time the first prescription can be repeated. No other remedy can be given.

21. Remember a prescription that changes the image of the sickness is a cause for suppression.

22. Complementary remedy is the one that completes the case.

23. When the properly selected first prescription fails to cure permanently think of its complementary.

Aphorisms & Precepts

1. It is better to do nothing at all than to do something useless; it is better to watch and wait than do something wrong.
2. All prescriptions that change the image of a case cause suppression.
3. Never leave a remedy until you have tested it in a higher potency, if it has benefited the patient.
4. Principle teaches you to avoid suppression. A homoeopath cannot temporize. The sufferings are necessary sometimes to show forth sickness in order that a remedy may be found.
5. You cannot depend on lucky shots and guess work; everything depends on long study of each individual case.
6. Anything, which looks away from exactitude, is unscientific. The physician must be classical; everything must be methodical. Science ceases to be scientific when disorderly application of law is made.
7. You must be able to recognize every ambassador of the internal man.
8. Now when a person becomes sick, he becomes susceptible to a certain remedy, which will affect him in its highest potency; while upon a healthy person it will have no effect.
9. When a man thinks from the microscope, and his neighbor's opinion, he thinks falsely. Nothing good can come from this.
10. The sharper the edge of the tool you fool with, the more harm you can do. So it is with high potencies in unskilled hands.
11. A disease may be suppressed by a medicine as well as by a stronger dissimilar disease.
12. The whole aim of homoeopathy is to cure.

13. The symptoms, themselves, point to the thing, which the individual is sensitive to, and every one is susceptible in just this way to the remedy that will cure. That which he most wants, is that which Nature has provided him with the means of reaching out after by the symptoms.
14. That which we call disease, is but a change in the vital force expressed by the totality of the symptoms.
15. It is just as dangerous to suppress symptoms by drugs, as it is to remove them with the knife.
16. Diseases, themselves, cannot be suppressed, but the symptoms can. The totality of the symptoms must disappear in an orderly manner in order to constitute a cure.
17. The man who thinks it rests in the size of the dose does not know homoeopathy. One who lives in his sensorium thinks that way.
18. The physician will never grow stronger and wise, as long as he thinks there can be a substitute for the remedy.
19. When a man takes a remedy in too large a dose, *he* feels worse and his symptoms are worse; with a higher potency, *he* feels better, though his symptoms may be aggravated.
20. We must think what makes the patient sick; not what causes changes in his liver, his kidneys and other organs.
21. A cure is not a cure unless it destroys the internal or dynamic cause of disease. A tumor, if removed, does not cure the patient because its cause still continues to exist.
22. So far there is morbid anatomy to account for symptoms, so far it is unimportant as a symptom, for if no other symptoms are present you can find no remedy.
23. The word disease really means the signs or symptoms, before organic disease has taken place.

24. The physician must penetrate the inner recesses of symptomatology. The very life of the patient must be opened. Learn the fears, instincts, desires and the aversions of the patient. The remedy often crops out through affections.
25. The flopping about, and not waiting for the remedy to cure is abominable. There are periods of improvement and periods of failure. Let the life force go on as long as it can, and repeat only when the original symptoms come back to stay.
26. Every action in homoeopathy must be based on a positive principle.
27. Confusion comes from losing one's head, prescribing on few indications and giving medicine when no medicine should be given.
28. The increase of conditions shows increase of sickness; the increase of symptoms often shows diminution of disease.
29. It is worse than useless to give a second dose until the effects of the first dose have ceased.
30. The limit of drug action is symptomatology.
31. When a remedy has benefited a patient satisfactorily, never in your life change your remedy, but repeat that remedy as long as you can benefit the patient. Do not regard the symptoms that have come up.
32. The remedy has actually led to a change. Don't reason that if you had given a certain remedy in the beginning you could have cured the patient. The masked symptoms come out as a result of the remedy.
33. Unless the inner nature of the remedy corresponds with the inner nature of the disease the remedy will not cure the disease but simply remove the symptoms which it covers; that is suppress them.

Lecture - XXXVI

34. In advanced phthisis with pathological symptoms, if you prescribe for the old symptoms, which should have prescribed for some years before, you kill your patient.

35. All things that change the aspect of a case should be avoided.

36. When a case comes back in a few days with all the symptoms changed, unless they are old symptoms, the prescription was inaccurate and unfortunate.

37. The knowledge of complementary remedies is necessary of the nearest remedy in its nature and not in a few symptoms. Thus a series of complementary remedies, the conditions must be there as well as the symptoms.

38. Keep in a series of complementary remedies. We can never cure if we select a remedy for a part of the symptoms and as others come up, give a remedy that is not the complement.

39. Never leave a remedy until you have tested it in a higher potency if it has benefited the patient.

Lecture - XXXVII

Difficult and Incurable Cases - Palliation

This is our last lecture in this series of 'HOMOEOPATHY PHILOSOPHY'. In all our earlier lectures we have been repeatedly saying often that homoeopathy is a God given gift to humanity. It is a great science of truth; since it has been the blessing of the Providence it is perfect in all respects. It cannot be otherwise. It is complete. However, as in many other sciences the partial truth alone is known. The truth itself is Divine. The knowledge belongs to the man.

A truth has to be built brick by brick. It is not offered or does not come in a silver platter. One has to work to fully understand it. It is not achieved in a day or two. It takes a lot of time.

We all have heard the axiom, 'Catch them young'. Whenever we have to impart something of great value it is to be trained right from the younger age. The child is to be brought up in that consciousness. The seed has to be well planted in the child's mind, so that as child grows the seed that we planted in its mind also grows. Ultimately the consciousness is so well planted that it lights up the child's day-to-day living. The principle would have to sink into the mind so deeply that it is reflected in the thought, speech and act of the child. That is the way to do it.

They say that in Switzerland the children have been raised for centuries with the awareness of bringing out an excellent watch of 'world class'. They are constantly brought up in this atmosphere, in this thought and thereby build up the country's prestige.

Today, we know about Sony of Japan. It is said that any Japanese will be proud to link his name with Sony's products. They are taught to constantly think of the product they bring out and at each level the worker is encouraged to present his smallest idea to the management that can improve the product. That is Japanese Management.

So, from the above we see the great importance of educating a person right from his core about what we want him to do, think and speak. So is it with the truth. All this does take time and discipline. When living, they are able to know many more things that we might not know now.

When homoeopathy is several hundred years old, the little ones grow up in this awareness and knowledge of homoeopathy and observe and practice it, our successors will be much more knowledgeable than us. They will know and talk of many things we might have been ignorant of, today. As man thinks harmoniously the things are bound to become brighter.

The more we keep together the better it will be. Then the more we think as one the better it will be.

We have on our hands a wonderful truth. We cannot deny it. With this awareness can we afford to have any differences of opinions? This great truth will bind us into one and should all of us not stand united and feel 'all for one and one for all'. Think about it.

Let us go through our Materia Medica. There are several medicines with their characteristics mentioned therein. All these are proving given out by true and sincere volunteers. All these provings contain characteristic features of a case. This has been

Lecture - XXXVII

so right from the day Dr. Hahnemann compiled his first Materia Medica and all those who had helped prepare the voluminous Materia Medica have maintained this principle.

Almost every physician makes use of the Materia Medica, whoever is the author. But this is one step that all the beginners most certainly do take, to find remedies. They rely very much on these repertories. The process of finding the similimum is so easy with the repertories. We are able to find one remedy after another.

Consider what we said about a hundred years later from now on. We said that there would be a better understanding most definitely. All the symptoms become more definite and striking and more clearly understood. This understanding has become better than what it was during the days of Dr. Hahnemann. They are better understood now. This is bound to get still better in the years to come.

We have seen certain cases where the patient keeps on coming to the physician for years together. Such patients have a great confidence in the doctor. They may fly out to some other doctor - but that will only be temporary. They will come back to the first doctor. Over the years, in this case several medicines would have been administered - the patient would have improved in small stages, but the improvement is definite. Such patients approach the physician in a very cooperative and positive manner. They have a lot of confidence in their physician.

This great confidence they have in the physician is contagious. The doctor also trusts the patient and appreciates the co-operation afforded by the patient. The feedback from the patient is excellent and the doctor is able to plan his next step on how to deal with the case. So the doctor has a great confidence in himself to pick up the correct remedy since he is very well acquainted with the patient and his problems. The physician's mind is calm and composed - no agitation whatsoever reflecting the improved confidence; his working is also eased up and more accurate. The patient's confidence sharpens the physician's intelligence.

Very closely analogous to the above cases are cases, which could be referred to as alternating or one-sided complaints. These show only one side of the patient's malady. A coin has two sides - almost everything in nature comes like that only. Some examples could be 'hot, cold', 'dark, light'; etc. Similarly we have these complaints also. How does these examples justify their part here? We said alternating or one-sided complaints. When can one be alternating? Anything can alternate only when there are two things. Otherwise there can be no alternating.

Keeping this in mind we shall see a patient with two problems. While one manifests the other lies low. Say, eye symptoms could be prominent when the stomach symptoms may not be present. For the eye problems in this case *Euphrasia* could be the medicine. There might be an antipsoric that may fit the whole case. Similarly for the stomach symptoms exhibited *Pulsatilla* could be ideal. Again there will be one antipsoric remedy, which will fit the whole case. But remember here that one antipsoric that will suit the whole patient. That antipsoric will fit better because of the generals. We discussed the generals in an earlier lecture.

Now, in these cases we do administer medicines that fit a group of symptoms. Now what happens? The constitutional state of the patient is riveted upon the patient. What does this mean? There the disease becomes incurable. What does this teach us? It is always wise on the part of the physician and better for the patient that the doctor carefully analyses the case and chooses the correct fitting remedy for the case. A little time taken in this direction will definitely pay dividends.

It may appear that using several medicines will work out better as each medicine appears to suit individual groups of symptoms. But consider the fact that when a single remedy is chosen properly, it goes and hits squarely at the base of disease in the center thereby trying to affect a complete cure. In these cases where the remedy hits the epicenter of the disease, the economy is restored. In process the patient will be put to a great suffering and turmoil. They are dreadful to manage. Where the symptoms appear as ultimate on the surface or the extremities the patient will be really frightened and even run away from you. Principle-wise this correction from center or within out is good. But can the patient withstand it. We must consider his state also in such cases.

Incurable complaints are always very difficult and trouble every physician coming across it. Let us take the case of allopathy in incurable disease. The patient is given drugs that are strong. The patient is all the time under the belief that he is being benefited. But what is the real fact. The patient's condition is sinking internally all the while. Strong drugs will cause damage. Here they have acted as palliatives. Unfortunately some homoeopathic physicians follow this line. They do not realize palliatives are extremely detrimental to the patient.

Reproduced below is a portion of Aphorism — "But what authority have you to hush the cries of the patient, if by palliating you do away with the ability to heal him."

"Unless the inner nature of the remedy corresponds with the inner nature of the disease but will simply remove the symptoms which it covers; that is suppress them"

We have been speaking about the law and doctrines of homoeopathy very often in almost every lecture. We have also been stressing on one single remedy of minimal dose, etc. The physician who has practiced on the law of single potentized remedy will easily be convinced that there is no other way of palliation that holds out a permanent hope for the patient.

Let us take the case of *Opium*. *Opium* relieves pain, stops diarrhea and drives away cough - but then woe to the patient. *Opium* annuls reaction and there are no development of the symptoms. For the homoeopathic physician the symptoms are the language of nature. He cannot do anything in its absence. Now here, that is missing. So we have lost track and we do not know the remedy the patient needs. Of course, *Opium* will cure the pains. In this case the patient is not cured. We have talked about *Opium* only here. But this holds true for almost all painkillers in homoeopathy. When an opiate must be given please remember the cure of this patient is abandoned. So, handle the painkillers on a very guarded fashion.

Can any thoughtful homoeopathic physician abandon the expectation of a cure during painful sickness so long as life endures? Cancer, consumption and other coasting diseases are diseases, with painful symptoms. Painkillers may look like a boon here. It is a forlorn hope that tempts the abandonment of such remedies.

Summary

1. This is our last lecture on *Homoeopathy Philosophy* series.
2. Homoeopathy is a God given gift to humanity.
3. This is a complete science - but the humanity has learnt only the partial truth of homoeopathy.
4. Truth itself is Divine. The knowledge belongs to the man.
5. Several great people have worked meticulously to present this to us in this level. It is yet to be developed to blossom out fully.
6. It is for the younger generation to build this. We have to educate our younger generation to make this achievement possible.
7. Here, a quote by The Mother of Shri. Arabindo Ashram, Pondicherry, India will not be out of place.

"With confidence we shall advance; with certitude we shall wait."

Lecture - XXXVII

8. The Materia Medica contains so many medicines. Each one has characteristics that have been proved. Wherever the proving is not complete it is said so.
9. Materia Medica is indispensable to our profession.
10. A patient could be under treatment for years. Several medicines would have been administered in such cases. These patients have a lot of confidence in their physicians.
11. When the patient has a lot of confidence on the part of his physician, there is reciprocation from the doctor's end also. This helps the physician in the right choice of the medicine for that patient.
12. There are alternating or one-sided complaints. The patient may have two symptoms, which manifest alternatively. When one is manifested the other lies low.
13. A patient may come in with several symptoms. On a quick look it will appear as if each group of symptoms be treated with a suitable medicine.
14. Here we have not attacked the root cause. The disease remains. It is as if we have dealt with only the branches and not the tree completely.
15. It is not wise to do it. We should take time to choose the most appropriate remedy for the totality of the symptoms. Then, such a remedy penetrate deep enough and attacks the epicenter of the disease. The economy is set in order. But in achieving this settlement a great turmoil is set up which is dreadful. The patient may be frightened.
16. Incurable diseases are always very troublesome. We have to handle this very carefully. The patient is sinking all the while; we should consider this while deciding the strength of the remedy. In these case palliation alone will be proper. But the palliative means suppression. That is a double-edged sword.

17. Be wary of using opiates, and other painkillers. These will kill the pain, but cause a block for remedy. Though under painful circumstances these may appear to be a boon, never never be careless with them.

18. With this we come to end of our lectures on homoeopathy philosophy. As a closing quote, we provide below the saying of Shri. Arabindo. Contemplate on it.

19. "For those who have within them a sincere call for the Divine, however the mind or vital may present difficulties or attacks come or progress be slow and painful, even if they fall back or fall away from the path for a time, the psychic always prevails in the end and Divine help proves effective. Trust in that and persevere - then the goal is sure."

20. We wish every one of you who have gone through these lectures understand them and follow what is suggested here. Each one of you must be an efficient homoeopath and do remarkable service to the humanity and thereby discharge your duty creditably. Consecrate your action, speech and thought to the cause of homoeopathy — TO CURE GENTLY, RAPIDLY AND PERMANENTLY.

Aphorisms & Precepts

1. In Epilepsy, as long as Bromides suppress, nature is paying more attention to the disease of Bromides than the disease of Epilepsy.

2. Principle teaches you to avoid suppression. A homoeopath cannot temporize. The sufferings are necessary sometimes to show forth sickness in order that a remedy may be found.

3. A disease may be suppressed by a medicine as well as by a stronger dissimilar disease.

4. This physician spoils his case when he prescribes for the local symptoms and neglects the patient.
5. It is just as dangerous to suppress symptoms by drugs, as it is to remove them with knife.
6. Diseases themselves cannot be suppressed, but symptoms can. The totality of the symptoms must disappear in an orderly manner in order to constitute a cure.
7. All physicians recognize that suppressing an acute rash is dangerous, but all are not far sighted enough to see that such is the case with chronic eruptions, excepting that the resulting symptoms come more slowly.
8. In the infant we see the father's history; in old age the history of youth. This enables us to look into the future to see whether a patient will recover, or die or be palliated.
9. This flopping about, and not waiting for the remedy to cure is abominable. There are periods of improvement and periods of failure. Let the Life Force go on as long as it can, and repeat only when the original symptoms come back to stay.

PART-II
BEYOND THE LECTURES

PART-II

BEYOND THE LECTURES

Chapter - 1

About Aphorisms and Precepts

In the foregoing chapters on Homoeopathy Philosophy, we have added at the end of each chapter (from fifth chapter onwards) a few pages of these Aphorisms and Precepts. *In Dr. Kent's lectures on Homeopathy Philosophy these Aphorisms and Precepts are not added.* You may ask why then have these been added in this book? Where is the necessity? Would not have Dr. Kent added these in his lectures themselves if he had thought it was necessary? Do the authors profess to have more homoeopathical knowledge and sense than Dr. Kent? Why did Dr. Kent add these in his Lessser Writings and not in his lectures on Homoeopathy Philosophy? Many questions of this sort may crop up in many of the readers' mind.

In this chapter we shall try to explain why we have added these Aphorisms and Precepts. We shall answer the questions to the best of our ability and as truly and honestly as possible. Before we proceed further let us understand what an Aphorism and Precepts are:

"Aphorism is a concrete support of a principle in any science. A brief pithy saying."

"Precept is a principle or maxim."

—**Chambers Twentieth Century Dictionary**

We understand a few things. Homoeopathy is a vast study. It is not a single time reading and acquiring its principles, laws and doctrines overnight after a single reading.

Here again, it is an Aphorism and Precept that comes to our minds. That is: "The Homeopathic Physician *must continue to study* in the art before he can become an expert. This will grow in him until he becomes increasingly astute and he will grow stronger and wiser in his selections for sick people."

Various lectures of Dr. Kent have been put together in an orderly form in the form of a book. After all a lecture is a lecture. In any lecture, from our small experience, the authors are yet to face a hundred percent involved complete audience. While about thirty percent of the audience are really involved hundred percent in the subject matter of the lecture, the balance has just gathered with a general interest in the topic of the lecture. They may make a note of a point here and there. For them the lecture is just another reminder of the points they are already aware of. They are not committed to polish their knowledge more and more, whereas the thirty percent mentioned are serious students who really want to gather as much more understanding as possible. Further several members of the audience do not have the patience even to sit through a complete lecture. Definitely they will not sit after the finish of the lecture. Sometimes when there is a small break, some of the audience does think that it is the end of the lecture and go away. So, these Aphorisms and Precepts were not added to the lectures. This is what we assume.

In the book this is not the case. The books are a different matter, altogether. They are records. They are always ready at hand - any time anywhere. These Aphorisms and Precepts are available to any one who can read and comprehend, on the bookshelf or on the table. Just waiting for the reader most

Chapter - 1

expectantly. While talking about books two things come to our mind.

One master homoeopath has said that there can be no books on the desk of scholars, historians and great literates. But it will be an unpardonable one if there are no books on a homoeopathic physicians table, which he will be constantly referring to.

Another master has said that homoeopathy has not become very popular because there are not many sincere practitioners due to lack of sufficient quantity of good quality books, capable of imparting good knowledge.

"It is due to lack of knowledge, that men err", says J.H. Allen.

"My people perish for lack of knowledge" is a quote from the Divine Book. This is true with many physicians of the day.

Remember the adage "to be the best learn from the best".

Keeping these things in the mind, the authors created this book. So, we wanted to give as much information as possible to the reader of this book. At the same time we desired to leave out the technicalities, kept the English simple and understandable. Before writing this book, the authors made a general survey amongst students and practitioners of homoeopathy and gauged what was the need of the hour.

The result of the survey was that some students said they entered the college for two things - they took this course just to be called a doctor and also to make some earnings. Some said that their parents forced them into this. What a sad thing and what a waste for the nation in churning out such so called physicians? Some said we have to read - we do not have easy-to-read books. The English is a hundred years old or more - our background is not that strong. We want easily readable and assimiable books to make good grades in our examinations.

Such students asked us about Organon - they asked what can a person with poor background of English do with a book of

Organon? Some books have been brought out in this subject - but yet they are lacking something. That is what they said.

While such a sad state of affairs was prevalent with students, our approach to the people already in profession told us a different story. Some of them said we have long since forgotten the laws and doctrines of homoeopathy, since our college days were over. In today's busy world, who has the time to sit down with the patient for hours together and collect his symptoms — then do the homework with the Repertory and Materia Medica? It is a laborious process and nobody pays us for the time we spend like that. In today's hurry burry we also want to make a fast buck. That is all there is to it. So, who cares about books? Every year there are hundreds of books churned out by the publishers. They are having a strong marketing support. What support do we have? Further when a patient comes in to the clinic and when he sees his doctor turning the pages of a Materia Medica or Repertory the patient feels - "I must have gone to some other doctor. See, this doctor knows nothing. Look at his table overflowing with books, which he refers constantly. Had he a sound knowledge he would not do it. His table would be clean with a calendar, prescription pad one or two pens and perhaps a thermometer in a glass of antiseptic!" These doctors unfortunately forgot what they learnt in their colleges: The Homeopath physician's first and foremost mission in life is to cure the patient.

Then we did get a few wonderful homoeopathic physicians. Their tables are with Repertories and Materia Medicas, sheats of paper, two or three different colored pens. They confirmed the need for more and more illustrative books on laws and doctrines of homoeopathy, Materia Medica, Repertory that suit the present day conditions. Of course they did hold Dr. Kent's Repertory very high. But they said some more practical and every day rubrics must also come in from experienced physicians. We need more and more reference books. That will be more helpful for the growth

Chapter - 1

of the profession Such doctors were service minded - spent a lot of time *intelligently* with the patients to take genuine care of those people. They were classical homoeopathic physicians who greatly respected the laws and doctrines of the science. They lived for the patients. May their tribe grow!

At this juncture we remember another Aphorism, "The time may come when Homoeopathy of the purer kind will be popular, but it s a very long time ahead."

Now we will get back to Aphorisms and Precepts where we left it after their meanings. We shall re-read it here.

Aphorism is a concrete support of a principle in any science - a pithy saying.

Precept is a principle or maxim.

In our present book on Homoeopathy Philosophy (Volume - 1) we wanted our statements to be properly supported. So in several places, in the book the reader will find our statements repeated also the corresponding support repeated. It is with a purpose we have done it. When you read, re-read and re-read a principle and also examples that helps the reader to comprehend the principle, retaining it in his mind and recalling it in the earliest manner becomes possible.

Memorizing cannot help.

Regarding memory:

"Memory is not knowledge until it is comprehended and used."

Comprehension and proper understanding is needed so as to use the knowledge in a successful and purposeful way of working. To put in the points into the head of a student or a reader it has got to be repeated and also explained sufficiently in several ways. In due course it will automatically become a second nature for him during his practice. So, we feel justified in repeating the statements, principles, laws, etc., as often as possible in different ways.

Do the authors think or feel that they are homoeopathically more knowledgeable than Dr. Kent? The authors most humbly say a big **"NO"**. One purpose with which this project was started by the authors was they wanted a better understanding of the homoeopathy philosophy. This is accomplished to a great extent.

Finally the authors wanted to do some service to homoeopathy. There appeared to be some solutions for this purpose. We did study each way that was open for us. We did realize our limitations in each of the pathways. Then the comment of a homoeopathy master that more and more good books on homoeopathy must be available for those interested in homoeopathy. We studied this from various angles and thought of what we should write and bring out. We felt there was a need to spread out more and more the principles, laws of this God given science, throughout the world. English was a language spoken, read and written in a greater part of the world. We also felt we had sufficiently sound English knowledge to attempt this. One more book on homoeopathy philosophy will help this cause. But we **needed** to make it more useful. So, we thought what all we could **do to achieve this,** we understood the soundness of repeating a **thing to make it** automatic in us. So we thought of making this book **on homoeopathy philosophy** slightly different from others. Hence we **have brought in two things.**

We provided a summary after each lecture. For those who do not have the patience or time they can go through the summary in a rush.

These people can read the lecture wherever they wanted to learn more on that topic. In addition the Aphorisms and Precepts provided will help any serious follower of homoeopathy to brush their knowledge in this aspect now and then. We have taken care in several places to bring in such Aphorisms and Precepts related to the topic of the lecture. It supports the various statements furnished in that particular lecture topic. Hence it is the firm conviction of the authors that this will be more useful to anyone serious in the ways of homoeopathy. It will definitely serve all the strata, who desire this knowledge.

We hope we have answered the various questions that were posed at the beginning of this chapter. We stand to correction in the various beliefs we have put forward. It is for the readers to assess this book. We sincerely feel that we have done a small portion for the cause of the homoeopathy through this book.

Chapter - 2

Susceptibility

Dr. Kent's lecture XIV on susceptibility ends here. As we are on an important subject we shall see whether we can gather any more information on this from any other source.

The difference in activities of a given remedy in the 30th and 10M upon the same constitution is most wonderful, and the difference in the 10M and CM is still more wonderful in some instances. *The very high potencies seldom require repetition, if clearly indicated, to produce a long curative action in chronic cases; but in severe acute sickness in robust constitution several doses in quick succession are most useful.*

It never matters whether the remedy is given in water in spoonful doses or given in a few pellets dry on the tongue - the result is the same.

The action or power of one pellet, if it acts at all is as great as ten.

When the medicine is given at intervals the curative power is increased and may be safe if it is discontinued with judgment. When a positive effect has been obtained the medicine should always be discontinued.

A correct observer will soon learn whether this is to be secured by a single dose or a series of doses.

In chronic diseases, for the first prescription the single dose dry on the tongue will be found even the best.

When the 30th and 200th potencies are used it is much often necessary to dissolve the medicines in water than when using higher potencies. These potencies have much milder curative action than the higher and highest potencies, and therefore, they are far more suitable to the very nervous and excitable women and children and to some men.

To suit all degrees of sensitivity in chronic diseases the Homoeopath must have at his commend deep acting remedies in 30th, 200th, 1000 and 10M, CM and MM potencies.

With many chronic patients, if the remedy fits the symptoms or the similimum, any potency will do all the curing in two or three doses at long intervals and a higher potency must be selected.

Giving very high potency to the feeble and extremely sensitive, we bring back old complaints and symptoms too violently and too hurriedly and fail to sustain the curative action long enough to eradicate the underlying miasm.

Medicine can be given during the day or night - it does not make any difference.

A deep acting chronic remedy should not be given in the midst of a paroxysm or exacerbation for it will aggravate the situation. So, it is better to administer it in the close of exacerbation or paroxysm.

Management of incurables differs widely.

When the symptoms change the remedy must be discontinued. (This has been explained in detail in the lecture).

It is unsafe for the beginner to indulge the desire to repeat too much — it should be restrained.

Plane of Disorder and Cure

We should lead our material mind to the realm of immaterial mind to understand this.

Simple substance must be recognized by reason. Material substance is fed and treated from the plane of nutrition, but immaterial substances are affected from the plane of disorder and cure.

The sunlight is attenuated in travel from the sun to the earth. We cannot conceive how much of it is attenuated. But we can see in it and do many things in it.

Sun ceased to be material substance when transformed into light. The light is a simple substance, at the beginning before getting attenuated.

Nutritive substances are material; curative substances are immaterial, simple substance.

Influx tends to be where simple substance is active.

When there is a disturbance in the inner plane of the individual's economy there is an influx, from the atmosphere, of some delirious simple substance.

When there is a curative immaterial substance it would be drawn in by influx and acts as an antidote.

When remedies are given on the plane of disturbance they will cure.

Man's every cell has all the planes. Every cell is what man is.

Crude drugs give opposite effects from the attenuated dose. The primary effect of a drug is that of a crude drug. The effect of the attenuated dose is similar to what would be experienced long after consuming the crude form.

If the bacteria could cause disease, we have to think of many things.

WAIT AND OBSERVE

Chapter - 3

Value of Symptoms

In our Homoeopathy Philosophy in lecture XXXII & XXXIII we have dealt with the Value of Symptoms exhaustively. Then why two lectures have been allotted to this topic. This chapter is only an extension of the above lectures. We have approached this subject here with practical suggestions to do our work more easily and of course with cent percent efficiency. Now, let us proceed.

Symptoms are the language of nature. The physician must be able to recognize ambassadors of nature and deal with them with proper care and attention.

Homoeopathy is a Science of Symptomatology.

Symptoms are the guideposts of the disease. They cannot be ignored.

We can say many more things about symptoms and flood several pages - each one as important as the other. We shall stop here and shall see what kind of symptoms are there.

Symptoms are of various types.

1. Unseen   -   Mental Symptoms.
2. Felt   -   Sensations - like pain, pressure, etc.

3.	Seen	-	Runny nose, eyes watering, red eyes, discharges, appearances
4.	Environmental	-	Living conditions, working conditions or causative, etc.

What is Totality of Symptoms?

Any deviation from perfect health
(i) Observed by the patient himself.
(ii) Observed by those around the patient.

This includes all disturbances of the functions, sensations, all alterations in the external appearances of the patient and all probable causative conditions.

In acute diseases the totality of symptoms can be easily compiled since the deviation from the health is generally well defined and sharp.

Some symptoms of a chronic disease existing in the patient may persist and be active during acute disease. Such symptoms are peculiar. These guide us to choose the remedy for the acute disease.

In chronic diseases we have to consider :—

(i) The present symptoms, which may not indicate the complete disease picture.

(ii) Many former symptoms, which may not be active now. There is always method and order running through all their illness provided we get a clue.

(iii) We must also consider the causative symptoms — like habits, occupation, living atmosphere, etc.

When we have excluded all such symptoms we will have several symptoms that can be ascribed only to the disease alone.

Grading of the Symptoms

We must learn as to how to **grade** the symptoms. There are two classes of symptoms in every case.

(i) Symptoms pertaining to disease, which are common or pathognomonic ones.

(ii) Symptoms pertaining to the patient.

In advanced cases there will be a third category of symptoms:—

(iii) They are those relating to the results of the disease or what we call ultimate.

We have to consider the symptoms, which pertain to the patient. The other two need not be considered.

We must place the importance on symptoms that signify the patient. *Our particular attention must be to those that are peculiar to or characteristic of the patient.* Symptoms common to the disease cannot guide us to the correct remedy. This is what we learnt in Organon paragraph 153.

In chronic cases the symptoms are complex in nature. It is difficult to separate the patient's symptoms (peculiar ones) from the common symptoms of the disease. (Organon Para 82 and 152).

When Cure is Practically Impossible

Many chronic diseases are long-standing ones. These patients might have also undergone allopathic treatment. Many of the original disease symptoms are either vanished or totally forgotten. Here the physician has difficulties. Sometimes the patient may not have any of the characteristic symptoms, but his ancestors might have had them. Such cases are practically incurable.

Peculiar Symptoms

There are some symptoms, which are peculiar to the particular patient. These are distinguished from the common symptoms of disease.

These are unusual symptoms. One example:

Great thirst (a common feature)

Every time he drinks he shivers (peculiar to the patient when he feels great thirst).

Here, modalities, changes of the patient's desires and aversions, loves and hates, etc. from the normal will also be important.

While taking into main consideration peculiar symptoms of the patient it is equally important to note the symptoms that signify the disease. Patients' peculiarities are the most important ones.

We may find that three or four remedies correspond to the peculiar symptoms, having approximately the same value. In such a case choose a remedy that has also the common symptoms.

Remember that there must be general correspondence between all the symptoms of the patient with that of the remedy.

However, peculiar symptoms are not the only criterion in choosing the correct remedy.

The so-called peculiar symptom must be well marked in the patient as well as in the remedy for us to consider it.

Chapter - 3

The Generals

The general symptoms affect the patient as a whole.

Wherever the patient conveys a symptom in first person it is a general.

E.g.: The patient says "I am thirsty", "I am sleepy", "I cannot swallow", etc.

We now give below a list of symptoms that can be branded as the generals. These will play a role in the selection of the remedy.

(1) **Mental state that reflects the condition of the innermost part of the man. This is of utmost importance.**

Symptoms of the will and affections including desires, aversions, are the most important as they relate to the innermost of man.

(2) **Effects of sleep and dream.**

(3) **The effect of the different temperatures upon the patient as a whole.**

The effects of temperature become valuable when one temperature, and some particular organ by the opposite temperature affect the body markedly. *That is the patient is exquisitely sensitive to both extremes of the temperature at the same time.*

E.g.: Patient shrinks from cold, but respiration relived by cold air- *"Ammonium carb."*.

(4) **Where aggravations from weather changes are expected - but not present or are absent.**

Though this is a general it has become peculiar due to the absence of the expected aggravation. This becomes an important symptom.

E.g.: Weather changes affect a rheumatic patient - where a rheumatic patient is not aggravated due to weather change.

(5) **Various positions.**

Positions of standing, sitting, lying down etc. *Strong aggravation due to this. Here the patient as a whole is affected. Such general symptoms are of great value.*

E.g.: (1) Standing hurts a *Sulphur* patient.

(2) Head symptoms aggravated while lying on right side — *Phos*. (This is a peculiar aggravation).

(6) **The tendency to affect particular parts of the body — like side or in oblique pattern, semi-laterally, etc.**

E.g.: (1) Semi-lateral: *Alumina, Kali-carb*. etc.

(2) Right side of body: *Apis, Bell,* and *Lyc.*,etc.

(3) Left side of body — *Arg.nit., Lach., Phos.,*etc.

(7) **Aggravation at a particular time, and periodicity.**

E.g.: Periodicity: *Cinchona off.*

(8) **Various craving and aversions. They depend upon some deep need in the body as a whole. Where outstanding and definite, they rank high.**

(9) **Eating. Where a patient states that eating influences him wholly - he feels better, or worse all over by eating this symptom ranks high.**

(10) **Smell — A sensation experienced by the patient, wholly.**

E.g.: Smell of food nauseates.

(11) A symptom or modality running through all the organs, which may be predicated of the patient himself.

(12) Symptom blended by all generals and particulars into one harmonious whole.

Particulars

We call the symptoms particulars when they relate to any particular organ in the body.

E.g.: An offensive smell in the nose. Here the symptom relates to a particular organ in the body - nose.

Compiling all the above together, we get the totality of the symptoms — **Characteristic totality of the case.**

The remedy must have an identical picture that corresponds to the characteristic totality of the disease. When this is so, the remedy can be a curative.

Chapter - 4

Selecting a Remedy

(1) Write down the patient's statements in his own words. This is done especially for comparative purposes.

(2) Now start searching for strange, rare and peculiar symptoms. For this purpose take the patient through his symptoms — ask him to amplify and qualify his statements.

In this process we can stumble upon one or two peculiar symptoms that may prove invaluable. Do not go in for the symptoms, which may be diagnostic of the sickness.

Leave out common symptoms. — For instance, breathlessness in asthma. This is a common symptom for all asthmatics.

But when the patient says, "I can breathe only when lying on my back or knee-elbow position", this is not common for all asthmatics. This symptom is peculiar to this patient. Underline this.

(3) Now make a note of definite and well-marked general symptoms that have been altered — like reactions to environments, mental and physical. The effects on him

of temperature, humidity and delicately probe for mental symptoms. Remember all these must be those, which have changed due to the patient's sickness. These details can be collected from the patient's friends, relatives and nurse. The doctor must also exercise his observations at the same time.

(4) In complicated and chronic diseases always record the past history of the patient.

(5) Family history must be noted down.

(6) Smallpox and Vaccination details to be collected. A dose of *Variolinum* should be given to this patient to improve his health, physical and even mental conditions.

(7) Check up for any T. B. manifestations, scars on neck, family history for T. B. For this remedies like *Tuberculinum* or *Drosera* will raise the resistance of the patient. Also you can think of *Phosphorus*, *Psorinum, Calcarea,* etc. according to the symptoms.

In case the above medicines are not prescribed to the patient we cannot benefit the patient permanently. (Variolinum, Tuberculinum, Drosera, Phosphorous, Psorinum, Calcarea, etc. - according to symptoms).

CAUTION: Do not prolong the drug. This drug can confuse the patient's symptoms. The whole case will become complex with the disease symptoms because of mixing with the already present disease symptoms.

To get maximum results you have to go to deep disturbing cause.

The one and the same drug in high potency can antidote itself in crude preparation.

Chapter - 4   577

> Drug symptoms may be due to toothpaste, douches, gargles, etc.
>
> A septic tooth may poison the patient.

Our case has been recorded to the needed extent. The next step after the case has been taken is:

> (i) We have noted the common symptoms also. Out of these, we have chosen and underlined the strange, rare and peculiar ones.
>
> (ii) Mental symptoms that are marked which have changed from his normalcy.

From the above, we have the complete disease picture of the patient.

Totality of the Symptoms

We might have noted down a hundred and one symptoms. This does not mean we have the totality of the symptoms. Then what does it mean by the totality of the symptoms? *Here, the Totality of symptoms means the totality of characteristic of the disease collected from the symptoms.*

We do not pay attention to the very common symptoms: symptoms that might be observed in almost all diseases. E.g.: No hunger, body paining all over, etc. But the same becomes important when qualified - say like body pains come at a fixed time and goes at a fixed time in the day, or only when in a fixed position, etc.

To select the proper remedy:

> (i) Compare the more prominent and peculiar (characteristic) symptoms of the disease particularly and more exclusively. There must be a great similitude between the two.

(ii) To select the remedy match the patient's mind and temperament. This plays the most decisive importance in the selection of the remedy.

(iii) Out of the symptoms noted down first choose or select carefully 3, 4, 5 or 6 or more, strange, peculiar and rare symptoms. These are the highest generals since they apply to the patient himself.

(iv) Now you have the first generals. From the Repertory choose the remedies suggested therein. Then with the help of Materia Medica look out the remedies taken off from the Repertory and see which of the remedies come very close to the patient's symptoms.

(v) Now crosscheck these medicines' symptoms; also correspond with the other common and particular symptoms of the patient.

(vi) Once you have the strong, strange, peculiar symptoms check and see that there are no generals in the case that oppose or contradict.

(vii) Where the remedy has the generals it is enough. Do not try to match the little symptoms.

Totality of the Symptoms

Here, we provide a chart giving us all limbs of the **Totality of Symptoms**. The purpose of this chart is to guide one to take the case. The physician can have this chart - preferably laminated - in front of him and check with each item the patient's various symptoms.

The same can be done for the drug symptoms with Materia Medica. By doing so, there will be a close correspondence with the disease symptoms covering all the symptoms you have noted down.

Both ways this chart can be made very useful - quick and reliable. The work will also be enjoyable and shorter.

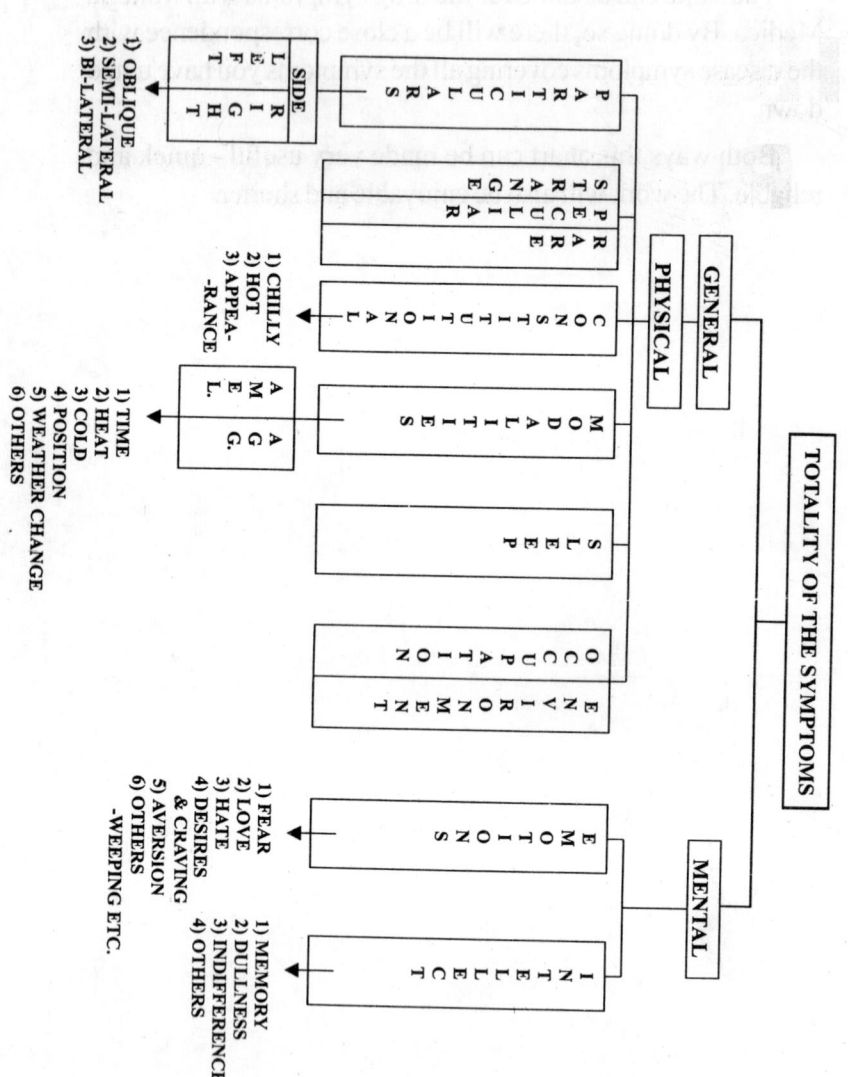